THE ALL-NEW
ATKINS ADVANTAGE

THE ALL-NEW
ATKINS ADVANTAGE

The 12-Week Low-Carb Program to Lose Weight, Achieve Peak Fitness and Health, and Maximize Your Willpower to Reach Life Goals

STUART L. TRAGER, M.D.
WITH COLETTE HEIMOWITZ, M.Sc.

ST. MARTIN'S PRESS ✖ NEW YORK

NOTE TO THE READER:

The information presented in this work is in no way intended as medical advice or as a substitute for medical counseling. The information should be used in conjunction with the guidance and care of your physician. Consult your physician before beginning this program as you would any weight loss or weight maintenance program. Your physician should be aware of all medical conditions that you may have as well as the medications and supplements you are taking. Those of you on diuretics or diabetes medications should proceed only under a doctor's supervision. As with any plan, the weight loss phases of this nutritional plan should not be used by patients on dialysis or by pregnant or nursing women or anyone under the age of eighteen.

www.stmartins.com

Book design by Gretchen Achilles
Illustrations by Wendy Wray/Vicki Morgan Associates, NYC

Trager, Stuart L.
The all-new Atkins advantage : the 12-week low-carb program to lose weight, achieve peak fitness and health, and maximize your willpower to reach life goals / Stuart L. Trager.—1st ed.
p. cm.
ISBN-13: 978-0-312-33129-0
ISBN-10: 0-312-33129-0
1. Low-carbohydrate diet.   2. Low-carbohydrate diet—Recipes.   3. Reducing exercises.   I. Title.

RM237.73 .T73 2006
613.2'5—dc22   2005044993

First Edition: January   2008

10 9 8 7 6 5 4 3 2 1

CONTENTS

ACKNOWLEDGMENTS

Writing *The All-New Atkins Advantage* has been much like running the final leg of a long-distance relay race. Almost forty years ago, Dr. Atkins ran the first lap, and many laps after that, introducing a groundbreaking approach to weight control and good health. He handed off the baton to gifted researchers and clinicians who continue to refine the message, affording important scientific support for Dr. Atkins's revolutionary approach. They are too numerous to name here, but their contributions were instrumental in creating the Advantage Program. Special thanks to Veronica Atkins, who, as the chair of the Dr. Robert C. Atkins Foundation, continues to fund important independent research in the field of nutrition and health. Special thanks are also due to Colette Heimowitz, M.Sc., R.D., whose vast nutritional expertise and experience, along with her appreciation of emerging research, have been invaluable to this project.

Laura Tucker, wordsmith extraordinaire, turned doctor-speak into prose and hunkered down in the trenches with me to help articulate the Atkins Advantage Program. My literary agent, Laurie Bernstein, also went above and beyond, offering help, guidance, and friendship each step of the way.

Dan Moser, Ph.D., offered expert input for the exercise portions of the Advantage Program. My training partners, especially coach Jeff Devlin, have each helped me to stay motivated and to always remember the important thing is training smarter, not harder.

Most of all, I am grateful for the support and understanding of my wife, Leslie, and my daughters, Samantha and Carly. Together they have given me the strength and motivation to complete this book as well as to reach so many other important finish lines.

—Stuart L. Trager, M.D.

PREFACE

STUART L. TRAGER, M.D.

How did I go from being the last kid picked for every team in grade school to competing in the Ultraman Triathlon World Championship— swimming more than 6 miles, biking another 261.4, and running for 52.4 miles through the lava fields of Hawaii?

Even having done it, it sounds pretty incredible to me, too. But as I discovered, when you have the right keys, you can open any doors.

My story has everything to do with being hungry. I love to eat, and I have a big appetite. I've struggled with my weight for most of my life. In college I started counting calories and watching my fat intake. In medical school I started exercising, not for fun but so I could eat whatever I wanted. I remember doing one 15-mile run so I could justify dining on a friend's homemade buffalo chicken wings.

Adhering to a low-fat, low-calorie diet was really painful. I was either hungry because I hadn't eaten enough or guilty because I had eaten too much. I was constantly torn between eating enough to satisfy myself and fuel my workouts, or going without in an effort to manage my weight.

Still, I wasn't seeing results. My energy level was low, my weight was holding me back in terms of my running performance, and I couldn't shed those extra pounds. I was following all the rules—I *did* eat less, and I *did* exercise more—but I was still coming up short. It wasn't the number of pounds I had to lose that made the struggle so overwhelming; I am well aware that there are many people with bigger weight challenges. But like everyone who battles the bulge, those extra pounds were standing between me and my goals. The constant pressure to slim down was zapping my energy. Finally I found the right tools for the job. After struggling through my third or fourth marathon in the fall of 1999, I wanted to get to the next level by qualifying for the prestigious Boston Marathon, which meant I'd have to shave about 15 minutes off my best time—and that meant losing weight. I increased my training and renewed my commitment to curb calories. Despite running close to 60 miles a week, I was still struggling to get in better shape.

Then my luck turned. During the spring of 2000, my wife and I went on a boating vacation on Chesapeake Bay with a doctor friend and his family. My friend had lost 20 pounds in two months doing Atkins and had never looked or felt better. I couldn't believe what he was eating—guilt-free! He dug into crabs, ham-and-cheese omelets, peanuts, and spareribs—while I tried to keep hunger at bay nibbling on celery sticks and low-fat pretzels. As soon as our holiday was over, I ran out to buy *Dr. Atkins' New Diet Revolution.*

Not only did I manage to lose the pounds (and take another 20 minutes off my marathon time), but the weight loss was just the tip of the iceberg. I suddenly had tons more energy for my work and my family, was recovering faster from my workouts and, for the first time I could remember, wasn't ravenous all the time!

But the transformation I experienced went deeper than improved energy and performance. By changing the way I ate, I found myself finally in control of my appetite, my weight, and my energy level. I satisfied my hunger instead of ignoring it, and that gave me the fuel to feed my other passions as well. Once I wasn't struggling to balance hunger and weight control, my world opened up.

Feeling better about myself than I could ever remember, I wanted to see how far the low-carb lifestyle could take me. I signed up for my first Ironman race—an event that combines swimming for 2.4 miles, then bicycling for 112, capped off by a full marathon (26.2 miles)! When I got to the event and saw the fierce competition, I thought, "I'll be lucky to finish." I'm happy to report I did better than that: I finished 286 out of almost 1,800 competitors, and 61 out of the 282 men in my age group.

As a physician I was so amazed by what had happened to my body—and to my life—that I got in touch with Dr. Atkins. When I met with him and other people in the organization, I learned about the emerging science supporting a low-carb nutritional approach, and I was hugely impressed by what I saw. I became a consultant to the company, helping deliver Dr. Atkins' message while learning more about how the Atkins program transforms people's lives in myriad ways.

That first Ironman was just the beginning for me. I now have eight Ironman finishes under my belt, including two world championship races, and I've even pushed further, completing the Ultraman, a three-day race that culminates in a double marathon. I'm not alone.

As an athlete I consider Atkins an essential part of my fitness training. As a physician I celebrate the health benefits this approach can offer. The program design in this book promises not only to leave you slimmer but empowered to embark on the life you've always dreamed could and should be yours.

In the years I've been associated with Atkins, I've met many people whose lives have been changed, just as mine was. The idea for this book germinated in meetings and discussions with other health and nutrition professionals at Atkins who worked with people whose stories you're about to read. As a physician my job is to create a prescription for correcting a condition. If I could take the Atkins Nutritional Approach and codify it into a program based on the experiences of the most successful Atkins followers, would it not give everyone a better chance at success? And by success I mean not just shedding excess pounds and becoming fitter but changing lives. The people who have acquired the tools to move beyond weight loss to total empowerment, what we call the Atkins Advantage, became my instructors—as did those individuals who were unable to maintain the momentum necessary to achieve permanent results.

In coming to understand the differences between the two groups, I was able to craft the 12-week guided program that should allow *everyone* the best shot at success. As you meet some of the many individuals who inspired *The All-New Atkins Advantage*—we call them the Atkins Achievers—I'm sure that you will find their accomplishments as motivational as I did.

By combining my own experience with those of many Atkins Achievers, as well as the most up-to-date clinical research, we have created a step-by-step program that will help you not only shed pounds but change your life, just as mine was changed. We are passing along the key to help you unlock the gateway to your own dreams and goals . . . to gain the Atkins Advantage.

PREFACE

COLETTE HEIMOWITZ, M.Sc.

The principles of the Atkins Advantage not only have stood the test of time, they also are continually being confirmed in new research. I truly believe that even if a modest portion of the population follows the Atkins Advantage basic nutrition principles, we could have a healthier population. Dr. Atkins worked tirelessly to help others understand how to incorporate these principles into their lives. His legacy lives on in more than a dozen books he and his team have written and in the Robert C. Atkins Foundation's fine work in supporting research. The spirit and energy of all who have benefited from his innovative thinking are certainly evident. Now, more and more independent research trials are confirming his basic principles.

There has been more than thirty years of independent research on low-carbohydrate diets with more than 3,000 subjects; thirty years of clinical experience and now four years of trials looking specifically at the Atkins protocol, all of which have consistently demonstrated safety and effectiveness.

In one of the more recently published studies, the prestigious *Journal of the American Medical Association* released results of a year-long weight loss and health study conducted by Stanford University researchers among more than 300 overweight, pre-menopausal women. These women were randomly assigned to follow the Atkins, Zone, Ornish, or LEARN diet for the year.

According to the results of this year-long weight loss and health study:

- The Atkins weight loss program proved significantly more effective than the other leading weight loss programs tested, and lowered risk factors associated with cardiovascular disease.

- The women who followed the Atkins weight loss program lost on average 40 percent more weight than the women on the next-best plan.

- The best news was that women following the Atkins program also experienced the most favorable results in their "good" cholesterol levels (HDL), blood triglycerides, and blood pressure.

Studies of such magnitude, and the addition of the stringent peer reviews that take place before publication in JAMA, provide another level of credibility to the report. Also important to note is that the support was provided by grants from the National Institutes of Health, an agency of the U.S. Department of Health and Human Services.

Given the complexity of the research and the difficulty in reaching conclusions that everyone can agree on, are there any basic principles that we can extract from the mass of data available? Are there any clear "lessons learned"? And just how well do the general principles of the Atkins Advantage hold up?

Actually, the Atkins Program holds up very well indeed. Several basic "lessons learned" have clearly emerged and have been supported by a significant amount of research. These basic points—all principles of the Atkins Advantage—are both easy to apply to real life situations and can be used to help maintain a healthy weight and a healthy body.

THE FIVE PRINCIPLES OF THE ALL-NEW ATKINS ADVANTAGE PROGRAM

PRINCIPLE NUMBER ONE: HIGHER PROTEIN

If you keep calories in different nutritional approaches the same, diets that limit carbohydrate content have more protein and fat than the "high-carb" or low-fat diet. In the last several years, dozens of studies have investigated "low-carb" diets (which by definition are higher protein) for their effect on weight loss, triglycerides, inflammation, body composition, insulin resistance, and glycemic control. The results have been almost universally positive. Across the board, one conclusion that it is fair to make is this: if you're interested in losing fat, a diet with a higher proportion of calories from protein is the way to go. Such diets have fared very well in the research and seem to have an advantage over diets with a higher proportion of carbohydrates.

Evidence is accumulating that higher protein intake, within reason, has other far-reaching benefits besides its positive effect on weight management. For example, higher protein intake can actually create stronger bones.

Lesson learned: protein at every meal—and especially at breakfast—is one surefire way to get the Atkins Advantage of higher protein.

PRINCIPLE NUMBER TWO: GOOD FAT

Despite an overwhelming amount of research showing the vital importance of good fats in the diet, and despite a turn-around on the subject of fat by many of the country's top dietitians, nutritionists, and doctors, many people remain fat-phobic, a holdover from the 1980s when anything with fat was considered taboo. Astonishingly, many people still shun foods like salmon and nuts and whole eggs because of their fat content. Yet the research on "good fats" is abundantly clear and not at all ambiguous: We need fat for optimal health.

Though there has been much debate about "good fats" and "bad fats," the emerging truth is that the biggest villains in the fat family are a type of fat about which little research was done until only a decade or so ago: trans fats. Conversely, the emerging truth is that the undeniable heroes of the fat family are omega-3s.

Omega-3 fats have been found to reduce inflammation, maintain the fluidity of cell membranes, lower the amount of lipids like cholesterol and triglycerides circulating in the bloodstream, and reduce the risk of becoming obese. They also improve the body's ability to respond to insulin and are one of the most highly recommended supplements for diabetics.

The bottom line: fat in reasonable amounts is a vital part of a healthy diet. It has virtually no effect on blood sugar or insulin, making higher-fat snacks ideal from a blood-sugar control point of view. When the fat eaten is the right kind of fat—and doesn't result in an excessive amount of calories consumed—there is nothing at all to be afraid of.

The Atkins Advantage has always recommended a high intake of omega-3 fats and a proportional, reasonable intake of other healthy fats.

Lesson learned: healthy fat belongs in every diet, a confirmation of another of the basic principles of the Atkins Advantage.

PRINCIPLE NUMBER THREE: LOW SUGAR

One of the central foundational pillars of the Atkins Advantage has always been "carbs from vegetables," supplemented with low-sugar fruits and some whole grains.

From the very beginning, Dr. Atkins was a fan of fibrous vegetables. They remain the cornerstone of any good dietary program and are one of the few foods all nutritionists and doctors across the board agree upon. The new catchword "smart carbs" is just popular terminology for carbs that don't raise blood sugar quickly and is pretty much synonymous with carbs from nonrefined sources. Vegetables are high on the list, but so are low-sugar, high-fiber fruits, and, for many people, high-fiber whole grains. What is not on the list is junk food: highly refined cereals, white pastas, cakes, cookies, soft drinks, and other staples of the American diet. These are largely responsible for the surge in obesity and diabetes and are increasingly being implicated in a host of other health disasters.

Simple: if a food is highly processed with refined flour and high-sugar content, it's probably not good for you. If a food is high in refined sugar or low in fiber and protein, stay away.

Research on glycemic impact is proliferating, and it is confirming the basic principle of the Atkins Advantage: favor foods with low amounts of sugar, which don't cause large fluctuations in blood sugar and insulin.

Lesson learned: get your carbs from low-sugar, unrefined sources, and avoid fast-acting sugars and foods that contain them.

PRINCIPLE NUMBER FOUR: HIGH FIBER

The best health and weight management benefits accrue to those eating a low-sugar diet, but the other half of that equation is high fiber. Fibrous vegetables are almost always low in sugar but they are also high in fiber. A cornerstone of the Atkins Advantage is high fiber. Our Paleolithic, or cavemen, ancestors routinely got between 50 to 100 grams in their daily diet, and even the relatively conservative Dietary Guidelines for Americans recommend at least 25 grams a day. Why is fiber so important? For one thing, it slows the rate at which food empties from the GI tract into the bloodstream, blunting the spikes of blood sugar and insulin that can occur when fiber isn't present. This makes it the ideal "tool" for those interested in weight management. In addition, many studies have suggested a role for fiber in the prevention of cardiovascular disease and colorectal cancer.

Lesson learned: get more fiber! It's an Atkins Advantage principle that virtually everyone agrees on and that guarantees health and weight management benefits!

PRINCIPLE NUMBER FIVE: GET ADEQUATE VITAMINS AND MINERALS

There is no longer any serious disagreement that vitamins, minerals, antioxidants, phytonutrients, and all the other wonderful compounds found in foods and nature do incredible things for your body. Unfortunately, most of us get the bare minimum. A number of dietary surveys have suggested that Americans do not consume recommended amounts of magnesium, a mineral that has important roles in both carbohydrate metabolism and in the regulation of blood pressure. And literally dozens of studies have documented the health benefits of antioxidants and other vitamin and mineral supplements.

Lesson learned: foods and on-the-go nutrition snacks with the most vitamins and minerals give you the most bang for your nutritional buck.

WHAT WE CAN ALL AGREE ON: WHAT YOU NEED TO KNOW

Protein at every meal (higher protein) helps with weight loss, appetite control, and improves lean body mass; eating the right fats helps lowers risk of certain diseases like diabetes and contributes to cardiovascular health; avoiding the wrong ones (trans fats) does the same thing. High sugar and refined carbohydrate consumption is your worst enemy when it comes to weight management, and may well be your worst enemy when it comes to general health. And vitamins, minerals, and fiber are an essential part of every diet, so products and food that contain more are almost always preferable to those that contain less.

Atkins Advantage nutrition principles are all about proactive nutrition: providing you the information and inspiration you need to take charge of your health and enjoy your active life to the fullest. These principles are easy to understand and follow once you know the basics. When it comes to eating right for increased health and energy, this book will steer you in the right direction.

The five principles of the Atkins Advantage are simple, but following them will give you a huge advantage in attaining your goals both from the point of view of weight management and from the point of view of better health! It is simply better for you.

Based on feedback we have gotten over the years from those of you attempting to follow Atkins, we have created this book. The underlying principle is how to do Atkins right and how to make it simpler to understand and make it a way of life. The results will ultimately be better energy, not only to take on challenges for the day but also to maintain vitality for life.

Come with us on a 12-week journey. This book will give you the tools to reach your health goals. Thanks to Dr. Trager, *The All-New Atkins Advantage* covers subjects that have not been adequately explained in previous books. Those subjects are covered in more detail to keep you focused and motivated to help ensure success.

INTRODUCTION

People come to Atkins for weight loss, but they gain something more: *empowerment*. That's one of the many Atkins advantages that gave this book its title. It is also why the success that people experience doing Atkins is unrivaled and why so many of them are thrilled when they talk about how their lives have changed.

On Atkins, people don't just become trimmer, they take charge of their lives—sometimes for the first time. Doing Atkins is like discovering that the race you're running is all downhill, and this feeling will take you to the winner's circle. That's why empowerment has been put front and center in this book.

This intangible force was always a by-product of doing Atkins, but now the All-New Atkins Advantage Program is specifically designed to demystify—and magnify—that energy so that it reaches into every area of your life. Millions of people have used the Atkins Nutritional Approach (ANA) to successfully lose weight; now the All-New Atkins Advantage Program builds upon the ANA, offering you the opportunity to make success your watchword, not only with respect to controlling your weight but in accomplishing all your goals.

One of the reasons traditional diets typically fail over the long run is that they ask you to swim against the forces of nature, against the body's fundamental physiology, and against the tide of plain old common sense. They ask you to do the impossible—such as not eat when you're hungry or exercise when you're drained of energy. So even if you lose weight, you'll more than likely gain it back—usually with extra pounds—because no one can be expected to deprive himself indefinitely.

The long-standing assumption that sacrifice is the true path to weight loss springs from a fundamental misunderstanding about *why* people become heavy and what is required to shed excess pounds. Shaking free of that mind-set is the first step toward true weight management and the beginning of empowerment.

Dr. Atkins showed the world that weight loss doesn't mean you have to starve as long as you break free from the stranglehold of eating too many carbohydrates—or the wrong ones—which programs our bodies to produce and to store more fat.

The tenets of the ANA are not just principles to lose weight by but ones to live your life by. Dr. Atkins based his entire approach to weight loss and weight management on a simple but radical departure from the established orthodoxy: Better health and weight loss results come when you work *with* your body, not against it.

In sports the advantage that comes from working with the elements is called "free speed." It is the extra boost that comes from swimming with the current. It is why a cyclist wears clothes that cling to his body: By reducing drag from the wind, he can actually shave precious seconds off his time without expending any additional effort.

Dr. Atkins revolutionized weight loss by bringing free speed into the dietary equation. We call it the Atkins Advantage. This is what happens when you do Atkins:

- Your body burns fat instead of storing it.

- You no longer crave unhealthy foods because you stabilize your blood sugar, eliminating such cravings for good.

- Most important, after you are no longer controlled by food, you are free to pursue your life's dreams.

Atkins has always harnessed free speed to help you lose weight. Now, with the Atkins Advantage, we take it a step further by helping you maximize free speed in all your endeavors.

Instead of the collateral damage you may have experienced with low-fat or low-calorie diets, with Atkins you will actually experience a collateral *advantage*. With the All-New Atkins Advantage Program you will learn how to channel this sense of empowerment into all areas of your life.

HOW TO USE THIS BOOK

One of the defining characteristics of the Atkins Nutritional Approach (ANA) is that each person can individualize it to his or her own needs and tastes. Regardless of whether you have a high metabolism and lose weight relatively easily or are a "slow burner," Atkins can be tailored to your needs. If you are willing to have your weight loss journey take a little longer in return for enjoying a wider variety of foods than you might otherwise, you can do so. Alternatively, if you need to lose a lot of pounds and are willing to stick with a more restricted menu for a longer period of time, you can speed up your progress—by lowering your carb intake or upping your exercise time and intensity, or both. Finally, whether you like nothing better than a rare steak or you're a confirmed vegetarian, you can do Atkins *your* way.

Part I introduces the basics of how to do Atkins and its four increasingly liberal phases, offers a brief discussion of the metabolic processes that make it work, and prepares you for the 12-week journey ahead of you. The Whys and Hows of Atkins includes everything from a list of foods you'll want to have on hand to fuel your body to some mental exercises to get your head in the right place.

Part II is comprised of the actual 12-week Atkins Advantage Program. Because of the individualization inherent in the ANA, many of you will be starting in the first phase, known as Induction, while others will begin in Ongoing Weight Loss or Pre-Maintenance. (The final phase is Lifetime Maintenance.) The decision about where to start will be yours, but you will be provided with plenty of advice on how to make the right choice.

Although the 12 weeks progress from Induction to Lifetime Maintenance, there is absolutely no expectation that everyone will reach that ultimate phase. In fact, depending on your weight loss goals and your body's metabolism, you may not get beyond Induction by the end of the 12 weeks. Not to worry: The program is designed to allow you to move at your own pace, and the chapters include information for people at all levels. Likewise, the fitness component of the book is set up so that regardless of whether you are a confirmed couch potato or a gym rat, you can design a workout that is appropriate for you.

Nowhere is the individualization more apparent that in the meal plans, which constitute **Part III**. When you do Atkins, you count the grams of carbohydrates you consume each day. This section includes 12 weeks' worth of daily meal plans at net carb levels ranging from 20 grams to 80 grams daily.

To decide each week whether to move from one phase to another or from one level of carb intake to another within that phase, you simply go to the Meal Plans and find the appropriate carb level. There are four weeks' worth of meal plans at 20 grams of net carbs; beyond that we offer one week at each level. If you stay at one level more than a week, simply repeat the week's plan. Feel free to modify the meal plans to suit your needs and tastes while staying at the right number of daily grams.

The References section is in two parts: Studies and Sources. The first offers a listing of approximately 40 studies that have contributed information pertinent to the Atkins Advantage Program. The second offers works that have been referred to in the chapters of this work. We hope that you will find additional data and assistance in these publications.

PART 1

THE WHYS AND HOWS OF ATKINS

ONE

WHAT YOU CAN ACHIEVE: DOING ATKINS CAN CHANGE MORE THAN YOUR PANTS SIZE

Congratulations on embarking on this 12-week journey. As you move through the nutrition, fitness, and motivation segments of the Atkins Advantage Program, you will be embarking on a journey toward better health, permanent weight loss, and personal fulfillment. Make no mistake about it: This is a *global* approach to weight loss, one that will change not only the shape of your body but the quality of your life. In the weeks to come you will lose pounds, get healthier, and become more fit, but also build the mental "muscle" you'll need to reap the fullest advantages from the All-New Atkins Advantage Program—and from life.

Empowerment is the engine that drives success in any endeavor. Many Atkins followers have found that empowerment starts with weight loss and have caught and ridden the wave into other areas of their lives. The goal of this book is to enable everyone who does Atkins to experience this effect. Taking control of your life is not a chance by-product of the Atkins Advantage Program but its very essence.

Changing the way you eat is key to being healthier, slimmer, and happier—but on its own it is rarely enough to produce permanent changes. The Atkins Nutritional

Approach (ANA) has always embraced fitness and stressed the importance of tending to your spiritual and emotional well-being, but until now it has not delivered an Atkins-appropriate fitness and motivational program.

A COMPLETE PROGRAM

The Atkins Advantage Program has three parts designed to work in concert: Nutrition, Motivation, and Fitness. Each week you'll proceed through all aspects of the program. Can you lose weight by using only one or two? Sure. But the surest and fastest way to your goal is to employ all three in unison. They work in tandem as you progress through the program, gradually building to the experience of *empowerment*.

NUTRITION: THE HEART OF THE MATTER

Dr. Atkins' revolutionary low-carbohydrate eating plan, founded on a single fundamentally empowering principle of saying yes, is at the heart and soul of the Atkins Advantage Program. When you do Atkins, you don't do without, you do different. We think you'll be delighted to discover that many of the foods you can eat in the first phase of Atkins are the same ones you couldn't eat when you were trying to lose weight in the past. That is the Atkins way. Get ready to dine on roast chicken complete with crispy skin, or lamb chops accompanied by tasty broccoli and a salad topped with avocado slices and creamy Caesar dressing. Moreover, when you cut out refined carbs in the form of processed foods containing bleached white flour and white sugars, you'll not only lose weight but reduce your risk factors for many chronic diseases.

Controlling carb intake is a crucial part of the answer to the nationwide epidemic of obesity and can be the solution to your personal struggle in the battle of the bulge, but it must be done correctly to reap the rewards. With the Atkins Advantage you'll be on the right track from day one, and your results will show it.

MOTIVATION: THE WINNER'S EDGE

As you stand at the threshold of a new beginning, you will likely find yourself filled with optimism and determination. Take note of this feeling—that's *motivation*. But as you probably know, sustaining this feeling of hope, energy, and optimism is the hard part. You may have felt hopeful and excited about other supposedly life-changing diets and fitness programs, only to find that none of them gave you the tools to maintain that enthusiasm long enough to see lasting results.

Changing your body means changing your mind, which is every bit as crucial as increasing your physical activity and improving your eating habits. Think of motivation as the key in the ignition: Without it, you can't even start the engine, let alone go the distance.

Each week we'll introduce targeted mental exercises that draw upon the best of sports medicine and motivational training.

You'll learn to set realistic but challenging goals that will help you achieve all your dreams. You'll give those goals a concrete shape by "seeing" yourself attaining them in guided visualizations. You'll learn to replace the habit of negative self-talk with positive, personalized, verbalized self-reinforcement in the form of affirmations. Guided journaling activities will allow you to monitor your progress, refine your approach, and celebrate each milestone on your journey toward lifelong weight management and optimal health.

With the All-New Atkins Advantage Program you'll achieve not just a new body but a new outlook—one that will enable you to reach out and embrace life to the fullest. These skills will empower you to eliminate excess pounds and rid yourself of the encumbrances that have held you back from realizing many of your dreams.

FITNESS: THE BEST YOU

Moving—and getting fit—is a prescription for a happier, healthier, more active and fulfilling life. But if you have tried to lose weight by exercise alone, you might have a very different perspective on exercise; you may recall the hours spent sweating on a treadmill, only to see little or no difference on the scale at the end of the week.

If you've tried exercise before and been disappointed, it'll be different as part of the Atkins Advantage Program. Here's why:

- You'll look better. Working out promotes better posture and more toned muscles.

- Your results will be better. Research shows that most people who maintain their weight loss exercise regularly, and most people who regain weight loss do not. Muscle burns more calories at rest than fat, so the more muscular you are, the more fat you burn even when not exercising! Exercise helps you stay focused when weight loss inevitably slows.

- You'll feel better. Exercise increases your coordination, stability, and physical confidence—a boon if you no longer want to wake up feeling stiff and creaky or simply want to move more gracefully. It improves mood, decreasing depression, anger, and stress, alleviates sleep complaints, and has a calming effect on our minds and bodies. Exercise actually replenishes your energy reserves and makes you stronger so that you can more easily handle the activities of daily life.

- Your overall health will be better. Weight-bearing exercise increases bone density. Even moderate exercise boosts the immune system.

The All-New Atkins Advantage brings unique benefits that not only improve overall health, but deliver these benefits through proven techniques.

Diminish your disease risks. Physical inactivity is a major independent risk factor for coronary heart disease. Exercise has been shown to lower total cholesterol, LDL ("bad" cholesterol), triglycerides, blood pressure, and amount of body fat, all risk factors for heart attacks, stroke, and Type 2 diabetes. It can also normalize blood clotting factors and also increase insulin sensitivity (a good thing) and HDL ("good" cholesterol). A study that followed more than 70,000 postmenopausal women for about three years found that those who exercised at least two and a half hours a week had a 30 percent lower risk of heart-related problems than the least active women. Another study of 2,600 elderly men found an average 15 percent decrease in risk of heart disease for every half mile the men walked each day. It doesn't take a lot of exercise to make a difference. One study revealed that of all cardiac risk factors, the most significant indicator of risk of death is an individual's exercise capacity.

You can eat more carbs! Anyone can tell you to control carbs, but only Atkins individualizes it so you eat the maximum amount of healthy carbohydrate foods your metabolism can handle while still losing weight. The Atkins Advantage Program includes a Fitness Rewards Chart (page 202) that offsets the time and effort you expend working out with additional grams of carbs you can eat.

This doesn't mean jogging eight miles to burn off an ice-cream sundae. But would a piece of whole grain bread jazz up your lunchtime turkey and cheese roll-up? By focusing on carbs, not calories, and by looking at exercise to help you raise your carb threshold, the rewards become meaningful and the goals become achievable.

It's individualized. The fitness component of this 12-week program has been designed specifically so that no one will be left behind. In the same way that Atkins can help you lose weight no matter how far away you are from your goal weight, the fitness component of the Atkins Advantage Program will help you get into better shape—whether you already work out regularly or haven't made regular fitness part of your routine. Whether your goal is to walk briskly for 30 minutes a day or run a marathon, *you* decide how high to set the bar.

It's full spectrum. The Atkins Advantage Program offers you a fitness plan that incorporates stretching, cardiovascular (aerobic) exercise, and strength (resistance) training, encouraging you to increase your overall activity. A study that followed middle-aged men for seven years found that those who engaged in moderate activities ranging from tennis to gardening had a 20 to 30 percent reduced risk of dying compared to those with less active lifestyles. Those who expended even more calories further reduced their risk. According to the American College of Sports Medicine, a program should build strong habits, not just strong muscles.

In the weeks to come, think of this book as your coach, giving you professional, around-the-clock, personalized, hands-on care and attention—and the encouragement you need—to make fitness an integral part of your healthy lifestyle.

It's fun! Even the best-designed program in the world won't make you fit unless you *do* it. And you won't do it unless you enjoy it. This program is fun, productive, and satisfying, because that's the only way to ensure you'll stick with it. After all, the objective isn't simply exercise but adopting a more active lifestyle.

WHY A WEEK-BY-WEEK PROGRAM?

Have you ever envied those celebrities who jet off to a secluded location to receive personalized care from a world-class trainer, sports physiologist, life coach, chef, and nutritionist to get them in shape for their next role? Well, now it's your turn. This is your chance to have the hands-on, seven-days-a-week support you'll need, not just to finally get in shape but to feel empowerment in every area of your life.

The weekly format also allows you to further individualize the program. For example, once you leave Induction, you may be willing to trade less variety in your meals in order to see the pounds fall off more quickly. Or perhaps you can handle losing a little more slowly in exchange for incorporating some carbohydrate foods sooner rather than later. This flexibility puts you in control.

WHY 12 WEEKS?

Research has shown that 12 weeks is the minimum amount of time it generally takes to replace old habits with new ones. The All-New Atkins Advantage Program is designed to help you weave these new habits seamlessly into the fabric of your life so that eventually they become second nature.

The 12-week period does not mean everybody should or will reach his or her goal weight in that time or will cycle through the first three phases of Atkins and reach Lifetime Maintenance in that time. It all depends on how many pounds you have to lose and the pace at which you lose them, but as long as you successfully complete the 12-week program, you will have acquired the skills and mind-set necessary to place yourself securely on the path to achieving your target weight and other goals. In fact, at the end of the 12 weeks you will be embarking on a journey that will last a lifetime.

So get out your calendar, open it to 12 weeks from today, and circle the date with a bright red marker. In that short time you will be rounding the corner to a new you, someone who will look and feel better than you even dared dream possible.

TWO

WHY ATKINS WORKS: WHAT YOU NEED TO KNOW ABOUT CARBOHYDRATES, PROTEIN, AND FAT

Humans aren't designed to be overweight by nature, nor are we designed to eat the way we do. Our modern diet, loaded with sugar and other refined carbs at the expense of protein and natural fats, has sabotaged our body chemistry. In one year the average American consumes:

- 156 pounds of caloric sweeteners (sugar, corn syrup, honey, and so on), an increase of 30.1 pounds over the last 30 years.

- 61 gallons of sweetened beverages alone, a rise of 36 gallons between 1970 and 1997.

- 200 pounds of flour and cereal products, an increase of an amazing 64.3 pounds in the same period.

Ironically, it is our "super-size" culture of five-ounce bagels and 20-ounce beverages that is the reason we are constantly unsatisfied and craving another "fix." Lack of satisfaction and our inability to distinguish cravings from true hunger, coupled with decreased physical activity, in large part are responsible for this country's obesity epidemic—to say nothing of the skyrocketing rates of related diseases such as Type 2 diabetes, heart disease, and certain forms of cancer.

Too many carbs can not only make you fat but can make you sick. Studies from major medical centers, funded by organizations such as the American Heart Association, the National Institutes of Health, and the Philadelphia Veterans Hospital, have shown that a high-glycemic diet can actually be bad for your heart. For instance, the Nurses' Health Study found that "a high intake of rapidly digested and absorbed carbohydrate increases the risk of coronary heart disease *independent* of conventional coronary disease risk factors."

The current low-fat, high-carbohydrate diet that is routinely recommended in the United States for people with heart disease (and those trying to prevent it) may not be optimal if you can't limit your calories and portion sizes.

THE COMPLICATED CARBOHYDRATE

As pleasurable as food is, the purpose of eating is to fuel your body. A major component of the American diet is carbohydrate, one of the three macronutrients—the other two are fat and protein—that your body converts to energy. Indeed, carbohydrate is the first energy source the body turns to.

When you eat foods that contain carbs, your body converts them directly to blood glucose, also known as glucose or blood sugar, which it uses for energy. Regardless of whether you eat spinach, a pear, pasta, bread, potato chips, jelly doughnuts, or a chocolate bar, it is converted to blood glucose. The end result may be the same, but there are huge differences among carbohydrate foods in terms of how rapidly the glucose enters the bloodstream and the benefits or risks they provide.

The Atkins eating plan emphasizes the benefits of protein and natural fats—and nutrient-rich carbohydrates. Although Dr. Atkins was the first to draw attention to the dangers of too many carbs—and the wrong ones—the ANA is not anti-carb. Yes, some foods are off-limits in the earlier phases, but there is room for all whole food carbohydrates when you do Atkins. From day one you will eat at least five servings of vegetables and even some fruits. From the start you can enjoy salad greens, asparagus, string beans, broccoli, cauliflower, and many other vegetables (for a complete list see Acceptable Foods in Induction on page 27).

The goal is to eat as many "good" carbohydrates as your body can tolerate without interfering with weight loss or getting your blood sugar out of whack. You will *control* carbohydrates, not eliminate them. And you will choose healthy, satisfying whole foods, ones that provide nutrients and fiber.

Refined carbohydrates are not only significantly lower in nutrients and fiber than whole foods but they also break down more rapidly into glucose and enter your bloodstream far faster than vegetables and other low-glycemic carbohydrates. So when you eat refined carbohydrate foods, your blood sugar skyrockets. Think of how you feel after having a so-called healthy high-carb breakfast of orange juice, cereal, and skim milk. By mid-morning you're probably dragging and already "starving" for lunch. When you have pasta for dinner with some garlic bread on the side, you're probably snoring in front of the television by 9:00 p.m. Or if you're awake, you're sneaking into the kitchen for a snack at every station break.

When you eat meals full of refined carbs, the result is a super-charged elevation in blood sugar. In response, your pancreas releases excessive amounts of the hormone insulin, which sops up some of that extra blood sugar by moving it from the blood into the muscles and liver, where it is stored as a fuel reserve. What is not used for energy is stored in fat cells. That flood of insulin causes your blood sugar to plummet, along with your energy level and mood. Low blood sugar is a signal that your body is low on fuel and needs to restock by eating. The food your body screams for is more of the same: sweet and starchy, setting up the cycle of "addiction."

Have you ever felt compelled to finish a dessert you didn't really want in the first place? Have you ever found yourself at the bottom of a bag of potato chips after you had promised you'd have just a few? If that sugar-filled mid-afternoon pick-me-up from the vending machine feels more like a necessity than a treat, you've had a brush with the blood sugar roller coaster.

Unstable blood sugar caused by too many refined carbs wreaks havoc with your energy level and mood, and makes you feel hungry again soon after you eat such foods. Succumbing to a craving doesn't mean you lack willpower; it's a bona fide biochemical compulsion. Just as with any other "addiction," there's a biological component that can vanquish the best of intentions, which is why you've probably lost this battle in the past. It's not your fault but your biology: Unless you provide your body with a steady energy source—stabilizing your blood sugar—you'll always feel compelled to seek a new quick fix once the effects of your previous high-carb meal or snack have worn off.

Mood swings and hunger are only two signs of unstable blood sugar. Another is weight gain. Transporting blood sugar isn't insulin's only role. It also signals the body to burn carbohydrates for fuel and to store fat, so releasing too much insulin on a regular basis may be contributing to your weight problem. This surge of insulin also directs your body to use blood sugar as fuel instead of your body fat. Worse, when there is too much fuel available, it tells your body to store that excess glucose as *more* fat, which is why insulin is known as the fat-promoting hormone.

That's not all. When your blood sugar dips, the body is stimulated to release a hormone called cortisol, also known as "the stress hormone." High levels of this hormone have been linked to premature aging as well as a number of diseases.

The long-term effects of a diet high in refined carbohydrates are serious because the vicious cycle can lead to long-term disease:

- Blood sugar spikes and plummets become the norm.

- In an effort to stabilize blood sugar, the pancreas dumps more and more insulin into the bloodstream.

- As the cells' receptors become desensitized to the effects of more insulin, they require ever increasing amounts to have any effect on blood sugar, a condition called insulin resistance.

- Insulin resistance is the precursor to the metabolic syndrome and Type 2 diabetes.

CHOOSING THE RIGHT CARBS

Whole, unrefined carbohydrate foods take longer to digest because they are higher in fiber, which acts as a brake on the rise in blood sugar absorption. This, in turn, prompts a much more moderate release of insulin (imagine a faucet's slow drip instead of a flood) which is how your metabolism is supposed to function. These slow-release carbs are the ones you'll be eating when you do Atkins.

A carbohydrate food's impact on blood sugar can be measured, providing you with the information you need to make smart carb choices. A piece of white bread, for instance, causes an immediate, dramatic, and short-lived spike in blood sugar and insulin production. Nuts, on the other hand, take longer for the body to break down, so their effects are felt much more gradually, keeping blood sugar on an even keel. The extent and rate of a food's impact on blood sugar is known as its glycemic impact.

Scientists use two methods to determine glycemic impact. One is a ranking called the glycemic index (GI), which compares the effect a food has on blood sugar to the standard, which is pure glucose (in the form of a sugar solution) or white bread, both given values of 100. Foods high on the glycemic index, such as doughnuts, bananas, and fruit juices, can cause a surge in the blood sugar level and a rush of insulin, followed by an equally rapid drop. Lower GI foods, such as vegetables and nuts, have a less dramatic effect on blood sugar, insulin, and energy levels, and are therefore much healthier.

Unfortunately, by itself the GI isn't a great tool for making day-to-day food choices because the calculations aren't based on normal portion sizes. Rather, the amounts must contain 50 grams of carbohydrate. So, for example, carrots have a high GI ranking because the calculation is based on six cups of the vegetable, although a normal serving of half a cup would have a minimal impact on blood sugar.

A more sophisticated measure of the impact of a certain food on blood sugar is called the glycemic load (GL), which takes typical portion sizes into account. The GL is an improvement over the GI but is still hard to use when selecting foods. As you can see below, there are significant differences between the GI and the GL rankings of the same food.

GLYCEMIC INDEX VERSUS GLYCEMIC LOAD

The glycemic index (GI) considers foods that rank between 0 and 55 as low GI foods; those that fall between 56 and 69 are considered medium GI; those that rank at 70 or above are regarded as high GI.

The rankings for glycemic load differ: A GL of 10 or below is considered low; 11 to 19 is medium; and 20 or more is considered high.

Here is a comparison of GI and GL ratings for several common foods. Note that GI values use white bread as the reference food.

FOOD	GI	GL
POPCORN (PLAIN, COOKED IN MICROWAVE)	103	8
WATERMELON	103	4
CARROTS	68	3

These measures tell only half the story, neglecting important considerations such as nutrient density and the ability to fill you up, due in part to fiber content. They also don't factor in other foods (and their macronutrient makeup) eaten at the same time, which can moderate or aggravate the glycemic impact; fat and protein, for example, slow down the absorption of blood glucose. So while you may be hearing a lot about high- and low-glycemic foods, you needn't worry about glycemic impact. Instead, in the weight loss phases of Atkins, you'll simply count carbs and follow the Atkins Carbohydrate Ladder that follows. When you get close to your goal weight or are maintaining your weight, we'll introduce you to the Atkins Glycemic Ranking (AGR) (page 223), which helps you decide which carbohydrate foods to eat more frequently and which to go easy on, depending on both their glycemic index and their glycemic load.

THE ATKINS CARBOHYDRATE LADDER

The food groups in the Carbohydrate Ladder are presented in the order in which they are meant to be reintroduced once you move beyond Induction. The foods on the first rungs, such as vegetables, nuts, and seeds, contain the nutrient-rich carbs that have the least impact on blood sugar. Beginning with these will give your body a chance to adjust to a slightly higher carbohydrate level without overwhelming and stalling your metabolism.

1. salad and other low-glycemic vegetables, such as asparagus, spinach, tomatoes, onions, etc.

2. seeds and nuts: almonds, walnuts, pecans, Brazil nuts, macadamias, pignolias, hazelnuts; sunflower, pumpkin, and sesame seeds

3. berries: strawberries, blueberries, raspberries, gooseberries, and cranberries

4. legumes, such as lentils, chickpeas, kidney beans, soybeans

5. fruits other than berries, such as oranges, apples, grapes, kiwi, grapefruit, etc.

6. starchy vegetables, such as carrots, sweet potatoes, peas, and parsnips

7. whole grains, such as oats, brown rice, barley, millet, and buckwheat groats

The question of how high up you can climb on the ladder—and when you can do so—will depend entirely on your metabolism and your activity level. Some people can climb quite high—and those individuals will be able to enjoy legumes, whole grains, and starchier vegetables in later phases of the program. A few lucky individuals can even enjoy some of these foods in Ongoing Weight Loss (OWL). Others may find that in Lifetime Maintenance, they cannot or rarely tolerate items at the top of the Carbohydrate Ladder. The point is that everyone needs to ascend gradually in order to find what he or she can tolerate without instigating weight gain or cravings.

THE IMPORTANCE OF NET CARBS

On Atkins, when you eat whole foods, you count grams of net carbs, not of total carbs. Net carbs are those that have a significant impact on your blood sugar. They are also sometimes referred to as "impact carbs" or "effective carbs." Interestingly, although fats and proteins can be assayed or measured, in the United States anything that is not protein, fat, water, or ash (minerals) in a food is considered a carbohydrate. That means fiber, which passes through your body with negligible impact on blood sugar, is treated as a carbohydrate on food labels. (European countries and Australia don't consider fiber a carbohydrate.) However, when following the ANA, fiber is not tallied in the net carb count because it does not impact blood sugar.

In order to determine how many grams of net carbs are in a whole food, such as vegetables, simply subtract the grams of fiber from the grams of total carbs. For example, four spears of asparagus have 2.5 grams of total carbs and 1 gram of fiber. Subtract the fiber from the total carbs, to arrive at 1.5 grams of net carbs.

In packaged foods the Nutrition Facts panel on the label lists fiber grams as a component of total carb grams; simply subtract the fiber, and you'll have the number of grams of net carbs.

You'll also find net carb claims on packages of low-carb food products. In these cases, fiber often isn't the only thing that's subtracted. Glycerine, polydextrose, and most sugar alcohols are also considered carbohydrates in the United States, but because they have minimal impact on most people's blood sugar, they are subtracted as well in order to arrive at the net carb count. Please be aware that not all companies calculate net carbs the same way, which means that the net carb count indicated on the package may not be accurate. Atkins, however, uses a clinically validated method to determine the equivalent number of grams that impact blood sugar, known as the Net Atkins Count.

For more information on low-carb products, see pages 27 through 31.

PROTEIN: THE BUILDING BLOCK

Consider these facts about protein, the mainstay of the Atkins Nutritional Approach and the macronutrient on which every human diet relies. Protein

- maintains normal metabolism

- is essential to make enzymes and hormones

- grows and repairs all tissues

- keeps you satiated longer (feeling full)

Protein comes from poultry, meat, fish and shellfish, eggs, and soy foods such as tofu (bean curd). Nuts and seeds also contain protein, as does cheese, milk, and some other dairy products, along with fat and carbohydrate. Additionally, legumes such as lentils and grains such as brown rice and quinoa contain some protein.

Only animal sources of protein are *complete*, meaning they contain all the essential amino acids that the body needs but cannot manufacture on its own. Vegetable sources of protein contain some but not all or enough of the essential aminos; a good vegetarian diet combines the proper vegetable sources to make complete proteins.

WHAT YOU NEED TO KNOW ABOUT PROTEIN

Eating adequate protein is essential for achieving your health goals. Protein is made up of amino acids, also known as the "building blocks of protein." We get protein primarily from poultry, beef, lamb, pork, and other animal products, including almost anything that swims. We also get it from animal by-products such as eggs, milk, and cheese. Protein comes in vegetable form, most notably soy, and from seeds/nuts as well.

WHY DO I NEED PROTEIN?

Protein furnishes the raw materials your body needs to make muscles, organs, hair, neurotransmitters, enzymes, and just about anything else necessary to keep it running like a well-oiled machine. Simply put, without protein you would die. (The same cannot be said, by the way, of carbohydrate, but that's another story.) Protein also plays a role in weight loss or weight management. Compared to carbohydrate, consuming protein has less of an effect on insulin (which drives fat storage), a greater effect on glucagon (which drives fat release), and a considerably greater increase in metabolic rate. Several studies demonstrate greater body-fat loss on a high-protein diet than on a high-carb one. Increasing intake of protein relative to carbohydrates fills you up more, so you wind up eating less. A recent study showed that even eating snacks with a higher protein and lower carbohydrate composition can reduce the amount of food you eat at the next meal by 5 percent. And eating protein boosts your metabolic rate—the technical term is thermogenesis. In fact, one study showed that healthy young women experienced 100 percent higher thermogenesis after eating high-protein meals—even two and a half hours later—than when they ate a "conventional" high-carbohydrate meal.

HOW MUCH PROTEIN DO I NEED?

Many nutritionists recommend that individuals consume about half a gram of protein per pound of body weight, but other nutritionists feel that figure is far too low. For example, a 145-pound person would need at least 70 grams daily, which translates to roughly 10 ounces, or about two and a half small chicken breasts. Athletes need more, as do muscular people, those under stress, and pregnant or nursing women. It's worth noting that Atkins guidelines call for at least 6 ounces of (weighed uncooked) protein at each meal.

Because older adults don't use protein as efficiently, they need at least 15 percent more than younger people. Researcher Ronni Chernoff, Ph.D., R.D., recently stated, "The importance of dietary protein cannot be underestimated in the diets of older adults; inadequate protein intake contributes to . . . increased skin fragility, decreased immune function, poorer healing, and longer recuperation from illness."

HOW CAN I BE SURE TO GET ENOUGH PROTEIN?

Protein bars and shakes are an easy way to get high-quality protein into your diet. In addition to adding variety to the menu of protein choices, both are especially convenient when you are on the run or just don't feel like sitting down to a meal. But all bars and shakes are not created equal. As a meal replacement, products should contain at least 12 grams of protein per serving.

No matter where you get your protein, be sure to balance it with the appropriate amount of nutrient- and fiber-rich carbs and healthy natural fats, as well as plenty of muscle-building and cardio-enhancing exercise.

FAT: FRIEND, NOT FOE

Fat is often and incorrectly cast as the bad guy in the nutritional drama. "Mainstream nutritional science has demonized dietary fat, yet 50 years and hundreds of millions of dollars of research have failed to prove that eating a low-fat diet will help you live longer," wrote Gary Taubes in *Science* magazine. In a later *New York Times Magazine* article, Taubes wrote that the failure to separate the effects of eating a lot of fat in combination with a lot of carbs *as part of a high-calorie diet* has led to an incorrect conclusion with devastating consequences for our national health. By misreading the clues we have spent the last 30 years barking up the wrong tree while stuffing ourselves with the real culprit: excessive carbs. Walter Willett, the chairman of the Department of Nutrition at Harvard's School of Public Health, is quoted in the *Times* article as saying, "The exclusive focus on adverse effects of fat may have contributed to the obesity epidemic."

> ### YOU NEED CHOLESTEROL TO LIVE
>
> Contrary to what most people think, cholesterol is not a fat although it is found in some fat. Rather, it is a waxy substance attached to protein and carried in the blood. Cholesterol is necessary to maintain cell membranes and brain function and to insulate nerves, and it is a building block for many of our most important hormones, including estrogen and testosterone. The main source of cholesterol is not your diet. Although some of the foods you eat do supply cholesterol, most people manufacture three times as much in their body, particularly the liver, than they get from cholesterol-containing foods. The percentage of dietary cholesterol that is absorbed by your body may depend on how much your body makes, which in turn may depend on how much is absorbed. In large part this is a result of your genetic makeup. This means that cutting down on dietary cholesterol won't necessarily lower your blood cholesterol.

Natural fats, including saturated fats, are vital to good health. Fat is an essential nutrient and a backup energy source. Fat also protects our organs from injury and our cells from the cold.

Fat plays an important role in helping your body transport and absorb some of the fat-soluble vitamins obtained from foods, especially if the food is low in fat, as is the case with vegetables and fruits. For instance, without fat your body can't process the vitamin A in dark green vegetables, such as spinach and broccoli, or in orange or yellow vegetables, such as pumpkin and carrots. A drizzle of olive oil or a pat of butter helps transport fat-soluble nutrients such as vitamins A, D, E, and K to your cells.

Fat is also essential to satiety (a comfortable sense of fullness that helps you eat mindfully and with control) and dining pleasure. Fat carries flavor and contributes to what chefs call "mouth feel," the texture and the way food feels in your mouth and on your tongue. For example, think of the difference in feel between heavy cream and water.

When fat is removed or reduced, as is the case in many low-fat "diet" products, something has to replace the missing flavor. That something is usually sugar in one form or another, often as high-fructose corn syrup. The calorie content doesn't necessarily drop, but nutrient value definitely does. The result is that these supposedly healthier foods can actually make us fatter without making us full.

Insufficient fat is a key reason that many people cannot stick with calorie-controlled diets, which translates to a low-fat, high-carbohydrate diet. Without that feeling of satisfaction they binge on sugary, starchy foods.

The bottom line is that when you control carb intake, you can enjoy foods such as avocado, olives, meat, and shellfish without guilt and without damage to your health. As you gradually incorporate more carbohydrates into your diet and rely less on burning fat for energy, you slowly moderate your intake of fat.

A FAT PRIMER

Monounsaturated fats are found in avocados; olives and olive oil; peanuts, cashews, almonds, and other nuts; and vegetable oils including canola and peanut oil. They have been shown to lower LDL ("bad") cholesterol and to raise HDL ("good") cholesterol.

Polyunsaturated fats are found in vegetables, vegetable oils, tofu, and fatty fish (and other protein sources such as meat to a lesser degree). Avocados, olives, walnuts, and salmon are all terrific sources.

There are different types of polyunsaturated fats:

Omega-3 fatty acids, found in fatty fish such as salmon, flaxseed oil, algae, and nuts, lower triglycerides and reduce platelet stickiness (the buildup of plaque on cell walls of arteries), two of the major risk factors for heart attack. Omega-3 and omega-6 fatty acids, plus omega-9s, are also known as essential fatty acids.

Omega-6 fatty acids, found in vegetable oils, are too prevalent in the standard American diet. Replace the refined corn, safflower, and "vegetable" oils in your pantry with cold-pressed flaxseed oil, canola oil, and olive oil to achieve a desirable ratio of omega-6 to omega-3 of 1 to 1. (Because these fats are so important, we also recommend that you take a supplement containing the essential fatty acids, as explained on page 36.)

Omega-9 fatty acids are also found in canola and olive oil.

Saturated fat is found in meat, eggs, butter, and other animal products as well as in coconut oil and palm oil. Contrary to what you may have heard, these fats also play a role in good health. They enhance the immune system, support liver function, and are an essential component of every cell. Because they are saturated (more solid at room temperature), they are more stable during cooking and less likely to get rancid than other fats, preserving antioxidant levels in the body. Emerging research indicates that saturated fat may not be to blame for high cholesterol linked to heart disease.

Because monounsaturated, polyunsaturated, and saturated fat play different roles in maintaining our health, it is important to make sure you are getting a balance of these natural fats from a variety of sources. This will happen effortlessly when you eat an array of whole foods, as you do when you do Atkins. Indeed, most of the protein foods you'll be eating when you do Atkins naturally contain a balance of different types of natural fats. So although beef is usually considered high in saturated fat, it actually contains more than 50 percent mono- and polyunsaturated fats. In fact, only 17 percent of the calories in a porterhouse steak comes from saturated fat.

HOW TO BALANCE YOUR FATS

Here's how to ensure you're getting a healthy balance of mono- and polyunsaturated fats, saturated fat, and essential fatty acids:

- vary your protein choices

- dress salads and cooked vegetables with olive oil

- decrease the use of corn and other vegetable oils

- consume avocados, olives, nuts, and seeds regularly

- take an essential fatty acids supplement

TRANS FATS: THE REAL BAD GUYS

Highly processed foods rely on hydrogenated or partially hydrogenated oils (also called manufactured trans fats). To make them, food chemists take natural fats, heat them to extremely high temperatures, and add hydrogen. (Trans fats also occur naturally in small amounts in the human intestines as well as in meat and dairy products.) Manufactured fats were very popular in the food industry because

- They're inexpensive to produce.

- When used in baked goods, they keep the product from crumbling.

- They don't get rancid, meaning they have a significantly longer shelf life than foods made with natural fats.

As many as 40 percent of the foods on supermarket shelves contain manufactured fats. Almost all packaged baked goods contain them. Along with margarine (unless it's labeled trans-fat free) and almost all vegetable shortening, manufactured trans fats turn up in some strange places—such as in jarred marinated artichoke hearts and in pasta and rice mixes. So check food labels carefully. Most fast-food products are fried in them, and many fast-food restaurants use them as their primary cooking oil. You'll also find partially hydrogenated oil in many "diet" and some low-carb food products and in many products marketed to children.

Unlike other kinds of fats, manufactured trans fats are bad for you. How bad? Hydrogenated fats have been shown to raise triglycerides, LDL ("bad") cholesterol, and other heart disease risk factors, and to lower HDL ("good") cholesterol; they have also been linked to an elevated risk of heart disease and death from heart attack.

In the Nurses' Health Study of 85,000 women, those who had the highest dietary intake of trans fats had a 50 percent higher risk of heart attack compared to women who consumed the least amount. One Food and Drug Administration (FDA) expert estimates that removing all trans fats from margarine and 3 percent from baked goods would prevent more than 17,000 heart attacks and more than 5,000 heart-related deaths a year. Researchers at the Harvard School of Public Health suggest that replacing trans fats in the diet with polyunsaturated fats can reduce diabetes risk by as much as 40 percent. A review study concluded that no amount of manufactured trans fats in the diet can be considered safe.

The FDA has ruled that by January 2006 all products containing manufactured trans fats must be labeled accordingly. As long as you concentrate on eating whole foods, as the ANA recommends, and strictly avoid highly processed choices, you will bypass the foods most likely to contain trans fats. By reading the nutritional information on the labels for everything else, you can avoid these dangerous fats altogether.

THREE

ATKINS 101: HOW TO DO IT RIGHT

For many of you the Atkins Nutritional Approach (ANA) represents a new way of thinking about what you eat and how you control your weight. It is a nutritional approach designed to help you achieve a healthy weight and stay there. If you want to shed a quick 15 pounds for your high school reunion or your daughter's wedding and then revert to your old habits, Atkins is not for you. Remember that the eating plan is only one of the three parts of the Atkins Advantage Program. Motivation and fitness are the other two.

THE FOUR PHASES

The ANA allows for the gradual reintroduction of healthy carbs into your diet so that you and your metabolism can adjust to this healthy new way of eating. Moving through the first three phases, which culminate in the fourth and final phase that is really a permanent lifestyle, allows your new culinary habits to become second nature.

Following is an overview of the principles behind each of the phases. We'll explain the rules specific to each phase in the appropriate weeks in Part II. Of course, you may not be moving into the next phase of the program in the week that phase is described; in fact, you may spend the whole 12 weeks in the first two phases. That's just fine. By reading about all four phases you'll know what is ahead and where to look when you are ready to progress to the next phase. If you have more than a few pounds to lose, moving from Induction to Lifetime Maintenance is essential for long-term success.

PHASE 1: INDUCTION

Induction is a powerful tool and your first step toward weight loss and a lifetime of better health. During this phase you'll switch your metabolism from one that burns carbohydrates to one that burns primarily fat. By controlling carb intake you'll stabilize your blood sugar and insulin levels, which enables you to escape the cravings and energy dips that can make it nearly impossible to control your weight. You will be consuming daily about 20 grams of net carbs. The foods you can and cannot eat are listed under Acceptable Foods in Induction on page 26.

Because Induction requires some psychological and physical energy, it is important that you choose the right time to begin. Don't start the program during a period of great stress or under unusual circumstances such as on a vacation.

Don't overextend yourself physically or otherwise; this is a time to take good care of yourself and to honor the hard work your body is doing.

In some respects, Induction is the most rewarding phase of the program: Most people find it extremely liberating to be free of their dependence on refined carbohydrates and are richly rewarded after the first few days by an energy surge typically accompanied by quick weight loss.

Induction is a very important part of the ANA, but it's not the whole story and most definitely is not the way you'll be eating for the rest of your life. We recommend that people do Induction for a minimum of 14 days, because that's how long it usually takes to break your body's addictions. If you have a significant amount of weight to lose, you may choose to stay in this phase longer; in fact, for most people it is perfectly safe to stay in Induction for up to six months. It is important to have your lipid profile checked again 8 to 12 weeks into the program. If you have been following the program correctly, you can expect to see improvement or at least learn that no adverse effects have occurred. On occasion an individual will see an unusual result that will require follow-up with the doctor.

In Ongoing Weight Loss (OWL) you add more and a greater variety of carbohydrate foods to your meals. You'll do so slowly, in small increments and in a certain order, so as to minimize the impact they have on your blood sugar. In the process you'll discover how many grams of carbohydrates you can eat while continuing to lose weight steadily.

You'll add carbs in increments of 5 grams daily every week until your weight loss slows to a crawl or stalls altogether. To resume weight loss or pick up the pace, usually all you have to do is cut back slightly on your carb intake until weight loss resumes. This number, expressed in grams of net carbs, is your Critical Carbohydrate Level for Losing (CCLL). A number of factors determine your CCLL, including your genes, metabolism, and level of activity. Finding your CCLL allows you to individualize Atkins to your needs and tastes, which is key to achieving success.

IS IT SAFE TO BURN FAT?

You may have heard the term *ketosis,* which is really a shortened version of lipolysis/ketosis or benign dietary ketosis. Lipolysis simply means that you're burning fat, and ketosis means that you're producing ketones, the by-products of fat burning. Ketone production is not exclusive to doing Atkins. Other weight loss methods also stimulate the production of ketones, and your body makes ketones in the hours you fast between dinner and breakfast. Whenever your body turns to fat for energy, ketones are burned.

Ketosis isn't, and shouldn't be confused with, a dangerous condition called ketoacidosis that is experienced by uncontrolled diabetics, severe alcoholics, and seriously malnourished individuals. Ketosis is simply chemical evidence that your body is burning fat, its backup fuel, which is why we prefer to use the term "burning fat" instead of ketosis. No matter what you call it, it is a completely safe and normal process.

OWL is an opportunity to learn about your own personal parameters, as the most successful Atkins Achievers have. How many grams of carbs can you eat while still losing weight? What types of new foods can you add without beginning to see a significant slowdown in the pace of your weight loss? You'll stay in OWL until you have only 5 to 10 pounds left to lose to reach your goal weight.

PHASE 3: PRE-MAINTENANCE

During this phase you'll increase your daily carb intake by 10 grams each week as long as you keep shedding pounds and/or inches. Your weight loss will slow to a crawl. This might feel like a setback, and you might be tempted to cut out those extra carbs—but please don't. If your goal is permanent weight control, it won't help you to sprint to the finish line. This phase retrains your body for a lifetime of weight management and good health.

Another challenge most people experience in this phase is slightly increased appetite, the result of cycling back and forth between burning primarily fat and burning carbs for fuel. This won't be a problem as long as you continue to control your carb intake and to consume carbs with adequate amounts of protein and fat. It is also very important during this phase not to become overly hungry by going too long between meals.

During Pre-Maintenance you'll reach your goal weight. Once you reach this milestone, you'll experiment with finding the number of grams of net carbs you can eat without either losing or gaining weight. This is called your Atkins Carbohydrate Equilibrium (ACE), your personal threshold for carb intake. Once you have maintained your goal weight for a month, your ACE is the number of daily grams that will accompany you into the next phase.

PHASE 4: LIFETIME MAINTENANCE

The previous three phases present the tools you need to lose weight—and practice keeping it off. Lifetime Maintenance really isn't a phase at all; it is a permanent way of eating.

We recommend that once you've reached your goal weight, you monitor your weight closely, being careful never to gain more than 5 pounds. Typically, all that involves is staying at or slightly below your ACE. However, if you do regain pounds and your behavior and eating habits haven't changed, and you're still keeping your carbohydrate consumption at or just under your ACE, it may be time for a bit of adjustment. This can happen for many reasons, including reduced physical activity, hormonal shifts, a new medication, or the aging process itself. If it does happen, you'll find that regaining your footing isn't difficult because you have all the tools you need at your disposal. You'll simply slowly decrease your carbohydrate intake until you've lost any weight you've gained back, and then find your new ACE. The good news is that this is a two-way street. If you take up running or otherwise become more physically active, you may be able to raise your ACE. For more on this, see the Fitness Rewards Chart on page 202.

DOING ATKINS IN THE REAL WORLD

Here are some things you'll want to keep in mind as you shop and plan meals:

At the core of Atkins is a commitment to whole foods. It's one thing to snack on a bar or a shake, or even to use a product as an occasional meal replacement; it's quite another to spend your day eating one low-carb product after another. Instead, integrate low-sugar, high-protein, fibrous products into your daily meals and plan intelligently to make sure you are not skimping on whole foods. It is worth remembering that quality low-sugar foods can be good sources of protein, vitamins, minerals, and fiber.

Not all products are created equal. As of this writing there are no government guidelines for what constitutes low carb, so you must study the Nutrition Facts panel to determine how low a certain "low-carb" or low-sugar product really is. Nor are "low carb" and "lower carb" the same thing. In particular watch out for the so-called low-carb or low-sugar versions of popular products such as candy bars and sodas. A lower-sugar soda may contain half the carbs or sugar found in the regular version, but it still may be high in sugar or high-fructose corn syrup. You must read carefully both the Nutrition Facts panel and the list of ingredients on the label.

Not all products are made with good nutrition in mind. Worse, major food companies are jumping on the low-carb bandwagon regardless of whether they really understand the Atkins approach. Some products may be lower carb than the conventional alternative but still contain high levels of sugars, trans fats, bleached white flour, and other nutrient-empty ingredients.

Many low-carb products use sugar alcohols such as maltitol, sorbitol, and isomalt (a combination of the first two) in low-carb products as sweeteners and to add structure that sugar normally provides. Despite their name, sugar alcohols, also called polyols, are not alcohol and have a limited impact on most healthy people's blood sugar. (However, people with diabetes should test their blood sugar 90 minutes after eating products that contain sugar alcohols.) If you are not diabetic but find that you are having trouble losing weight, try eliminating products that contain these substances (especially those containing maltitol syrup) for a week or two to determine if this is the case for you. Some people find that eating more than 20 grams of sugar alcohols in a day gives them gas, cramping, or diarrhea. (Some people get symptoms at lower doses.) Compare products to find those with the lowest levels of sugar alcohols.

ACCEPTABLE FOODS IN INDUCTION

The chart on the next page shows the foods you may eat liberally during Induction.

ALL FISH, INCLUDING . . .	ALL FOWL, INCLUDING . . .	ALL SHELLFISH, INCLUDING . . .	ALL MEAT, INCLUDING . . .	ALL EGGS, INCLUDING . . .
TUNA	CHICKEN	OYSTERS*	BEEF	SCRAMBLED
SALMON	TURKEY	MUSSELS*	PORK	FRIED
SOLE	DUCK	DUCK	LAMB	POACHED
TROUT	GOOSE	CLAMS	BACON[†]	SOFT-BOILED
FLOUNDER	CORNISH HEN	SQUID	VEAL	HARD-BOILED
SARDINES	QUAIL	SHRIMP	HAM[†]	DEVILED
HERRING	PHEASANT	CRABMEAT	VENISON	OMELETS

OTHER FOODS THAT ARE ACCEPTABLE DURING INDUCTION

Cheese. You can consume 3 to 4 ounces daily of the following full-fat, firm, soft, and semisoft aged cheeses,[‡] including:

cheddar

cow, sheep, and goat cheese

cream cheese

Gouda

mozzarella

Roquefort and other blue cheeses

Swiss

* Oysters and mussels are higher in carbs than other shellfish, so limit them to 4 ounces per day.

† Processed meats, such as ham, bacon, pepperoni, salami, hot dogs, and other luncheon meats—and some fish—may be cured with added sugar and will contribute carbs. Try to avoid meat and fish products cured with nitrates, which are known carcinogens. Also beware of products that are not exclusively meat, fish, or fowl, such as imitation fish, meatloaf, and breaded foods. Finally, do not consume more than 4 ounces of organ meats a day.

‡ All cheeses have some carbohydrate content. The quantity you eat should be governed by that knowledge. The rule of thumb is to count 1 ounce of cheese as equivalent to 1 gram of carbohydrate. Note that cottage cheese, farmer's cheese, and other fresh cheeses are not permitted during Induction. No "diet" cheese, cheese spreads, or whey cheeses are permitted. Individuals with known yeast symptoms, dairy allergy, or cheese intolerance must avoid cheese. Imitation cheese products are not allowed, except for soy or rice cheese—but check the carbohydrate content.

Vegetables. You should eat 12 to 15 net carbs a day of vegetables. These salad vegetables are high in phytonutrients and provide a good source of fiber:

alfalfa sprouts	daikon	mâche
arugula	endive	mushrooms
bok choy	escarole	parsley
celery	fennel	peppers
chicory	jicama	radicchio
chives	lettuce	radishes
cucumber	lettuce, romaine	sorrel

Other Vegetables: Within the 12 to 15 net carb daily vegetable requirement, these vegetables are slightly higher in carbohydrate content than the salad vegetables listed above, but they also provide important nutrients and add variety to your daily food intake:

artichoke	chard	sauerkraut
artichoke hearts	collard greens	scallions
asparagus	dandelion greens	snow peas
bamboo shoots	eggplant	spaghetti squash
bean sprouts	hearts of palm	spinach
beet greens	kale	string or wax beans
broccoli	kohlrabi	summer squash
broccoli rabe	leeks	tomato
Brussels sprouts	okra	turnips
cabbage	onion	water chestnuts
cauliflower	pumpkin*	zucchini
celery root	rhubarb	

* technically a fruit

If a vegetable, such as spinach or tomato, cooks down significantly, it must be measured raw so as not to under-estimate its carb count.

Salad Garnishes

    crumbled crisp bacon

    grated cheese

    minced hard-boiled egg

    sautéed mushrooms

    sour cream

Spices. All spices and herbs to taste, but make sure none contain added sugar.

basil	garlic	rosemary
cayenne pepper	ginger	sage
cilantro	oregano	tarragon
dill	pepper	thyme

For salad dressing, use oil and vinegar or lemon juice and herbs and spices. Prepared salad dressings without added sugar and no more than two carbs per tablespoon serving are also fine.

ACCEPTABLE FATS AND OILS

Many fats, especially certain oils, are essential to good nutrition. Olive oil is particularly valuable. All other vegetable oils are allowed, the best being canola, walnut, soybean, grapeseed, sesame, sunflower, and safflower oils, especially if they are labeled "cold-pressed" or "expeller-pressed." Do not cook polyunsaturated oils, such as corn, soybean, and sunflower oil, at high temperatures or allow to brown or smoke.

Butter is allowed. Margarine should be avoided, not because of its carbohydrate content, but because it is usually made of trans fats (hydrogenated oils), which are a health hazard. (Some nonhydrogenated margarines are now available.)

You don't have to remove the skin and fat from meat or fowl. Salmon and other cold-water fish are an excellent source of omega-3 fatty acids.

Remember that trying to do a low-fat version of the Atkins Nutritional Approach may interfere with fat burning and derail your weight loss.

ARTIFICIAL SWEETENERS

You must determine which artificial sweeteners agree with you, but the following are allowed: sucralose (marketed as Splenda), saccharin, cyclamate, and acesulfame-K. Natural sweeteners ending in the suffix "-ose," such as maltose, etc., should be avoided. However, most sugar alcohols have a minimal effect on blood sugar and are acceptable. Saccharin has been extensively studied, and harmful effects were produced in the lab when fed to rats only in extremely high doses. The Food and Drug Administration (FDA) has removed saccharin from its list of carcinogens, basing its decision upon a thorough review of the medical literature and the National Institute of Science's statement that there is "no clear association between saccharin and human cancer." It can be safely consumed in moderation, meaning no more than three packets a day. Saccharin is marketed as Sweet'n Low.

The Atkins preference, however, is sucralose (Splenda), the only sweetener made from sugar. Sucralose is safe, noncaloric, and does not raise blood sugar. It has been used in Canada for years, and the FDA approved it after reviewing more than 100 studies conducted over the past 20 years. Note that each packet of sugar substitute contains about 1 gram of carbohydrate, so don't forget to include the amount in your daily totals.

ACCEPTABLE BEVERAGES

Be sure to drink a minimum of eight 8-ounce glasses of water each day, including filtered water, mineral water, spring water, and tap water.

Additionally, you can have the following beverages:

clear broth/bouillon (not all brands; read the label)

club soda

cream, heavy or light (limit to 2 to 3 tablespoons a day; note carbohydrate content)

decaffeinated or regular coffee or tea*

* Caffeine can cause cravings or blood-sugar spikes with some people. If you're one of them, you should drink only decaffeinated beverages. If you don't have a problem with caffeine, you may drink one or two caffeinated beverages a day, because evolving research indicates there may actually be health benefits to a limited amount of caffeine. However, if you have a true caffeine addiction, it will be best to break it during Induction, because any food addiction can cause problems if it isn't taken care of. Once you've broken the addiction and moved on to OWL, you can carefully try adding caffeinated beverages back into your food intake, as long as it doesn't trigger the addiction again.

diet soda made with sucralose (Splenda); be sure to count the carbs

essence-flavored seltzer (must say "no calories")

herb tea (without barley or any fruit sugar added)

lemon juice or lime juice (note that each contains 2.8 grams carbohydrate per ounce); limit to 2 to 3 tablespoons

SPECIAL CATEGORY FOODS

To add variety, each day you can also eat 10 to 20 olives, half a small avocado, an ounce of sour cream, or three ounces of unsweetened heavy cream, as well as 2 to 3 tablespoons of lemon juice or lime juice. But be aware that these foods occasionally slow down weight loss in some people, and may need to be avoided in the first two weeks. If you seem to be losing slowly, moderate your intake of these foods.

CONVENIENCE FOODS

Although it is important that you eat primarily unprocessed foods, some controlled-carb food products can come in handy when you are unable to find appropriate food, can't take time for a meal, or need a quick snack. More and more companies are creating healthy food products that can be eaten during the Induction phase of Atkins. Just remember two things:

1. Not all convenience food products are the same, so check labels and carbohydrate content.

2. While any of these foods can make doing Atkins easier, don't overdo it. Remember you must always follow the Rules of Induction.

FOUR

GET READY, GET SET: BEFORE YOU BEGIN

Before you begin your amazing journey, there are a few things you'll need to do.

Regardless of where this day falls in the calendar year, I'd like you to think of this as New Year's Eve. You're preparing for a new beginning—as you do when you bid adieu to the old year. Likewise, this should be a joyful time, one full of hope for the future.

OUT WITH THE OLD

In ancient Rome on New Year's Eve, people would throw out their old furniture in order to make room for a new and better future. In the same spirit let's perform a purification ritual on your kitchen: Get out a heavy-duty garbage bag and let the tossing begin!

Think of this as a mission to discard the junk food that is making you heavy and unhealthy. Ultimately, the program will help you curb your desire for these unhealthy foods, and after the first or second week your cravings for them will naturally subside. For now, having them out of sight will help keep them out of mind.

Here's what should go in the trash bag:

- all sugars—granulated, confectioner's, and brown

- all sweet syrups including honey, molasses, maple, and corn

- bleached white flour and all products containing it, including crackers, bread, and conventional pastas

- all products containing added trans fats. Look on the label for hydrogenated or partially hydrogenated oils or shortening. Store-bought pastries, doughnuts, crackers, and cookies are likely suspects.

- snack food: chips, cookies, ice cream, and so on

- soda and other beverages sweetened with sugar or high-fructose corn syrup

---

FAMILY ISSUES

Get your family on your team by talking to them about the principles of smart nutrition—high protein, fiber, and low sugar. Even if they're not doing the program, they can support you and learn common-sense nutritional principles—whether it's helping with grocery shopping, joining you on a walk, or picking up some housekeeping duties so that you have time to exercise. Enlist their support and answer any questions they might have.

What should you do if you encounter resistance from your family when you ditch unhealthy foods? Ask if they'd mind living without these products in the house, at least for the next month or so to help ensure your success. If you meet with tremendous resistance, don't fight it but ask what your significant other or housemates are willing to do.

If all else fails, designate a single junk food cupboard, one that will be off-limits to you.

Atkins can be highly contagious, especially when the person doing Atkins is also the chef. Once the rest of the family sees how good you feel and look (and how delicious the food is), don't be surprised if they ask to come aboard. Even if they don't join you on your low-carb voyage, you can ensure that they are eating the best carbs available. They'll like whole grain breads and crackers, whole wheat pasta, and grains such as quinoa and brown rice instead of instant white rice. After all, everyone can benefit from avoiding high sugar intake and trans fats as well as refined products, and replacing them with whole foods full of the nutrients we all need—especially growing children. (Note: Anyone under the age of 18 should not follow the weight loss phases of Atkins or any weight loss program unless monitored by a physician.)

As you put all those unhealthy food items into that bag, be mindful of why you are doing it. How do you feel about these foods that have compromised your health and caused you to be overweight? As you work your way through the refrigerator and cabinets, remember that not only can you live without all this unhealthy food, but you'll thrive without it.

Finally, because a new start is about ushering out the old and bringing in the new, you might want to discard one more item. Choose something emblematic of the "old you," something you'd like to leave behind. It could be that big bowl you used for large portions of ice cream or cereal. Perhaps it's a recent photo of yourself—the one that made you decide to slim down—or an article of clothing that you hated having to buy in your current size. By ceremoniously discarding this token along with all those boxes of cookies, crackers, and chips, you will be letting go of the "old you."

What you do with the items is up to you. Toss them in the trash or give them to neighbors. Give unopened packages to a food bank or homeless shelter, and give discarded clothing to a church sale or the Salvation Army.

IN WITH THE NEW

Being prepared saves you time and energy so that you'll have more of each when it really matters. You won't need many *things* (besides the right foods and motivation, commitment, and dedication) to follow the All-New Atkins Advantage Program, but you will need to have these few items on hand:

- a soft measuring tape

- an accurate bathroom scale

- a notebook or blank journal. This will become your Atkins Advantage Journal, a private place for you to record your progress and do the journaling activities required of you in this program.

- a carbohydrate gram counter, such as Dr. Atkins' New Carbohydrate Gram Counter, which contains lists of common foods and their net carb counts. With one of these in your pocket, you will always know the number of grams of net carbs contained in what you're eating.

THE ATKINS PANTRY

To restock those pantry and refrigerator shelves, refer to the list of Acceptable Foods in Induction in Chapter 3 and make your own shopping list to take to the grocery store.

It's not just what you eat that counts but what happens to the food before it reaches your table. Making healthy food choices starts at the market, long before your fork is on the way to your mouth.

- Whenever possible, choose organic foods that have been grown without artificial fertilizers and treated with the minimum of pesticides.

- Choose meat and dairy products from animals that have not been treated with hormones or antibiotics.

- Avoid nitrates, other preservatives, and colorings that are used in meats such as salami, bologna, pepperoni, cured ham, and smoked fish.

HAVE YOUR SUPPLEMENTS READY

Although whole foods are the heart of Atkins, supplements are an important reinforcement to give you the boost you need to look, feel, and perform your best. While your body needs certain vitamins and minerals, and must get many from the foods you eat, your diet may need supplementation for many reasons. Food grown in overharvested or polluted soil and shipped great distances is inherently less nutritious; cooking may further deplete its nutritional value. Also, even the best of us don't eat picture-perfect meals every single day.

We recommend that you take three supplements every day: a multivitamin, essential fatty acids, and fiber. We'll also introduce you to a few other nutrients that have helped many people who have done Atkins successfully. You can make an educated decision about whether these supplements are right for you.

Please speak to your doctor before starting any kind of supplement program, especially if you're taking prescription medication.

THE ALL-IMPORTANT MULTIVITAMIN

A good multivitamin is crucial for a well-balanced diet. (We refer to this supplement as a multivitamin, although it should contain minerals as well.) There is compelling evidence that taking a multivitamin improves health; in fact, a report published by two Harvard Medical School physicians recommends that all adults take one every day. Their recommendation was based on the research that taking a multivitamin helps reduce risk factors for a number of chronic diseases, including heart disease, some cancers, and osteoporosis.

For women who are pregnant or planning to become pregnant, a daily multivitamin also prevents neural tube birth defects caused by folate deficiency in the first trimester in pregnancy, which is why the American Medical Association recommends that all women of childbearing age or who are pregnant should take a multivitamin.

A 2003 study showed that 43 percent of people who took a daily multivitamin had an infectious disease such as a cold or flu over the course of a year compared to 73 percent of those taking a placebo. The most startling results were in the 51 participants who had diabetes: 93 percent of those in the placebo group got sick, compared to 17 percent who were taking multivitamins. So while a multivitamin is preventative for everyone, it seems to be especially important for people with diabetes.

All multivitamins aren't created equal. To get a quality product, make sure your multivitamin doesn't contain any of the following:

iron (unless your doctor has specifically said that you require iron supplementation)	wax	starch
	yeast	artificial colors or flavors
	corn	
	wheat or gluten	preservatives
sugar		digestible plastics
	salt	
hydrogenated oils		fillers

Follow the package instructions and take them with meals to encourage maximum absorption. Multivitamins taken in divided doses rather than just once a day make water-soluble nutrients available throughout the day.

ESSENTIAL FATTY ACIDS (EFAs)

These oils are called essential because they are needed to maintain vital bodily functions, but they must be supplied by foods or supplements. The omega-3 fatty acids, found in various plants and in fatty cold-water fish, have tremendous benefits for our health. The foods you eat when doing Atkins will provide more of these than you would get on a lower-fat diet, but to ensure that your body has the EFAs in the proper balance that it needs to run properly, we suggest you take an EFA supplement.

Omega-3 fatty acids, found in eggs, cold-water fish such as salmon and mackerel, nuts, seeds, algae, and flaxseed oil, are further divided into alpha-linolenic acid

(ALA), docosahexaenoic acid (DHA), and eicosapentanoic acid (EPA). The three omega-3 fatty acids lower inflammation and levels of triglycerides and blood pressure, all significant risk factors for heart disease.

Omega-6 fatty acids include gamma-linoleic acid (GLA) and also have beneficial effects on levels of triglyceride and blood pressure, along with important anti-inflammatory benefits. They are found in various vegetable oils, including borage and primrose oils.

Many processed foods contain omega-6 in the form of refined soy and corn oils, but excessive intake of these processed oils skews the balance of essential fatty acids. Our bodies work best when omega-3 and omega-6 fatty acids are in a 1 to 1 ratio; the typical American eats a ratio closer to 1 to 16!

Researchers believe that this imbalance may contribute to ailments such as heart disease, cancer, and autoimmune and inflammatory diseases. It is important to rebalance the ratio of omega-3 to omega-6 fatty acids. You can reduce the amount of omega-6s you consume by eating fewer processed foods (as you naturally do on Atkins) and by replacing corn, safflower, and other vegetable oils with cold-pressed canola or olive oil, which contain a better ratio of these fats.

Note: If you're on blood-thinning medication, consult your doctor before beginning a supplement that contains EFAs.

FIBER

New dietary guidelines from the Institute of Medicine recommend that women consume 21 to 25 grams of fiber a day, and men 30 to 38. Unfortunately, the average American consumes only about 16 grams daily. Based on these new guidelines and emerging research showing the numerous benefits of fiber, we recommend that everyone who does Atkins take a fiber supplement. Because some high-fiber foods such as whole grains, legumes, and starchy vegetables are concentrated sources of carbohydrate, their consumption will interfere with fat burning and should not be consumed in the early weight loss phases of the ANA.

Dietary fiber helps make food filling, and fiber-rich foods tend to be rich in vitamins, minerals, and other valuable nutrients. Fiber also has innumerable health benefits.

Fiber has a stabilizing influence on blood sugar because it slows the rate at which glucose from food enters the bloodstream. Although fiber is technically considered a carbohydrate, it has a negligible effect on blood sugar.

Fiber reduces levels of cholesterol and triglycerides, two of the major risk factors for heart disease.

Fiber reduces the body's exposure to toxins from certain foods by moving them quickly through the digestive system, which may reduce the risk of stomach and colon cancers.

Fiber is good for your gastrointestinal tract. Increasing your dietary fiber can help prevent diverticulosis, relieve constipation and hemorrhoids, and improve on-going regularity. This is especially useful when your body is adjusting to a new way of eating.

Note: If you are experiencing constipation, make sure you are drinking at least eight glasses of water a day and exercising in addition to supplementing with fiber.

A Variety of Ways to Take Fiber Supplements. You can choose from several fiber supplements and ways to take them:

- Ground flaxseed, found in the refrigerated section at health food stores, can be stirred into a protein drink, herbal iced tea, or soup. You can also sprinkle it on salads or cooked vegetables. If you wish to grind seeds yourself, be sure to use them immediately because they can quickly become rancid once ground.

- Psyllium husks and products made from them are readily available under brand names such as Fiberall and Metamucil. Make sure you use a product that does not contain sugar. Mix the husks in a glass of water and drink at about the same time every day.

- Unsweetened unprocessed oat or wheat bran is also available at health food stores. Sprinkle it on vegetables or salad, or mix with a little low-sugar yogurt.

Consume a minimum of 2 teaspoons of ground flaxseed, unprocessed bran, or psyllium husks daily. With fiber it is always a good idea to start small and to increase your dose incrementally so that your body has a chance to become accustomed to it. (Too much fiber and too little water can actually cause constipation.) Otherwise, you may experience digestive distress, such as bloating, gas, cramping, or diarrhea.

MAPPING YOUR JOURNEY:
WHERE YOU ARE AND WHERE YOU ARE GOING

To map your journey effectively you first have to find the "you are here" point on the map by assessing your risk factors, that is, your baseline blood chemistry, weight, and measurements.

Check with your physician before making any significant lifestyle changes—even beneficial ones. Before you begin the Atkins Advantage Program:

- Make sure your doctor understands that the Atkins Advantage Program has a fitness component, and ask if there are any restrictions or modifications you need to take into account.

- If you regularly take a medication, ask your doctor if the one you are on is likely to interfere with weight loss. (See pages 156–57 for a list of some that may slow your metabolism.)

- Have your blood pressure taken and record the results in your journal.

- Have your fasting blood levels done (only water for 8 to 12 hours prior). They should include total cholesterol, HDL, LDL, triglycerides, glucose, and uric acid levels as well as other routine blood chemistry tests. (If you have had complete lab work done within the last three months and your weight has remained stable, you

don't have to get these tests again.) When your blood work is completed, be sure to have a copy of the results sent to you for your records.

> ## REASONS TO DO ATKINS DIFFERENTLY—OR NOT AT ALL
>
> The following conditions would make it imperative that you proceed *only* with medical supervision because your doctor can help you modify the program so that it works for you:
>
> **You have kidney disease.** Do not do any phase of Atkins unless advised to do so and supervised by your physician.
>
> **You are pregnant or nursing.** You can follow Phase 4: Lifetime Maintenance but not any of the weight loss phases.
>
> **You are taking medications for blood sugar or blood pressure.** You'll need to consult with your doctor before you begin so that you can plan a strategy to adjust your medications as needed. You will need less as your blood sugar stabilizes.
>
> **You have a history of gout or high uric acid.** You should be careful when following any weight loss plan. Monitor your uric acid levels, stay well hydrated, and deliberately moderate the rate of weight loss to decrease the possibility of a gout attack.
>
> **You are under the age of 18.** You should not do any of the weight loss phases of Atkins unless supervised by your physician.

It is best to have these tests done before changing your diet. They can still be done during the first week of doing Atkins, however; they will serve as your baseline. Repeating these tests after 8 to 12 weeks on the program, along with your weight loss and how you feel, will be an indication of how you're responding. People who start

To get the most accurate measurement when weighing yourself:

Always weigh yourself at the same time. Your weight can fluctuate over the course of a day. You'll get the most accurate measurement by weighing yourself first thing in the morning without clothing.

Women should stay clear of the scale just before and during their period. The same water retention that makes you feel bloated will make a difference on the scale. The time just after your period is the most accurate time to check your weight.

Resist the impulse to weigh yourself too often. Once a week is sufficient.

Measure whenever you weigh yourself. Inches lost count as much if not more than the number on the scale.

out with high triglycerides or high LDL cholesterol numbers can usually see a dramatic improvement even in just 8 weeks. If you need to make a course correction, the numbers will tell you that, too. (Note: Unless your first round of tests reveals an abnormal result, your medical insurance may not pay for retesting within this time frame. If your baseline results are in the normal range and paying for a new set of tests in 8 weeks would cause you financial hardship, you can wait three months to be retested.

ESTABLISHING YOUR BASELINE WEIGHT

Record your weight in your Atkins Advantage Journal. (Mark the top of the page "Baseline Weight and Measurement," and add the date.) Include your blood pressure and blood work results on this page.

ESTABLISHING YOUR BASELINE MEASUREMENTS
Using your soft measuring tape, measure your:

upper arm at the widest point of your dominant arm, and do so each time

chest around the nipples

waist—the tape should meet at your belly button

hips—position the tape on the top knob of your hipbone, approximately 8 inches below your waist

thigh at the widest point on your dominant side

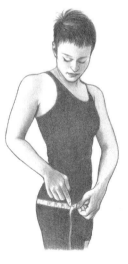

Record each of these measurements in your Atkins Advantage Journal, on the same page as your baseline weight.

When you are finished, look at the numbers you've recorded in your journal and then close the book on them. They may have been weighing you down for years, but that's about to change. Over the next 12 weeks you will get all the tools and support you need to change those numbers into ones that will make you proud and give you a greater sense of personal empowerment than you've ever known.

YOUR FOCUS STRING

There is one more activity that I'd like you to do as part of your "New Diet" celebration.

Last year when training for an Ironman, I just couldn't seem to achieve the level of concentration and focus I had been able to marshal when I was working to qualify for the event. The solution came from an unlikely quarter: my ten-year-old daughter. Imagining my daughters at the finish line is always a major motivator for me, but they wouldn't be at the Ironman because of school. So when Samantha asked me to help her tie a piece of blue string around her wrist as a "friendship bracelet," I asked if I could use the leftover string as a "focus" string of my own.

We tied it around my ankle, and I saw it every morning in the shower, every night before I went to bed, and every time I changed into my running shoes or into scrubs to operate. It became a meaningful visual reminder of my commitment, and it helped me turn my mental performance around—both during training and in the race itself when it made me feel that Samantha and Carly were with me even though they were thousands of miles away.

This trick can also give you the focus you'll need for the weeks ahead. Everyone has a part of their body they're not happy with—a big belly or wobbly thighs, for example. Take that troublesome body part, "measure" it with a piece of string, and cut the string at that length. Over the next 12 weeks keep that piece of string somewhere prominent—coiled in a pocket, wrapped around your ankle or wrist, or draped over the dresser mirror or the rearview mirror of your car—so that it serves as a constant reminder of your commitment to this program.

When you see it, reaffirm your commitment to feeling and looking better. Reassure yourself that you're on the right track and that all you have to do is follow the program to see results. When you find yourself distracted, take a moment to focus on the string and renew your commitment. In the final week of this program you'll remeasure that body part with that same piece of string, and I think you'll be surprised and pleased with the results.

—Stuart L. Trager, M.D.

Now that you know where you are, your next task is to figure out your destination point: a realistic, healthy goal weight.

Dr. Atkins didn't believe in a one-size-fits-all approach to weight loss. He thought that your goal weight should be the one at which you feel comfortable and attractive and able to enjoy life. Have you ever been at a weight that made you feel that way? Perhaps in high school or college or on your wedding day? Do you remember how much you weighed or what size you wore? Be realistic: If too many years have elapsed, that goal weight may not be achievable or maintainable as part of a healthy lifestyle.

The Body Mass Index (BMI) chart for adults can help you determine a healthy weight range (see http://www.nhlbi.nih.gov/guidelines/obesity/bmi_tbl.htm). All you need to know to use this index is your height in inches and your weight. If you wish to perform the calculation yourself, the BMI formula is weight in pounds/(height in inches)×(height in inches)×703. A BMI between 20 and 24.9 is what the government considers within a healthy range. Your BMI should fall within those parameters.

These are simply guidelines. For instance, a slightly higher BMI is perfectly okay if you're very muscular. If you are older, a BMI that is on the low side may mean you are poorly nourished.

Mark your target weight and BMI in your Atkins Advantage Journal under the baseline measurements you've already recorded.

ONE LAST SPLURGE?

People often ask, "Can I enjoy one last blowout before I start the program?" The answer is no, and we believe it's an answer you'll come to of your own accord when you examine why you want this last hurrah.

The urge to binge is probably a holdover from other times you've tried to lose weight, when you've desperately tried to "stock up" on energy and food that tasted good before going into a period of hunger and deprivation, like a bear going into hibernation. That may have been appropriate behavior then, but it's not necessary now. You're not going on a diet tomorrow; you're doing Atkins.

Atkins is a lifestyle, a way of eating that you'll be happy to incorporate in your life, not one that deprives you of foods that you love. Unlike those other times, we'll never ask you to go hungry, so you have no reason to stock up tonight. And there is no time like the present to give up those old unsuccessful habits.

WHAT HAVE YOU BEEN EATING?

This activity will make you think twice about having one last binge of your favorite high-carb foods. In your Atkins Advantage Journal, list your ten favorite foods, whether whole foods such as baked potatoes, sweets such as Rocky Road ice cream or Strawberry Twizzlers, or snack foods such as caramel popcorn or rice cakes. Be honest; no one else needs to see this list.

Create two columns next to each item. Estimate the portion size you tend to eat at one sitting and enter that in the first column. Then find the net carb gram count for each food, taking portion size into consideration. In the case of whole foods, use a carb gram counter (there is one at www.atkins.com/carb-counter). With packaged foods or snacks, which are unlikely to be included in the carb gram counter, check the label or the manufacturer's Web site for the information. You will see total grams of carbohydrate. Simply deduct the grams of fiber to get the number of net carbs, taking serving size into consideration. (If, for example, half a cup of a snack food contains 20 grams of net carbs and you usually eat two cups, the actual number will be 80 grams.) Put that number in the second column. Unless your favorite foods are hamburgers, omelets, and vegetables, chances are you will be shocked by the numbers beside your favorite foods.

Remember these numbers when you need a little added motivation in the weeks to come.

MAKE A "NEW YOU" RESOLUTION

Every one of us has made New Year's resolutions; most fell by the wayside before January was finished. This time you're not going to pledge to eat less or go to the gym more or be nicer to your colleagues or more patient with your children or call your mother more often. There will be plenty of time for all of that later. For now you only have to make one single promise: to faithfully complete this program. Simply by making this one resolution you'll see the rest fall into place. Twelve weeks from today you'll be glad you made this leap of faith.

Take out a piece of paper and an envelope, and on the piece of paper write: *"I pledge that for the next 12 weeks I will trust in the Atkins Advantage Program and follow it faithfully. If I work the program, it will work for me."*

When you sign your name on this document, you are entering into a contract with yourself. The program will require an investment of time and energy—in other words, a genuine commitment on your part. Like all investments it may not always be comfortable or easy to stick to. But if you hold up your end of the bargain, this particular investment is likely to pay a spectacularly high rate of return.

After you have signed your name, folded the paper, and sealed it in the envelope, put the envelope in a safe place; you will need it again later.

You're all set to begin. Get a good night's sleep knowing that the new you is now within reach.

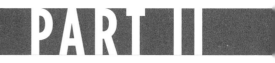

PART II

THE 12-WEEK PLAN

FIVE

WEEK ONE: INDUCTION—FLIPPING THE SWITCH

Congratulations. You've taken the first and most important step toward becoming slimmer, happier, and healthier.

Over the course of the next twelve weeks you're going to experience your power to change the way you feel, the way you look, and even the way you think about many things. When you've completed the program, you'll have developed a skill set that will enable you to capitalize on the momentum you've built. This momentum will carry you through week thirteen and beyond, to achievements that you never thought possible.

You're about to experience the All-New Atkins Advantage. Change, even for the better, is rarely easy, so this week we're not only going to introduce you to the powerful tools you need to change—including a way of eating that will actually change your body's chemistry—but also to the strategies you'll need to cope with those changes.

NUTRITION: THE HEART OF THE MATTER

PHASE ONE: INDUCTION

Induction kick-starts weight loss by changing your body's basic metabolism from burning carbohydrates to burning primarily fat for energy. Once Induction "flips the switch," you'll no longer be constantly tempted by cravings and weighed down by the mood swings and energy dips provoked by the typical high-carb diet.

Induction is the typical starting point for anyone embarking on the Atkins Program, but there are exceptions. If your goal is better health, relief from gastrointestinal complaints or other conditions, or a reduction in risk factors for diabetes and cardiovascular disease rather than weight loss, or if you need to lose only a small amount of weight, you can start at a higher daily carbohydrate level.

If you're within 10 pounds of your goal weight and eat a diet full of carbohydrates, start with Phase 2: Ongoing Weight Loss (OWL) (see page 24), at 30 grams daily of net carbs, which is low enough to reset your metabolism and get your cravings or preoccupation with a particular food under control.

If you're already at your goal weight (or within 10 pounds of it or are underweight, start with Phase 3: Pre-Maintenance (see page 24) at 60 grams daily of net carbs. You may need to adjust your intake up or down depending on whether you lose or gain weight the first week. (If you are underweight, make sure you're eating frequently and getting plenty of calories.)

If you are interested in starting in a later phase, read about OWL and/or Pre-Maintenance and then come back to Week One. *You will need to go through the 12-week program no matter what phase you start at.* Likewise, regardless of phase, you should be taking a daily multivitamin, a fiber supplement, and an essential fatty acids supplement.

THE RULES OF INDUCTION

- Consume approximately 20 grams of net carbs a day, primarily from salad and other vegetables.

- Eat only foods on the Acceptable Foods in Induction list (page 26).

- Eat at least 12 net carbs per day of acceptable vegetables.

- Spread your carb intake over the course of the day.

- Eat three regular meals or four or five small ones. Do not skip meals, especially breakfast, or go more than six waking hours without eating.

- Eat at least 6 ounces (the size of two decks of cards) of protein at every meal.

- Between meals eat an appropriate low-carb snack (see page 111) if you are hungry.

- Drink at least 64 ounces of water throughout the day.

- Take a daily multivitamin, a fiber supplement, and essential fatty acids.

- Stay on Induction for a minimum of two weeks.

GUIDELINES FOR SUCCESS

Keep these guidelines in mind as you move forward:

Eat until you're comfortably full but not stuffed. Atkins doesn't work through deprivation but by saying yes to delicious, healthy foods. Choose a variety of protein sources, which will also ensure that you get a balance of natural fats. Meat, poultry, fish, shellfish, and cheese all contain different natural fats (in various amounts) that your body needs to function optimally. You'll also obtain natural fats in olive oil and other vegetable, nut, and seed oils as well as in olives and avocados.

Eat a variety of vegetables. Recent research shows that the high fiber content of salad and other vegetables keeps the net carb count (see page 15) relatively low. You can eat a minimum of 12 net carbs or 4 cups of vegetables a day in Induction, three as salad and one as cooked vegetables on the Acceptable Foods in Induction list on page 26. If you select lower carb veggies such as lettuce, celery, or radishes and cut back on other carb foods such as cream and/or lemon juice, you can eat even more of them. (See Leave the Counting to Us on page 51.)

Don't skimp on fats. Natural fat is fine when it is not consumed with lots of carbs. The best meals and snacks combine acceptable carbohydrates with protein and fat (for instance, Caesar salad with chicken for lunch; celery sticks stuffed with cream cheese for a snack). These will lessen the impact of the carbs on your blood sugar.

Watch out for hidden carbs in gravy thickened with flour or cornstarch; barbecue, steak, and cranberry sauces, ketchup, and pickle relish, which usually have added sugars; and prepared salad dressings. Balsamic and some types of rice vinegar also contain added sugars. "Sugar-free" or "no-sugar-added" products may have a high carb count if the food is naturally high in sugar. Carbs can also lurk in deli salads such as coleslaw and in chewing gum, vitamins, breath mints, cough drops, and cough syrups.

Watch your caffeine intake. Caffeine can cause fluctuations in insulin and blood sugar levels, which can stimulate your appetite. For most people that takes a lot of caffeine, but others are more sensitive. If caffeine makes you hungry or jittery, avoid it in all its forms, including cola drinks, by switching to decaffeinated. If you are not caffeine-sensitive, however, feel free to have one or two servings of caffeinated beverages (including diet sodas) a day.

WHAT TO EXPECT

During the first week of Induction, you may experience powerful cravings for the high sugar or starchy foods that you are no longer eating. Your body is switching over from one main fuel source to another, and in the process it is severing a lifelong addiction to unhealthy foods. Stick with it. Getting through this period is critical to your success in the Program.

Some people also feel sluggish or tired, or experience headaches during the first few days. These symptoms can be due to withdrawal from caffeine and/or carbs. Don't worry if you have such symptoms. They are just more evidence that Atkins is working! Know these two things: You're doing the right thing for your health, and you won't feel like this forever. In fact, people often report a tremendous surge in energy once their body makes the metabolic conversion to burning primarily fat—and this may be as soon as the fourth day. If symptoms persist beyond the first week or are severe, you should consult a physician.

If you already exercise regularly, you may need to scale back this week until you feel a little more energetic. The relaxation, breathing, and mild stretching exercises found in this chapter are designed to help with the transition. Even if you feel some discomfort, know that fat is your body's natural backup fuel, and burning fat (as you do when you do Atkins) is absolutely safe. Many people feel no ill effects at all. If you're one of those fortunate folks, follow the rules of Induction and stick with your usual fitness routine.

Conquer Cravings. Ex-smokers can tell you that the worst thing about facing down a craving isn't just the intense desire for something but the fear that you'll *always* want it as intensely. Carbohydrate addiction is similar. Rest assured that once your body has switched to a fat metabolism, your cravings will diminish or even disappear. Meanwhile, if you find yourself at the mercy of a serious craving, try these tactics:

- Nibble on a low-carb alternative, such as a slice of turkey, a piece of cheese, some shrimp, or a few olives or avocado slices.

- Drink a full glass of water or a cup of broth or tea.

- Distract yourself by leaving the mental and physical space that's making you obsess about food. Get out of the kitchen or the mall. Read a book. Do the relaxation exercise on page 54, take a walk, play a computer game—whatever works for you.

- Reach out for support: call a friend or relative.

LEAVE THE COUNTING TO US

Doing Induction you'll consume 20 grams of net carbs a day, give or take a couple of grams, in addition to protein and fat. If you're happiest when you have a calculator in one pocket and a carb gram counter in another, by all means feel free to count your carbs during this phase. But if you'd prefer to have it done for you while you are getting familiar with Atkins, you're in luck. By choosing the types of foods and following the serving recommendations that follow, you'll automatically get the right carbs in the right amounts with no worry, no hassle, and no counting.

A well-balanced use of your 20 grams of net carbs from the Acceptable Foods in Induction (page 26) looks like this:

FOOD	NET CARBS (IN GRAMS)
MIXED SALAD GREENS: 3 CUPS	3
EGGS: 2	1
COOKED VEGETABLES: 1 CUP	4
CHEESE: 3 TO 4 OUNCES	3
AVOCADO: ½	2
OLIVES: 10	2
LEMON JUICE: 1 TABLESPOON	1.5
HEAVY CREAM: 1 TABLESPOON	0.5
SALAD DRESSING: 2 TABLESPOONS	2
SUGAR SUBSTITUTE: 1 PACKET	1
TOTAL	20

If you use any Induction-appropriate low-carb foods (no more than two a day), they can replace other carb foods, with the exception of salad and other vegetables, gram for gram. For a week's worth of meal plans at 20 grams of net carbs, see page 264. Meal plans at 30 grams for people starting in OWL begin on page 285. If you are starting in Pre-Maintenance at 60 grams of net carbs, see page 327.

DOING ATKINS AS A VEGETARIAN

Vegetarians need to do Atkins a little differently. Be sure that you are getting adequate protein—at least 6 ounces at every meal—from tofu, tempeh, seitan, eggs, and up to 4 ounces of cheese a day. We also recommend that you add at least 2 ounces of seeds or nuts a day, which will add roughly 4 grams of net carbs, putting you into Ongoing Weight Loss (OWL). Vegetarians should stay at this level for no longer than two weeks. Plant-based protein usually comes with carbohydrates, and you must make sure that you get enough protein. Once you progress further with OWL in Week Three, you can immediately add back legumes (lentils and black soybeans are among those lowest in carbs) in 5-gram increments. But be advised: That's just a few tablespoons at a time and not the typical half-cup serving size.

Alternatively, you can start at 30 grams of net carbs daily, with the extra carbs coming from more vegetables, nuts, seeds, and even small portions of legumes from the beginning.

At either of these levels you should still be able to stabilize your blood sugar and get cravings and hunger under control. Just remember that your rate of weight loss is likely to be slower than that of someone on Induction.

Vegetarians who are controlling their carbs have to be very careful to eat enough calories. If you find you need to be calorie conscious in addition to controlling carbs, a good rule of thumb is to limit your intake to 1,500 calories if you are a woman and 1,800 if you are a man. But no one should drop below 1,200 calories a day. We suggest consuming plenty of healthy fats such as those found in avocados and olives, to ensure that you are eating enough calories without adding excessive carbs. You'll find vegetarian selections in every week of the meal plans in this book. Since vegans do not eat dairy or eggs, it is very hard to get adequate nutrition while controlling carbs.

LOSING WEIGHT TOO FAST?

Rapid fluid and weight loss can result in electrolyte (mineral) loss. If your body is particularly responsive to controlling carbs, it's possible to lose weight too rapidly in the Induction phase of Atkins. If you develop any of the following symptoms by the end of the first week on Induction, you may need to slow down your weight loss.

- leg cramps, especially at night

- weakness when climbing stairs, known as ascent weakness

- lightheadedness or dizziness

- fatigue

- frequent urination along with any of the above symptoms

If you experience any of these symptoms, in addition to following the rules of Induction correctly, which means drinking at least 64 ounces of water daily and spreading your carb intake throughout the day, the following can help:

- Add a multimineral supplement (see What to Look for in a Multimineral, below) in addition to your multivitamin.

- Eat more frequently, making sure to have some protein, preferably something with a little fat in it (a boiled egg is perfect), every two hours.

- Replace the lost electrolytes by drinking a salty vegetable, chicken, or beef broth.

- Add salt to your food.

- Eat more iron-rich veggies such as spinach and Swiss chard.

If you have kept yourself well hydrated and followed these tips for several days but your symptoms and fluid loss continue, you will also need to increase your carbohydrate intake slightly to slow weight loss. Try adding an additional 5 grams of net carbs a day in the form of nuts and seeds or more vegetables.

Note: Be sure to talk with your doctor if you experience such complaints, especially if taking a multimineral does not make you feel better.

What to Look for in a Multimineral. There are three things you should look for: calcium, magnesium, and potassium.

Calcium, found in dairy products, nuts, dark green leafy vegetables such as spinach and broccoli, and tofu, keeps bones and teeth strong. Deficiencies in calcium—as well as in magnesium, boron, and vitamin D—can make you more prone to osteoporosis, or bone loss, a particular problem for postmenopausal women, although men can also develop it. Calcium also stimulates your pancreas to produce insulin, so adequate calcium plays a role in the proper regulation of blood sugar.

Magnesium is found in spinach, broccoli, tofu, chard, nuts, and pumpkin seeds. Like calcium, magnesium is vital for the health of bones and teeth. It also plays a role in energy production and cardiovascular health, which is why Dr. Atkins regarded it as the most important mineral for heart health. Low levels of magnesium are associated with diabetes, hypertension, and the formation of kidney stones. Loss of magnesium can occur with excessive consumption of sugar, alcohol, or caffeine.

Potassium, found in avocados, pumpkin, spinach, tomato, tofu, sunflower seeds, and wheat bran, is necessary to regulate water balance, heart rhythm, and electrical

Olives grow in many warm climates, which explains their importance in Mediterranean cuisines. Varieties abound, many of which are exported to the United States, including the Kalamata from Greece, Niçoise from France, and the Gaeta from Italy. Green and black olives are not different varieties; the former are harvested before they are ripe, while the latter are allowed to ripen on the vine. Many supermarkets now have "olive bars," with a selection of different types; a little experimentation can help you clarify which ones you prefer.

Olives (and their oil, made by pressing the fruit) are rich in monounsaturated fats and high in antioxidants. Olive oil lowers "bad" cholesterol and increases "good" cholesterol. Some olives are cured in salt, which makes them the perfect remedy for a salty snack craving. Others are packed in olive oil and herbs or in salt (they need to be rinsed before eating). Ten black or pimiento-stuffed green olives contain about 3 grams of net carbs. *Extra-virgin* olive oil comes from the first pressing of the fruit and is the purest; *virgin* indicates later pressings. Look for *cold-* or *expeller*-pressed olive oil. Buy it in relatively small quantities and store it away from light and heat so it stays fresh.

impulses to nerves and muscles. Potassium also helps regulate blood pressure; low levels contribute to hypertension. An excessively high or low level of this mineral can have serious consequences.

There are a variety of multimineral formulations; follow the recommended dose on the label.

MOTIVATION: THE WINNER'S EDGE

Starting something new can be disorienting or scary. The following relaxation technique and journaling activities will help you through the metabolic transition and the other life changes you are making.

RELAX!

The ability to truly let go is a skill that's increasingly hard to master in our fast-paced culture. Think about how you reacted the last time you were stuck in traffic, missed your train, or lost an argument with a colleague or your spouse. We do our bodies and our psyches an injustice by living in a constant state of tension; it robs us of our natural flexibility and makes us more likely to "snap." This feeling can make it especially hard to embrace new opportunities.

The following relaxation technique will ease you into the Program and give you a skill that you can use whenever you need a mini-vacation. While this 15-minute exercise can't remove the stress from your life, it can help relieve some of the toll it takes on you.

Before beginning, select a place where you will not be disturbed and will be free of such distractions as your computer, cell phone, or television. You will need enough room so you can lie down comfortably. Wear loose-fitting warm clothes or cover yourself with a lightweight cotton blanket. (Your body temperature drops when you lie still.) Note: Please read through all the steps and then set aside the book and give it a try.

1. Lie on your back on a mat or thick towel. Position your arms by your sides at a comfortable distance from your body. Your arms and hands should be relaxed, with a natural curl to the fingers, and palms facing up. Spread your legs slightly and let your feet fall outward. (If lying like this puts strain on your lower back, place a rolled towel underneath your knees or at the base of your spine for added support, or raise your knees and put your feet flat on the floor.) Breathe slowly and evenly.

2. Begin by tensing (as you inhale) and then releasing (as you exhale) every single part of your body at once. Point your toes, ball your fists, screw up your face, tighten your buttocks, and hold the squeeze as tightly as you can for five seconds. Release, then repeat.

3. When you have tensed and released twice, arch your lower back slightly and gently, squeezing your shoulder blades together toward the middle of your back so that your chest is fully open and both shoulder blades are lying flat on the floor. Roll your head from side to side. When you have found a comfortable position, stop and let your head settle comfortably on the floor.

4. Close your eyes. Consciously relax each muscle group you encounter as you move your focus of attention up your body. Feel each part of your body get heavy and settle more deeply onto the floor as you release the tension. Start with your toes, relaxing all the tightness from their joints. Work your way through the complex muscles connecting the toes to the rest of the foot. Feel the tricky area behind the knees and the powerful muscles of the upper thighs melt onto the floor. Pay attention to the muscular tension in your buttocks where many of us hold anxiety. See if letting out a deep exhale will allow them to loosen and get heavier, and allow your spine to settle a little more deeply against the floor. If you find a place that's particularly tight or resistant, clench the muscle tightly as you inhale, hold the clench briefly, and then exhale, releasing all the tension.

5. Continue all the way up your torso, through your back and the sides of the body, becoming aware that each body part becomes warmer and looser as you proceed. Work your way down your arms, feeling how they connect to the shoulders and upper back. Imagine them so heavy they're impossible to lift. Feel warmth in your elbows and wrists and at the base of each finger. Imagine that your hands are weighed down by two warm, heavy softballs, and feel the backs of your hands thaw in response.

6. Relax each of the muscles in your face, starting with the jaw. Let your lips part very gently and loosen your tongue—it's a muscle, too! Imagine two firm

fingers tracing the shape of your eyebrows, ironing the strain right out of them, and then circling your temples. Feel the stress leach out of your scalp as if someone were running their fingers through your hair. Let your eyes hang heavy in their sockets.

7. Now, simply enjoy the way your body feels. Pay attention to your breath entering and leaving your body. If thoughts enter your mind, simply observe them but then let them go. Your only job now is to pay attention to your breath. Stay here, enjoying the peaceful feeling for as long as you like.

8. When you feel that you have received the benefits of this relaxation technique, begin to bring some gentle movement back into your body by wiggling your fingers and toes. Move your ankles and wrists in a circle. Roll your head from side to side. You may want to rock yourself from side to side, giving your back a gentle massage against the floor. Give yourself plenty of time to rejoin the world. Keep the beautiful feeling of silence, stillness, and relaxation with you as long as you can. Roll over to your side and then into a sitting position before rising to avoid dizziness.

When you sit up, you will feel greatly refreshed, as if you had taken a nap. The more you do this relaxation exercise, the better you'll get at learning how to relax.

JOURNALING ACTIVITY: "BUT" BUSTERS

Winners in life and at doing Atkins don't let obstacles stop them. Instead of thinking, "I could do this but . . . ," they face the obstacle head-on and remove the "but." They change their thinking to, "I could do this if . . ."

This activity will help you root out your "buts" and bust them before they blast your chances of success.

The first step is to articulate your "buts" on paper. In your Atkins Advantage Journal write the following: "I want to slim down and get healthy by doing the Atkins Advantage Program, *but* . . ."

Make a list of the obstacles that might get in the way of your full participation in this program over the next 12 weeks. Nothing is too small and insignificant to matter; nothing is too big to solve.

For example, if Traci, a new mom, has made the commitment to herself to begin the Atkins Advantage Program, but is having a few doubts about her ability to follow through, here's how she might express her concerns: "I want to slim down and get healthy by doing the Atkins Advantage Program, *but* I've just had a baby. I feel as if I barely have enough time to feed and clothe myself, let alone exercise and shop for and cook healthy food."

The next step, after you've written down your concerns, is to transform them into a solution. List as many solutions as you can think of. Traci's list might look like this:

- get my husband to help more with household chores

- arrange for child care several hours a week

The idea is to see all the possible solutions, realistic or not. Then you can determine which ones will actually work for you and which may require some rethinking. When Traci talks to her husband, he will likely agree to help with chores because he knows how important it is to her to get her pre-baby body back.

Yet child care, which Traci also put on her list, isn't a viable alternative because she can't afford it. But is paying a sitter the only option, or are there other resources she can tap? Might her mother or trusted neighbor be called into service to provide babysitting while Traci exercises? Traci can always ask; they can decline if it's too big an imposition. But perhaps there is a gym in the area that has a babysitting service.

The point is to be as creative as possible. You may be surprised by what you come up with. Other ideas might include:

> **ATKINS ADVANTAGE TIP**
> If you prepare higher carb meals for your family and find you're still craving some of those foods, consider eating beforehand so that you're not hungry and apt to give in to temptation.

- making the baby part of the program by pushing the stroller during the walking portions of the fitness program or by doing Baby Lifts, using the baby as a "weight" during the strength portions of the program. Both Traci and her baby will enjoy this game!

- looking into yoga or other exercise ideas that can be done at home while the baby naps.

There were ways to fill in the gaps for Traci, and you will find the solutions to your own unique obstacles. None are insurmountable. The trick is to lay them out clearly, understanding that surrender is not an option. Your best solutions will be found now, before the obstacles themselves loom large.

JOURNALING ACTIVITY: SAY YES

Forget low-calorie diets in which you had to give up things you love in order to lose excess pounds. It will be different this time because on the All-New Atkins Advantage Program you'll be saying yes to a lifetime of better health.

Enjoy it! Open your Atkins Advantage Journal and make a list of the delicious foods you're looking forward to eating without guilt, such as blue cheese, whipped cream, and a flame-kissed steak. Atkins Achiever Gerald Godoy, who lost 26 pounds in three months, advises, "Keep your food list nearby. I've kept mine on my desk since the day I began Atkins so I have a constant reminder of everything I *can* eat, rather than allowing myself to focus on what I *can't*."

Imagine it! What will the slim new you be able to do that you can't do right now? Would you like to say yes to romping with your kids or grandkids? How about simple everyday things such as getting out of the car or the bathtub more easily, fitting into the seat on the bus more comfortably, or walking up a flight of stairs without huffing and puffing? Maybe the vision of yourself wearing the perfect sundress to a barbecue is motivation enough.

Believe it! Just because you can't change your genes doesn't mean you can't change your destiny. Some medical conditions, such as diabetes and heart disease, can have a strong genetic component, but your family history doesn't necessarily put you in the line of fire. Many factors contribute, including being overweight. You've taken the first step toward sidestepping risk factors for chronic disease simply by starting this program.

Say it! "Say Yes to Success" is your affirmation for this first week, one that will come in handy when you're finding it hard to make healthy choices. It's so important that we're going to ask you to record it in permanent marker directly on an article of clothing, preferably something you're looking forward to slimming yourself out of.

Frame it! Choose an article of clothing to inscribe with "Say Yes to Success." It will make a spectacular trophy when you hit your goal weight. Hang it inside your closet, and every time you'll see it, you'll think, "I can't believe that used to fit me!"

Or use a pair of sweats, shorts, or a T-shirt that you'll wear when you're working out. (If you're self-conscious about doing this, make the lettering small.) What better occasion to remind yourself that you've said yes to success?

Return to this page of yeses in your journal whenever you need to—either to list other desires you'd forgotten or new ones as you move through the Program.

Fitness: The Best You

FOCUS FOR THE WEEK: STRETCHING AND BREATHING AND USING THIS TIME TO HONOR YOURSELF AND YOUR BODY

Stretching ➔ 15–30 minutes ➔ 3 times

Your body is undergoing some significant changes. Think of the time you devote to the fitness component in this initial phase as a mental and physical warm-up for the fitness program to come that is designed to rejuvenate and soothe you. Use it to give yourself credit for the initial work you're doing, to refresh yourself mentally, and to begin tapping your internal reserves for the exciting changes ahead.

Note: If you're not feeling your best during the first week of Induction, you may not feel up to doing the fitness program. Since this week's exercises are designed specifically to address your symptoms, they may well help if you try them.

MAKING THE TIME

One of your goals as you do the Fitness portion of the program this week is to find out how to fit exercise into your life.

Be realistic. You may have the best intentions at bedtime, but if you're going to hit the snooze button and roll over when the alarm clock goes off at 5:00 a.m., you'll need to find another time. On the other hand, you may discover after a few days that your internal clock is easily reset and that you look forward to the peacefulness of the early morning. Many people find that it's easiest for them to stick to an exercise routine if it really *is* a routine, so they choose to work out at the same time every day.

Fitness is integral to making lifelong changes. Use this week to experiment by clearing your schedule at a particular time every day so that other activities won't interfere.

STRETCHING EXERCISES

The Atkins Advantage fitness program begins with stretching. You will learn the first four of the basic stretches this week. For now they are your warm-up to the program; in the weeks to come, they will be part of your workout. If you are already exercising but don't spend enough time stretching, add these flexibility exercises to your regular program.

Stretching plays an important role in overall fitness and can help preserve the range of motion that naturally diminishes as we age. Your joints lose some of their elasticity and become more brittle as you get older, but it's never too late to regain range of motion in the neck, shoulders, back, hips, knees, ankles, wrists, and other joints with stretching exercises.

> ## BUT I ALREADY WORK OUT!
>
> The goal of the Atkins Advantage Program is to give you the information and tools you need to develop your own safe, balanced, and effective fitness regimen. If you already have an exercise program, by all means continue what you're doing.
>
> Do read the Fitness sections each week anyway. You may find elements in our program that you'd like to incorporate in your own, and you'll doubtlessly benefit from participating in the nonexercise activities you'll find.

Some stretching basics:

- The best time to stretch is when your body is already a bit warmed up; your body will then have increased circulation and raised muscle temperature, preventing injury. Try brisk walking, light jogging, or even light weight lifting for five to ten minutes.

- For stretches you will do on the floor, it's advisable to add padding with a rug, mat, or thick towel.

- Never force a stretch! This isn't a competition. You should feel a stretch, but stretching should never hurt.

- Inhale through your nose as you go into the stretch, and exhale through your mouth. As you exhale, move just a little more deeply into the exercise.

- Don't hold your breath. If you can't breathe comfortably while you're holding the stretch, ease up until you can.

- When you've taken the stretch as far as you can, maintain the position for 10 to 30 seconds. Remember to keep inhaling slowly and exhaling.

- Avoid bouncing. It is traumatic to your muscles, tendons, and joints, and can cause injury.

- Perform each stretch three times, reaching a little bit further every time. You'll find that the repetition greatly increases your range of motion.

Determine Your Flexibility Level. Atkins allows for individualization, and that theme is as important in the stretching portion of the program as it is in everything else you do. In order to individualize the program most effectively, it's helpful to know where you're starting from so that you can begin at an appropriate level and then progress at your own pace. Be honest about your baseline, or you'll risk injury by putting unnecessary stress on your muscles and tendons.

The wonderful thing about stretching is that everyone can do it. Your own flexibility determines how deeply you take the stretch. To decide whether you're more Gumby or Tin Man, choose the level that best describes your flexibility. You'll find individualized advice targeted specifically for you within the stretches themselves.

LEVEL ONE   I can kneel on the ground.
I need to sit down to tie my shoes.

When I bend over to touch my toes, my hands are about two feet away from the floor.

LEVEL TWO   I can crawl on the ground.

I rest my foot on a stool to tie my shoes.

When I bend over to touch my toes, I can reach my shins.

LEVEL THREE   I can sit comfortably with my legs crossed on the ground.

I can tie my shoes from a standing position.

I can touch my toes with little or no need to bend my knees.

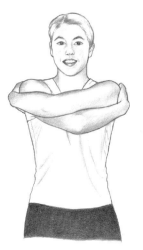

SHOULDER HUG

Begin with this stretch, which reinforces the important connection between breathing and stretching.

1. Stand comfortably with legs hip-width apart.

2. Reach to the opposite shoulder with each of your hands, hugging yourself. If you can, hold your shoulders gently; if not, simply cross your arms in front of your body.

3. Inhaling, lift your elbows slightly. Exhale and try to slide your hands around your back.

4. Feel the connection between your breath and the stretch. Breathe in and hold the stretch for a minimum of ten seconds.

5. Repeat, alternating the position of your arms so that the same one isn't always on top.

Number of Reps All Levels: three

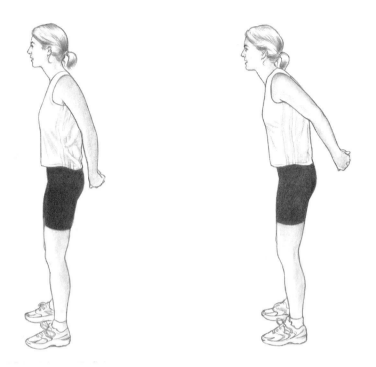

HEAD UP, CHEST OUT

This stretch will help you feel more open through your chest and the front of your shoulders. A more advanced variation will give you a neck stretch as well.

1. Pull your shoulder blades toward the center of your back, pushing your chest out. Move your arms behind your body so that both of your hands are behind you, palms facing one another.

2. If you can, bring your hands together and interlock your fingers.

To increase the stretch across the front of the chest, gently lift your arms while keeping your fingers interlocked. Breathe in and hold the stretch for at least ten seconds before exhaling.

Number of Reps All Levels: three

Modification: For Levels Two and Three, lift and extend your jaw outward so that you feel the stretch in your neck as well. Breathe in and hold the stretch for a minimum of ten seconds before exhaling.

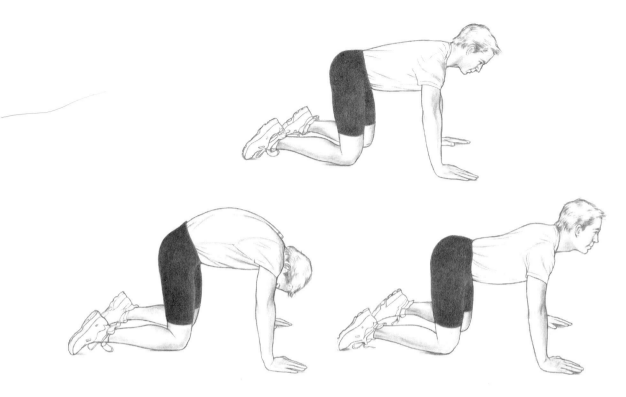

CAT AND DOG

This stretch gently warms up your entire spine.

1. Kneel on a mat or thick towel with your hands directly underneath your shoulders and your knees directly underneath your hips.

2. As you inhale, drop your head slightly, pulling your navel in and up, and curling your entire back toward the ceiling.

3. As you exhale, raise your head, lifting your chest and putting a slight arch in your back.

4. Continue to round your back on an inhale, arch and open your chest on an exhale.

Number of Reps All Levels: three breath cycles

Modification: For those in Level Three looking to advance this stretch, either walk or slide your hands forward, keeping arms straight and hands under shoulders as your bent knees progressively straighten. Breathe in and hold the stretch for a minimum of ten seconds before exhaling.

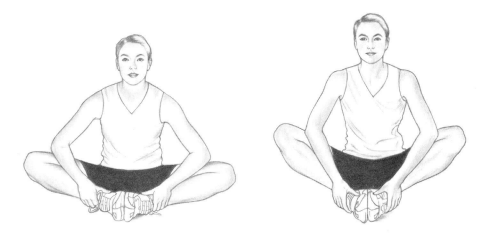

BUTTERFLY

While you open your inner thighs and hips with this stretch, energetically press the soles of your feet against each other.

1. Sit on the floor with the soles of your feet together. It doesn't matter how close your feet are to your body.

2. Clasp your feet with your hands as if trying to draw your feet a little closer to your body, lengthening the entire spine. Place your elbows on your inner thighs and gently push down to ease your knees toward the ground. Do not bounce. You should feel a mild stretch, not a pull.

3. Concentrate on keeping your back as straight as possible.

4. Breathe in and hold the stretch for a minimum of ten seconds before exhaling.

Number of Reps All Levels: three

ADVANTAGE CHECKPOINT: END OF WEEK ONE

If you started in Induction, congratulations! You've made it through the first week of what many people consider the most difficult period of the whole program. If you experienced signs of carb withdrawal this week, they should have lessened by now or will do so in the days ahead. As it is, you're well on the way to reprogramming your metabolism, and you'll be seeing—and feeling—the changes!

Get out your Atkins Advantage Journal, enter the date, and write down your answers to these questions:

Has your appetite decreased?

Are you experiencing fewer carb cravings?

Are you free of mood and energy swings?

Do you feel more energetic and focused?

Do your clothes feel looser?

If you answered yes to all these questions, you're already experiencing the Atkins Advantage. Don't worry if you said no to some of them. It's perfectly normal for your body to need a little longer to make the adjustment. That is why Induction lasts at least 14 days. Continue to follow the rules of Induction and give your body the opportunity to change.

> **ATKINS ADVANTAGE TIP**
> As a rule, women lose more slowly than men, so don't compare your progress with that of the men in your life.

When you weigh and measure yourself, do so at approximately the same time that you did before doing Atkins. (Remember to do your arms and thighs on the same side.) Record your new numbers in your journal.

If you lost weight and inches, continue at 20 grams of net carbs. You will find a second week of meal plans starting on page 271.

If you did not lose weight or inches or lost inches but not weight, continue as above. You may simply be resistant to weight loss, and it will take longer. Continue as above on about 20 grams of net carbs for another week.

If you lost weight too quickly and have symptoms mentioned on page 52, add another 5 grams daily of net carbs in the form of vegetables on the acceptable foods list or nuts and seeds. Once weight loss slows down, you can return to the 20 grams if you have a significant amount of weight to lose.

If you are close to your goal weight, move to OWL (see page 24).

If you gained weight, do not go below the Induction level of 20 grams of net carbs. Instead, do the following:

- Stay at 20 grams of net carbs for one more week; your metabolism might simply need more time to adjust.

- Check the rules of Induction on page 23 to make sure you're following the plan correctly.

- Enter everything you eat in your Atkins Advantage Journal.

- Be sure to read labels and avoid any products with unacceptable ingredients.

- If you have not yet begun the exercise component, do so now.

If you started in OWL or Pre-Maintenance, weigh and measure yourself as above.

If you lost desired weight, continue at the same level of net carbs for another week unless you are within 5 to 10 pounds of your goal weight, in which case you should move to Pre-Maintenance (see page 24).

If you were at your goal weight (or are underweight) and had unwanted weight loss (an initial loss of a pound or two of water weight is common at the start), increase your net carb intake by 5 grams (to 35 grams) if you are in OWL or by 10 grams (to 70 grams) if you are in Pre-Maintenance. Also see page 138 to learn how to find your carbohydrate threshold, known as your Critical Carbohydrate Level for Losing (CCLL).

If you gained some unwanted weight or your blood sugar symptoms and hunger or cravings have not improved, don't assume that Atkins isn't working for you or that you should return to Induction. It is important to complete two full weeks on OWL before adopting a course correction. One week simply isn't enough time to know if what you're seeing signifies a normal fluctuation or is a bigger issue. For that reason, complete two weeks in OWL before making any changes and do the following:

- Stay at your current carbohydrate level for one more week; your metabolism might simply need a little time to adjust.

- Check the rules of OWL (see page 86) to make sure you're following the plan correctly.

- Enter everything you eat in your Atkins Advantage Journal.

- Be sure to read labels and avoid any products with unacceptable ingredients.

- If you have not yet begun the exercise component, do so now.

SIX

WEEK TWO: ANYTHING IS POSSIBLE

This week the changes continuing to take place in your body will give rise to some exciting outward changes as well—pounds and inches vanishing. You now have proof that *change is possible!*

Tapping into positive results is the first key to empowerment. Allow your success to fuel your commitment to this life-changing journey. This week as you get healthier, happier, slimmer, and fitter, you'll learn how to leverage your success so you're not just meeting or exceeding your weight loss expectations but transforming your life in myriad other ways as well.

NUTRITION: THE HEART OF THE MATTER

Most of you will be continuing in Induction this week. For many of you the worst is over. Your cravings are gone, your energy level is up, and your waistband is already a little looser—all signs that you're on the right track.

You're no longer on the sugar roller coaster, and in order to continue feeling this way, make sure your kitchen is well stocked with the foods listed in Acceptable Foods in Induction on page 26. Also adhere strictly to the rules of Induction as laid out in

Week One. You'll have more flexibility as the Program continues, but right now you need to do Induction *to the letter* for it to work.

Note: By this time symptoms of carb withdrawal should be gone. If you are fatigued, suffer from muscle weakness or leg cramps, or are dizzy, you may be losing weight too fast. See page 52 for help.

Meal plans for Week Two of Induction start on page 271. If you started in Ongoing Weight Loss and are continuing at 30 grams daily of net carbs, simply repeat the meal plans for a second week, making some of the suggested modifications. If you lost weight and want to move on, plans for 35 grams of net carbs start on page 292. If you started in Pre-Maintenance and are continuing at the 60-gram level, repeat the week's meal plans, with modifications if you wish. If you started in Pre-Maintenance and are moving to 70 grams of net carbs, these meal plans start on page 334.

Regardless of whether you are in Induction, OWL, or Pre-Maintenance, continue taking your multivitamin, essential fatty acids (EFAs), and fiber supplement each day.

SOME COMMON PITFALLS

If you lost weight effortlessly in Week One and feel fine, the only thing you need to worry about is overconfidence. The first pounds, comprised in part of water, usually come off the fastest. If your results did not meet your expectations, remain patient and stay with the program. We all lose at different rates depending on metabolism, age, whether we are taking certain medications, and a host of other factors. Atkins Achievers have tipped us off to some common pitfalls you may encounter as you progress in the Program:

Don't cycle off and on. We've heard about dedicated carb counters who follow the Atkins Nutritional Approach (ANA) all week and then go off it on the weekend. Not surprisingly, their results aren't what they should be; insulin doesn't distinguish between Wednesday and Saturday! Remember, "just a bite" can undo your hard work, especially during Induction, and eating a higher-fat diet without controlling carbs won't work. The object is to rebalance your metabolism. Cycling back and forth between burning primarily fat for energy during the week and burning glucose on the weekends upsets this process. In fact, if you gorge on carbs over the weekend, your metabolism won't have switched over to burning fat until Wednesday or Thursday, by which time it is almost the weekend again. You'll eventually eat a wider array of healthy carbs on ANA, but don't jump the gun or you'll ruin your newfound control over cravings and sabotage your progress.

Don't forget that Atkins is based on whole foods. Use low-carb products to enhance your ability to stick with the program, but don't let them become a substitute for whole foods or good eating habits. Eating low-carb products without changing the other foods you eat will get you nowhere fast.

Water makes up 80 percent of our brains and 90 percent of our blood. The importance of staying well hydrated cannot be overstated. You lose somewhere between two and three quarts of water a day, and you must replace what's lost. Choose mineral, spring, or filtered tap water whenever possible. Remember the eight times eight rule: eight glasses of 8 ounces each. You should drink even more if you exercise regularly. Drinking enough water

- helps all the essential nutrients you're consuming in food and supplements make their way into your cells.
- removes waste products and toxins including the by-products of the body fat you're burning.
- minimizes muscle pain after exercise by helping to clear or dilute lactic acid buildup, as a result of working muscles.
- aids your digestive system to process food efficiently.
- plays an important role in preventing constipation.
- helps prevent bad breath.
- lubricates joints.
- assists in regulating your body temperature.
- improves the efficiency of your body's chemical reactions, which can help you lose weight as well as perform a host of other routine body functions.
- helps prevent overeating.

Don't stuff yourself. During Induction you are encouraged to eat as much of the right foods during meals as you need to feel satisfied. If you feel bloated and uncomfortable when leaving the table, you have gone beyond satisfying your hunger to overeating. The foods you eat during Induction provide slow-burning energy, and you can snack between meals, so you don't need to overeat at any given one. Keeping a log in your Atkins Advantage Journal can help you keep track of the amount you need to feel satisfied. To find that out, one of the Atkins Achievers told us that he used his old dieter's food scale to get an idea of what a reasonable portion of protein looked like.

Don't douse your food in fat. When you do Atkins, you can say yes to a balance of natural fats such as those found in meat, mayonnaise, butter, and olive oil (for more information about fats, see page 18). But that doesn't mean you should have equal parts of broccoli and butter on your plate.

You should have an appropriate amount of fat. Here are some tips:

- Use enough mayonnaise when making tuna, chicken, seafood, or other composed salads so that the mixture holds its shape and is neither too dry nor too moist. Use about 1 to 1½ tablespoons of mayo for a 6-ounce can of tuna.

- Drizzle—don't drown—vegetables with olive oil. If oil comes out of the bottle too rapidly, pour a small amount into the cap and dispense from there.

- Use just enough oil to sauté your food without burning it and without leaving oil in the pan.

Don't pig out on meat. Doing Atkins is not a license to eat only beef and bacon. Feel free to enjoy foods such as hamburgers (minus the bun, of course) and steaks, but also eat a variety of other proteins—and don't skimp on nutrient-rich vegetables.

MOTIVATION: THE WINNER'S EDGE

As you enjoy the exciting proof that you really can make change happen in your life, this week you're going to harness all that energy and good feeling, and use it to your advantage. Toss overboard the self-limiting patterns and behaviors that have held you back in the past, and while you're freeing yourself of all that excess baggage, we'll help you set the course for your dream destination. Remember, the sky's the limit!

FIND A "BUDDY"

Many Atkins Achievers report that one of the most effective tools for success was having a "buddy," someone—a friend, a family member, or a spouse—also on the Program. You can exercise together, cook

---

SPOTLIGHT ON AVOCADOS

If you're used to low-calorie, low-fat diets, you may still regard the avocado as a sinful indulgence. Not so when you do Atkins. Also known as the alligator pear, it has a buttery taste and rich, creamy texture. But the real reason this fruit—that's correct, it is not a vegetable—is an Atkins super food is its nutritional profile. Avocados are a good source of folate, vitamins A and B_6, potassium, iron, magnesium, copper, and riboflavin. They contain more vitamin E than any other fruit. They also contain lots of lutein, which fights macular degeneration; antioxidants, which neutralize free radicals and can help prevent cancer; and beta sitosterol, which helps lower blood cholesterol levels. Rich in fiber, avocados are also excellent sources of mono- and polyunsaturated fats.

Not all avocados are created equal. Hass avocados have a dark, pebbly skin. Fuerte avocados from Florida tend to be larger and have a shiny, bright green skin. They're lower in fat and higher in water, which tends to make them blander and less nutritious than the Hass variety, and they're also higher in carbs. These are the reasons we recommend Hass over Fuentes.

Half of a Hass avocado contains 7 grams of carbs but just 1.7 grams of net carbs once the fiber is taken into consideration.

together, share tips, tricks, and recipes, and, most important, use each other for support—both when the going's great and when you need a little extra encouragement.

If you don't know anyone close by who is interested in joining you, you can get much of the same support when you partner with someone even at a distance or someone you've met on-line.

Remember: Although a partner can be a terrific asset, you are the determining factor in your own success. Don't let your partner provide you with excuses; for example, just because he has a head cold and can't join you for your morning walk doesn't mean you shouldn't go. Make sure you're prepared to continue even if he drops out of the program entirely.

JOURNALING ACTIVITY: BAGGAGE CHECK

If you're like most people starting the Atkins Advantage Program, you've tried to lose weight before. In this activity, you'll look at those past attempts, to figure out what went wrong so you can eliminate that baggage from your life. Atkins is different from other weight loss programs because you work with your body, not against it, meaning that you don't ever have to go hungry. Still, unless you confront and correct your personal triggers, you could sabotage your efforts on Atkins.

Let's say that you were on track and losing weight until your promotion came through at work. Stressed and working late, you hit the vending machine instead of eating something healthy, and your waistline paid the price. Or maybe you did Atkins successfully before but found that "just a little" became "a lot," so that a bite of bagel turned into a bagel for breakfast every morning, and before long you returned to your previous size.

Take a moment now to describe your previous weight loss attempts in your Atkins Advantage Journal, listing the problems you encountered in the past. Don't feel discouraged or guilty. The point of this activity is simply to get to know yourself a bit better so that you can chart a new road this time out.

What happened to throw you off course? Were you hungry? Bored? Did you hit a plateau and become discouraged? Did an external event (an injury, pregnancy, professional disappointment, divorce) throw you off track? Did you lose speed and motivation before you made it to the finish line, or did your focus falter once you'd reached your goal weight?

Once you've isolated previous trouble spots, it's time to come up with preventative strategies to help you cope in the future. For instance, if you discover that you're a "stress snacker" when the pressure heats up at work, you'll need to be sure to have carb-appropriate snacks within reach at all times so that there's no reason to visit the vending machine while you're burning the midnight oil. If you have a tendency to bend the rules for a bite, you'll want to keep a food journal to make yourself accountable for every bite at meals and for snacks.

The good news is that Atkins can automatically offer support on many of the fronts that cause problems. Because of the way you are eating now, hunger and cravings simply won't be as much of an issue as they have been in the past, and the motivation activities you'll find in this book will help you anticipate stumbling blocks in advance so that this time you'll be playing to win.

JOURNALING ACTIVITY: SUCCESS SKILLS

Weight issues have a particular power. We've seen it over and over: A powerful and successful executive manages hundreds of people but experiences self-loathing because she can't manage her own waistline. A talented mechanic can fix anything except the ice cream cravings that get him up in the middle of the night.

To begin this activity, think of a "success scenario" in your past. Perhaps you kept a commitment despite the difficulties you encountered en route. Maybe you've become successful in business despite the lack of a formal education. Perhaps you put yourself through college by working nights and summers. Maybe you've brought your kids through the difficult teenage years with humor and grace, or you selflessly nursed an ill parent. The achievement should be one in which you take great personal pride.

Take a moment to record this achievement in your Atkins Advantage Journal. Review what you've written and ask yourself what the factors were that contributed to your success? What did you do right? Make a list of your answers. These are your Success Skills, and they might look something like these:

"I worked as hard as I could, even on the days I would rather have been doing anything else!"

"I put blinders on and didn't let anything take me off track."

"I was creative about figuring out solutions to problems."

"I never lost faith in myself; I always knew I could do it."

"I expected stumbling blocks and learned to overcome them rather than give up."

These Success Skills are the secret to your success on the Atkins Advantage Program. All you have to do is call them into service when you need them.

If your Success Skill was "doing what needed to be done" even when it meant passing up some fun along the way, you can use that same Success Skill to neutralize any excuse you might find yourself offering as you go forward on the Program, such as "I don't feel like going for a walk today." You may not have wanted to go on that business trip, but it was the only way to win that important and lucrative account. You enjoyed the rewards of that trip even when it meant that you spent the weekend on the road instead of relaxing with your family.

This activity is intended to be one you carry with you throughout the Atkins Advantage Program and beyond. You can use your Success Skills over and over again to achieve a new set of goals—including weight loss.

JOURNALING ACTIVITY: PERSONAL GOALS LIST

No activity in this program is more important than the one you're about to begin. This week you are going to create a Personal Goals List that will help you stay the course, both while you're on this program and well beyond.

Open your Atkins Advantage Journal to a new page and write: What are my personal goals?

Here are some rules to keep in mind as you're creating your list:

Write down everything you think of. There are no unrealistic dreams, just unrealistic ways to achieve them. Later you'll learn how small goals pave the way to success. If you don't shoot for the moon, you'll never make it over the fence. By the same token, don't hesitate to include something just because it seems trivial or silly. If it matters to you in your heart of hearts, record it.

State your goals in a positive way and make them specific. Instead of saying, for instance, that you want to "lose weight," narrow that down: "I want to hit my goal weight of 130 pounds and stay there permanently." Add as much detail as possible.

Don't restrict yourself to your weight loss goals. Your goal weight and fitness goals shouldn't be the sole focus of this list. Include dreams for all areas of your life. Do you want to learn to play tennis? Do you hope to meet your life partner? Do you wish you had more time to spend with your children? Do you aim to change career tracks?

Your Personal Goals List should feature no fewer than three and no more than five goals. If you find yourself at a loss, another way to think about this might be: "What are you no longer willing to settle for?" For instance, you might discover that you're no longer willing to make so little money that you live paycheck to paycheck and spend the end of every month stretched and miserable. Or you may decide that it's no longer acceptable to reject invitations for enjoyable activities because you're too shy and self-conscious about your weight to attend.

It's absolutely essential to write your goals on paper. The creation of a Personal Goals List formalizes the process of identifying your goals.

Fine-tune this list over the week to come and nurture your dreams. You'll be returning to this list again a little later.

In this activity, which should only be done after you've completed your Personal Goals List, you're going to take the list of goals and go one step further. One of the most effective reminders of a goal is a three-dimensional object that symbolizes and represents it. You're going to choose an object of desire. It can be anything that represents one of your personal goals and will inspire you. It can be as whimsical as you like, but it should be a powerful symbol to you of the dream you are hoping to achieve. If one of your goals is to travel more, you might choose a toy plane or a luggage tag. You can represent your weight loss goal with a pair of jeans you'd love to fit into again or the scuba mask you're going to wear as soon as you're fit enough to get certified. Hang it in a place where you'll see it every day, or carry it with you (attach that luggage tag to your key ring) so that you can reaffirm your goal every time your eyes land on it.

Fitness: The Best You

FOCUS FOR THE WEEK: WORKING ON YOUR BREATHING WHILE DOING THE FOUR STRETCHES FROM LAST WEEK PLUS FOUR NEW ONES.

Stretching → 30 minutes → 3 times

Do your stretches at a pace that is comfortable for you. These stretches may take you longer than half an hour.

The basic stretches you learned last week combined with the four basic stretches you'll learn this week are the foundation for the warm-ups and cooldowns that will become absolutely essential later in the Program when you're doing more vigorous exercise.

Stretching can help you counter the natural aging process in your joints by improving range of motion. Also, improved flexibility has been shown to help prevent injuries when participating in vigorous sport activities such as tennis, racquetball, and basketball—or any of the unexpected activities that may come your way.

We'll continue with stretching this week, but we'll begin with a breathing exercise. In the same way that the right foods fuel your body so that it can perform well, breathing properly gives your lungs the fuel they need to work at peak performance.

Over the course of this fitness program you will become aware of your breath, learning how to breathe fully and deeply as you perform certain movements. This basic breathing exercise will help bring your awareness to this elemental process and accustom you to the idea of linking movement to breath.

BREATHE DEEPLY AND MOVE

Throughout this exercise, breathe deeply and slowly through your nose, and connect your movement to your breathing.

1. Lying on your back on a thick towel or mat, bend your knees so your feet are flat on the floor and have your arms by your sides.

2. Keeping your arms straight, inhale as you bring your arms over your head in an extended position, so they rest on the floor. Your legs, torso, and arms should form a straight line.

3. Exhaling, slowly return your arms, with control, to your sides. Breathe deeply and slowly through your nose, and connect the movement to your breathing.

Number of Reps All Levels: three

STRETCHING EXERCISES

Now you're ready to continue with the stretching program you began last week. Use this new awareness of your breath to get a little deeper with every stretch. Begin with the following exercises, doing each one three times:

Shoulder Hug, page 62

Head Up, Chest Out, page 63

Cat and Dog, page 64

Butterfly, page 65

> **ATKINS ADVANTAGE TIP**
> If you tend to have constipation, twisting exercises may help relieve it.

Continue with the four new stretches that follow.

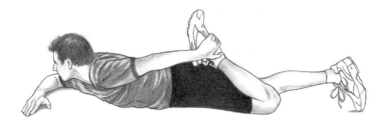

QUAD STRETCH

You should feel this stretch in the large muscles in the fronts of your thighs known as the quadriceps.

1. Lie on your stomach on a mat or thick towel. If this puts strain on your lower back, place a rolled-up towel beneath your hips.

2. Bend one knee at a time, bringing your foot toward your buttock. If you can, using a towel, reach behind you and loop the towel around your foot. Use it to gently encourage the foot to move closer. You may even be able to grab the foot with your hand.

3. Breathe in and hold the stretch for a minimum of 10 seconds before exhaling.

Number of Reps All Levels: three for each leg

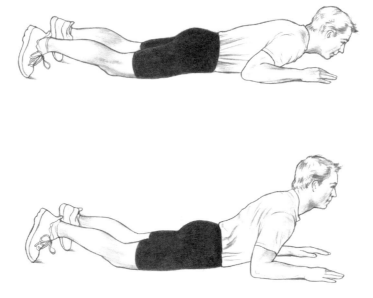

PRESS UP

This stretch has the dual benefit of strengthening the entire rear of your body, especially the upper back and hamstrings, while stretching the chest.

1. Lie on your stomach on a mat or thick towel. Place your hands next to your shoulders, with your elbows bent and on the ground.

2. Gently lift your upper body off the floor, keeping your forearms on the floor.

3. Breathe in and hold the stretch for a minimum of 10 seconds before exhaling.

Number of Reps All Levels: three

Modification: Those of you in Level Three can get a deeper stretch by beginning to straighten your arms in Step 3 so that more of your upper body moves off the floor.

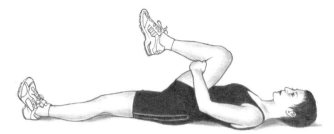

LOW BACK AND HAMSTRING COMBO STRETCH

You should feel a stretch in your lower back and in the backs of your legs.

1. Lie on your back with your legs extended and your hands behind one thigh.

2. Using your hands, pull your knee as close to your chest as possible, keeping your buttocks and back flat on the floor.

3. Breathe and hold the stretch for a minimum of 10 seconds.

4. Repeat Steps 2 and 3 with the other leg.

Number of Reps All Levels: three for each leg

Modification: If you are in Level Two or Three, begin to work toward stretching your hamstrings more deeply by repeating the above exercise with your leg extended, placing your hands behind your thigh or calf, and pulling your leg toward your chest.

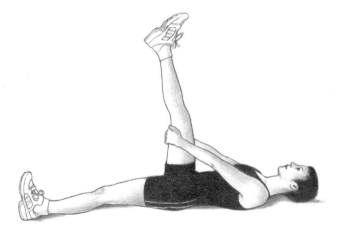

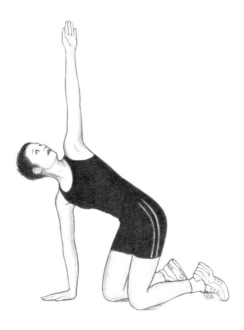

FOLLOW YOUR HAND

Twisting stretches like this one maintain the health of your spine and massage the internal organs to keep them functioning more efficiently.

1. Kneel on a mat or thick towel, placing your hands directly underneath your shoulders and your knees directly underneath your hips.

2. Inhale as you extend your left arm straight out to the side, at shoulder height.

3. Keeping your weight as evenly balanced on both knees as possible, exhale and begin to move your arm up, toward the ceiling. The twist should be gentle, and it should come from deep in the spine, not the shoulders. The trunk of your body should turn in one piece with your neck.

4. Follow your hand with your eyes, turning your head to look at the ceiling. (If this is not possible, look straight ahead or wherever is comfortable.)

5. Inhale and hold the stretch for a minimum of 10 seconds before exhaling. Return your left hand to the ground, extend your right arm, and repeat the exercise with your right arm.

Number of Reps All Levels: three on each side

If it has been some time since you last worked out, you may need to go shopping for appropriate clothing and shoes. Even if you already spend a lot of time in sweatpants and sneakers, we suggest that you reserve certain outfits exclusively for workouts so that when you change into those clothes, you are sending yourself a signal that it's time to get moving. You don't need a lot of gear, and it doesn't have to be fancy. Here's what to look for:

- Clothing should "breathe" and be machine washable. There are many good synthetic fabrics available now that wick moisture away from the skin.

- Your outfit should fit properly. Clothes that are too big can impede movement, and anything that pinches or binds will cause discomfort.

- For women only: A supportive sports bra is an absolute must. Evaluate the bra in the dressing room by jumping up and down; you should be able to move actively without discomfort. If you are large breasted, you may find it a challenge to find a good sports bra and may feel more comfortable in an ordinary, "minimizing" model.

- Choose a good pair of sneakers or running shoes that provide your feet with the proper support and cushioning. This is an absolute must if you want to stay injury-free.

When it comes to shoes, look for the following:

Get the right fit. It's best to have your shoes fitted by a professional. Ask for help at a sporting goods or running store. Some brands are better for different types of feet. Try on different brands and ask the salesperson to direct you. Many running and walking shoes have an extra set of eyelets that help them lace up tight, making for a better fit if you have narrow heels. Many stores that sell athletic shoes will let you walk around in them to try them out.

Shoes should feel good in the store. If they need "breaking in," they're too small or too narrow.

Replace shoes as needed. The rule of thumb for serious runners is that shoes last somewhere between 350 and 550 miles. Even if you're not a runner, when your shoes are more than a year old, chances are good that you need a new pair because they lose their cushioning with every step.

ADVANTAGE CHECKPOINT: END OF WEEK TWO

Weigh and measure yourself. Enter the results in your Atkins Advantage Journal and compare the results with last week's. If you are not experiencing the signs and symptoms of unstable blood sugar such as energy and mood swings and cravings for carbohydrate foods, if you are continuing to lose pounds or inches (or both!), if your clothes continue to feel looser, and if you feel good, take a bow. It's working! As early as it might seem in your journey, this is a major milestone. Change *is* possible.

ARE YOU READY TO LEAVE INDUCTION?

Completing the first two weeks of Atkins is a major milestone. It marks a period of significant change and renews the conviction that you can effect change in your life. For many of you it will mean the end of Induction and the beginning of Ongoing Weight Loss (OWL), when you'll begin to add some carbohydrates.

One of the most common misperceptions about Atkins is that it is synonymous with Induction. Atkins is a four-phase program, and it's important to move through all four phases so that you ultimately ease into a new and permanent way of eating. Most of you should stay in Induction for only 14 days. Some people may need to stay longer, and research has shown that it is perfectly safe to stay on Induction for up to six months.

The information below will help you determine whether staying in Induction or moving on to OWL is the right choice for you at this time.

First ask yourself how much weight you have lost. How about inches? Then consider whether any of the following apply:

- You've lost no weight or less than 4 pounds in two weeks.

- You are still very hungry between meals or are continuing to experience strong cravings for sweets and/or starchy foods.

- Your excess weight is causing or exacerbating health issues. (You will know this because you visited your physician before starting Atkins.) These issues include elevated blood pressure, joint problems, a blood sugar imbalance, pre-diabetes or Type 2 diabetes, huffing and puffing with mild exertion, sleep apnea, or a BMI of 30 or more (see page 42).

If any of these apply, you can consider staying in Induction a little longer. However, you can add an ounce of nuts or seeds as long as you stay at 20 grams of net carbs. If you're still hungry or see no reduction in cravings, or if you haven't lost weight, your metabolism has not yet switched to primarily burning fat for energy. That doesn't mean the Program doesn't work for you; it's just that your body needs a little more time to erase the effects of a lifetime of bad habits.

If you continue to have trouble losing weight in Induction, you may want to consider the following:

- Record everything you eat in your Atkins Advantage Journal.

- Be sure to keep cheese portions under 4 ounces.

- Make sure you're using cream or a reduced-carb dairy beverage instead of milk or half-and-half.

- Eliminate excessive amounts of caffeine; some of you may need to eliminate it altogether.

- Be sure you're not overconsuming low-carb products.

- If you aren't hungry between meals, don't snack.

Then ask yourself these questions:

Am I stuffing myself beyond what I need to feel satiated simply out of habit?

Am I eating in front of the television even though I'm not hungry?

Am I drinking alcohol because it's low in carbs?

Am I eating low-carb candy and ice cream products? Remember that these are not allowed on Induction.

Am I eating too many calories? (The range is 1,500 to 1,800 daily for women and 1,800 to 2,000 for men, but no one should eat less than 1,200 calories.)

Am I exercising enough?

Am I reading labels to be sure there are no hidden carbs slowing my progress?

Finally, review your journal to see if you can find any foods that you should not be eating. Even a few extra grams of carbs can destabilize blood sugar, so sneaking a few bites of forbidden foods may explain why you didn't lose more or why you're still feeling those cravings. You'd be surprised at how little it takes!

Cheating, especially during the Induction phase, can impede your body's ability to switch over to primarily burning fat and keeps your blood sugar on its roller coaster ride. Unless you break this pattern, you won't be able to overcome the cravings that are causing you to cheat. If you have not been faithful to Induction, regardless of your results you should continue in Induction for another week.

Even if you're seeing the pounds and inches disappearing, however, you may want to stay in Induction if you have a lot of weight to lose (a BMI of 30 or higher) or if the excess weight you're carrying is compromising your health. The rate at which you lose weight is greater (at least initially) in Induction than it is in later phases, and taking those extra pounds off quickly may prevent you from getting discouraged.

Staying in Induction doesn't mean that you shouldn't move on to Week Three. It simply means your nutritional requirements remain set at Induction.

MOVING TO OWL

If you're chafing under the restrictions of Induction, you may want to sacrifice speed of weight loss for a little more variety in your diet and move to OWL even if you do have a significant amount of weight to lose. However, you should move to OWL only if you no longer have cravings or out-of-control hunger or any of the other symptoms of unstable blood sugar. If you are experiencing any of these symptoms, stay in Induction a little longer.

If you do decide to move to OWL, you will increase your daily net carb intake to 25 grams, which you will learn about in the following chapter.

If you started the 12 weeks in Phase 2 (OWL) or Phase 3 (Pre-Maintenance), check in with your progress and adjust your net carbs accordingly.

If you have lost weight on OWL at a daily net carb level of 30 grams, be sure to read the Nutrition section of the next chapter now. It explains how to add an additional 5 grams of carbohydrate to your daily count.

If you started in Pre-Maintenance at a daily level of 60 grams of net carbs and have lost weight, turn to page 188, to learn how to add 10 more grams to your daily intake.

If you have not lost weight at your current level in OWL or Pre-Maintenance, decrease by 5 or 10 grams daily of net carbs, respectively. Stay at this level for one week. If you still do not lose weight, you will need to cut back again.

SEVEN

WEEK THREE: INTRODUCING ONGOING WEIGHT LOSS

Remember the parable of the tortoise and the hare? Likewise, when it comes to weight loss, enhanced fitness, and other life changes, slow and steady wins the race. Small but consistent steps are the way to secure big advances. The best way to reach your goals is with discipline and a measured expenditure of energy. Then, once the ball is rolling, it will take on its own momentum.

That's why the All-New Atkins Advantage Program provides you with stepping-stones, each one built on the foundation of those that came before and designed to support others in the future. That way you never have to claw your way up a mountain; instead, you build a staircase so that reaching your goals is never more difficult than putting one foot in front of the other.

NUTRITION: THE HEART OF THE MATTER

If you started the program in OWL at 30 grams of net carbs and are losing weight, you can move up another 5 grams this week. If you began in Pre-Maintenance and are losing, you can move up 10 grams as explained in Week Nine.

Even if you decide to stay in Induction in Week Three, you can begin to add nuts and seeds as part of your 20 grams daily of net carbs. Your choices include an ounce of almonds, walnuts, pecans, hazelnuts, macadamias, Brazil nuts, and filberts, as well as pumpkin, sunflower, and sesame seeds. Peanuts and cashews, which are not true nuts, are higher in carbs, so wait to introduce them until later in the program. Vegetables continue to comprise the majority of your carb intake. Those of you with the "I can't believe I ate the whole bag syndrome" should be careful with nuts and seeds because it can be hard to stop with just a handful.

> **ATKINS ADVANTAGE TIP**
>
> One sign of unstable blood sugar is waking in the early morning hours and not being able to go back to sleep. A small protein snack before bedtime can help.

If you are moving to OWL, turn to page 278 for a week's worth of meal plans at 25 grams of net carbs. If you are already in OWL or Pre-Maintenance, see the listings on page 278 and later to find meal plans appropriate for your daily net carb gram count.

WELCOME TO OWL

Ongoing Weight Loss (OWL) allows you to begin to tailor Atkins to your unique needs and tastes. Everyone has his or her own carbohydrate threshold, determined by many factors including genes, lifestyle, metabolism, age, the medications you're on, and so forth. Your journey toward that personalized number—the number of carb grams you can eat while still losing weight—begins in OWL. Adding carbs back *gradually* means you take the guesswork out of weight loss while gradually expanding the variety that makes sticking with the Program even easier.

In Induction you may have opted to "leave the counting to us" (page 51), but in OWL you'll learn to count for yourself so that you can be in control of your weight for life.

The Rules of OWL

- Begin with 25 grams of net carbs a day.

- Add 5 grams daily of net carbs each week as long as gradual weight loss continues, going from 25 to 30 a day, then 35, and so forth.

- In general, add carbohydrates in the order listed in the Atkins Carbohydrate Ladder (page 14), starting with more vegetables.

- Add foods from only one rung of the Carb Ladder each week.

- Add within the rung individually.

- Drop by 5 grams daily of net carbs for a week if your weight loss or inch loss stalls or if you regain weight.

Strategies for Success: Increasing Variety. If you started the program in Induction, you'll add 5 grams to begin OWL at 25 grams daily of net carbs. Following the Carb Ladder means that you'll add more vegetables this week. If you miss eating crunchy foods, another choice is to introduce nuts and seeds instead. They're a good source of protein, and most people can eat them without finding that they stimulate the blood sugar roller coaster. Again, stick to no more than 5 grams of net carbs from nuts per day.

Remember, protein helps keep your blood sugar stable, your energy up, and your appetite under control. Fat retards the time it takes for the stomach to empty, keeping you fuller longer. Have at least 6 ounces of protein (weighed uncooked) at every meal, and never go for more than six waking hours without eating!

IS ALCOHOL ALLOWED IN OWL?

You can have an occasional drink once you are out of Induction as long as you understand that adding a moderate amount of alcohol—no more than one drink a day—doesn't mean you get to choose a drink in lieu of adding nuts or more vegetables. Still, you can certainly have a glass of dry wine (a 4-ounce glass of dry white wine has 1 gram of net carbs; a glass of red wine has 2 grams) or a splash of spirits, such as vodka or gin, once you are a week or two into OWL. By the way, with the exception of sherry and other dessert wines, all wine is low in carbs; the low-carb wines presently being marketed are not significantly lower in carbs than any dry red or white wine. When choosing your drinks, keep these points in mind:

The higher the proof, the lower the carb count—and the more alcohol in the drink. If you are a beer fan, be sure to choose a light beer or one of the new low-carb brands.

Mixers count! Non-diet sodas and orange, cranberry, and grapefruit juice are filled with sugary carbs. Five ounces of tonic water—approximately the amount that would go into a gin and tonic—has a whopping 15 grams of carbs. Seltzer and sugar-free tonic are better choices.

Alcohol reduces inhibitions and clouds judgment, which might make it a little harder for you to keep your resolve not to overeat or wolf down the wrong things at the buffet table.

Don't drink on an empty stomach. Instead, have a snack high in protein or consume alcohol with a meal. If you sense that imbibing will compromise your commitment to the Program, choose a nonalcoholic beverage instead.

Your weight loss will naturally slow a little in this second phase; on average, you can expect weight loss of between 1 to 2 pounds per week in OWL, although individual rates vary and your own pace will vary from week to week. You'll find some variations to the standard rules of OWL in the Customizing OWL section (page 106).

No matter what phase you are in, continue to take a good multivitamin, a fiber supplement, and essential fatty acids.

MOTIVATION: THE WINNER'S EDGE

Novels aren't written in a single weekend; businesses aren't built overnight; and you can't qualify for the Olympics in two weeks even if you work really hard at it. The same holds true when it comes to achieving your personal goals. You can make significant progress if you keep at it every day and gradually build upon each achievement.

Think about the progress you've already made doing Atkins by following the easy, measured steps laid out for you here. The key is to see how what you're learning in the Nutrition portion of the program can help you in other areas of your life. Don't squander your time and energy focusing on the length of the trip. Start on your way to it now, and you'll be there before you know it.

JOURNALING ACTIVITY: CREATING AN ACTION PLAN OF SMALL STEPS

Last week you made a list of your personal goals. No matter how ambitious these may seem, they are not out of your reach. You simply need to see those big goals in doable chunks by creating an action plan and following it.

This week you'll choose one of your goals and promise yourself to take a small step every day toward that goal.

You're going to make a list of tasks, one per day, for the whole week. The tasks needn't be onerous or interrupt your busy schedule; in fact, they shouldn't. Remember that this isn't an exercise in moving mountains, so small steps are the best way to accomplish big dreams.

Let's say that one of your goals is to find a new job. You've felt stuck for a while, but the very idea of job hunting makes you feel stressed-out and fatigued. No wonder! You can't tackle the mountain all at once; you need to build toward that goal.

To begin, you have to look at it in a new way—in pieces instead of as a whole. What can you reasonably do in an already crowded day that will propel you toward your goal? Let's say you put "Networking" on your list. (Don't actually do anything just yet other than read this example. We'll get to finding solutions for your specific problem in a minute.) That entry is a start, but it doesn't really help; the task still feels overwhelming.

Break the entry down into smaller steps: Make a list of people who might be able to help. Go another step further by breaking that task down into two separate ones for two separate days. On the first day you'll make a list of the people in your field that you feel comfortable calling or e-mailing to tell about your search. The next day you'll list the people who might be tougher to reach but who might also be helpful.

Simply breaking the task down will make you feel better. Perhaps someone on the first list might help you connect with someone on the second. If the calls work out, someone might ask for your resume. So add "update resume" to your list as well.

As you review your list, you might realize for the first time that part of your anxiety about making these calls comes from not being entirely sure what to say once you're on the phone. You therefore might add "role-playing conversations with significant other or a friend" to the list. Before long you will have an action plan for the whole week.

In making this list you have taken some real steps toward accomplishing your goal. Everything will feel doable to you now even in the small amount of time you have to dedicate to this project every day. Nothing on your list should fill you with dread or make you feel anxious. Instead, you will replace that sense of dread and paralysis with a feeling of energy and focus, making you eager to start.

What happened? *You've just learned how to make momentum work for you.* You

> ## SPOTLIGHT ON WALNUTS
>
> Walnuts are high in protein, fat, and fiber, which is why it takes so few of them to fill you up. They're also a good source of magnesium, manganese, and copper. Walnuts contain sterols, which lower the level of LDL ("bad") cholesterol in the bloodstream, and a flavonoid called ellagic acid, which inhibits the growth of cancer cells. A diet high in walnuts also decreases C-reactive protein (CRP), a marker for inflammation strongly associated with heart disease. Walnuts contain more omega-3 fatty acids than any other nut and are particularly rich in alpha-linolenic acid (ALA), which protects against heart attacks; in fact, the amount in an ounce of walnuts a day is sufficient to produce these benefits.
>
> Of the two walnut varieties you're likely to find, the more common is English; the other one, the black walnut, has a very tough shell and a distinct cheeselike flavor. Because walnuts are higher in fat than other nuts, they go rancid easily. They should be kept in a cool, dark, dry place. In the shell they can keep for six months at room temperature; shelled walnuts should be kept in the refrigerator or freezer.
>
> Walnuts make a great "on the go" snack. When you're eating them at home, cracking the shells open should eliminate mindless consumption. It also helps to count out the number you can have and put the rest away. Fourteen walnut halves contain 3 grams of net carbs.

needed to break that mountain down into more easily scalable molehills. Those few phone calls might turn into an informational interview, an interview for a position, or people agreeing to make calls on your behalf. No matter what, you've taken a step in the right direction, and when you master this approach, the sky is the limit.

Take out your Personal Goals List and select one goal to tackle this week. You must choose something other than weight loss since you are already doing everything you need to do to achieve that personal goal.

Step One: Write your goal at the top of a new page in your Atkins Advantage Journal, being sure to state your goal in a positive way: "I want to become stronger," not "I'm tired of being weak."

Step Two: Break that big goal down into a series of smaller ones. What small tasks can you assign yourself that will help you toward this goal? Start dividing it and keep working on it until your list fits the following requirements:

- Nothing on the list fills you with anxiety or dread. If anything on your list has that effect, break it down or figure out how you can get help with it—and put that on the list!

- Nothing can be so big or time-consuming that it will disrupt your other obligations on a given day. If it does, the task you've assigned yourself is too big. Break it down further to spread it over more days.

Step Three: Write your tasks on your calendar. Follow-through is very important to complete this activity successfully. Cross off each task once you've accomplished it.

Keep track of the results of these initial efforts. You'll be surprised at the enormous ripple effect you'll see. This is a skill you can use in all areas of your life to tackle anything that seems too big and overwhelming to manage. The more you assign yourself these small, bite-sized tasks, the more accomplished you'll become at effectively realizing your goals and dreams—large and small.

JOURNALING ACTIVITY: CELEBRATE SMALL VICTORIES!

Atkins encourages mindfulness. You've spent the last two weeks learning to make healthy choices about what you put into your mouth. Similarly, you're bringing that same mindfulness to using your body more and to achieving your life's dreams. Commemorate those choices! It's as important to celebrate the daily victories as it is to celebrate the milestones. You deserve to be rewarded for the hard work you're doing, so every time you pass up a temptation, why not make a note of that small but significant victory in your journal?

Let's say you covet, but don't order, a croissant at breakfast. You passed a bagel store without even stopping for a whiff. You went to the gym even though you were tired, or you came up with a brand-new, Atkins-friendly snack. Give yourself credit in the form of a notation in your journal. Think of this as giving yourself a pat on the back, well-deserved recognition for the good work you're doing.

As you lose pounds and inches, you'll watch those entries in your Atkins Advantage Journal accumulate. Every single one of them represents a decision that you've made, a conscious choice to live and eat more healthfully. It will surely give you a boost—particularly in those moments when it's not so easy to do the right thing—to review the great choices you have made in the past, the choices that have brought you to a trimmer, slimmer body and to better health.

Fitness: The Best You

FOCUS FOR THE WEEK: BUILD MOMENTUM THROUGH A SERIES OF SMALL STEPS, INTRODUCING A STRENGTH TRAINING COMPONENT. DON'T FORGET TO PLAY AS MUCH AS POSSIBLE.

Stretching → 30 minutes → 2 times

Do your stretches at a pace that is comfortable for you. These stretches may take you longer than 30 minutes.

Strength training → 15–30 minutes → 3 times

Complete these exercises at a pace that is comfortable for you.

MOVE . . . MORE!

A well-balanced fitness program consists of cardio, which strengthens your heart and lungs; strength training, which strengthens your muscles and bones; and stretching, which increases your flexibility and may protect you from injury. But play is also an important and deliberate component of fitness. We've become a sedentary society, to the detriment of our health. Inactivity is not just bad for your physical health, it impacts mood as well. Regular exercise has been shown to enhance self-image and a sense of well-being, and to reduce stress and anxiety. Exercise has both physiological and psychological benefits. It can even help mitigate depression. By allowing yourself to play you can recapture the joy you experienced as a child when you felt your limbs in motion.

Your first assignment this week is to start moving more. Here are some ideas:

- Hide the remote control.

- Better yet, unplug the television and institute a new family tradition of a nature walk, hike, or a bike ride after dinner.

- Crank up the stereo and dance to a favorite song.

- Get off the bench when you go to the playground or park with your kids or grandkids. Get into the sandbox and in on the fun.

- Never drive when you can walk or bicycle even if that means factoring in a little extra time to get to your destination.

- Surprise your dog with a hike this weekend.

Whatever you choose to do, make it active and make it fun! Bringing more movement into your life will improve not only performance on the All-New Atkins Advantage Program but the quality of your life. These activities are natural stress busters, and exercise enhances mood.

You don't have to get on a treadmill to become more fit. I consider play, along with cardio and strength training, as equal key building blocks in the fitness portion of the Program. It's so important that you should substitute play for one of your fitness sessions every week.

STRETCHING EXERCISES

At least twice this week do the eight basic stretching exercises you've become familiar with over the last two weeks, but with a slight breathing modification. You should do them after performing a five-minute warm-up. Do each exercise three times.

Shoulder Hug, page 62

Head Up, Chest Out, page 63

Cat and Dog, page 64

Butterfly, page 65

Quad Stretch, page 77

Press Up, page 78

Low Back and Hamstring Combo Stretch, page 79

Follow Your Hand, page 80

In the spirit of momentum and the cumulative effect of small steps, use your breath to deepen each stretch ever so slightly. Here's how it works:

- As you inhale, concentrate by contracting the muscles and lengthening your spine.

- As you exhale, relax a little more deeply into the stretch.

Don't force yourself or overstretch. Be patient with your progress even if it feels as though not much is happening. Over the course of just a few breaths you'll find yourself much closer to your goal.

STRENGTH TRAINING

This week marks another exciting beginning: You're about to get stronger! Although you may shudder and make a face when you think about "lifting weights," it is not what you think. Muscle tone and strength are essential components in any fitness foundation and a gradual step toward total fitness. The work you do now will help you in the weeks to come. Think of it as getting in shape to get in shape.

While cardiovascular exercise should be the heart of any exercise program, strength training is necessary for maintaining or increasing muscle mass, which helps you burn more fat by increasing the amount you burn at rest. Even if you're only maintaining your muscle mass, you're helping to prevent the progressive decrease in muscle mass that typically occurs with age. It is estimated that you lose 2 to 5 percent of your muscle mass with every passing decade, starting in your twenties, so the impact can really add up. Sports science has shown that diminishing muscle mass is related to decreased muscle use, so strength training is the way to prevent—or at least minimize—this loss.

That's not all: Strength training will help you look better and feel better, and it will make it easier to complete your daily activities and stave off the aging process. Strength training has also been shown to increase bone density, improve blood sugar control, lower resting blood pressure, and even reduce the risk of constipation. If you think you are too old to build muscle and strength, think again: Studies on people as old as 80 have shown that strength training is safe and effective.

This week you will learn four basic strengthening exercises and then another four next week. These are the Essential Strengtheners, basic toning and strengthening exercises that will produce big changes with a minimum of gear and fuss. You will start with two upper and two lower body exercises.

Determine Your Strength Level. Like everything in the All-New Atkins Advantage Program, strength training is individualized. Using the information below, determine which level best describes you.

LEVEL ONE
I can carry an armload of laundry.
I use two hands to hold a gallon of milk.
I need assistance to get up from the floor.
I can't do a deep knee bend.
Walking up a flight of stairs leaves me winded.

LEVEL TWO
I can lift a gallon of milk with one hand.
I can get up from the floor by kneeling.
I can do one to three deep knee bends.
I usually walk up a flight of stairs instead of taking an elevator.

LEVEL THREE
I can carry a full laundry basket.
I can lift a gallon of milk over my head with one hand.
I can stand up from sitting on the ground without using my arms.
I can do more than three deep-knee bends.
I always choose the stairs and can climb three flights comfortably.

Once you have ascertained the level that best describes you, follow this level throughout the strength training program. If you notice that the assignments are becoming too easy, review this section to determine if you should move up to the next level.

What You Need. The only thing you'll need for the strength training aspect of the Program at this time is dumbbells or arm weights. If you don't have them (or belong to a gym that does), you can purchase them at a sporting goods store for around $10 a pair. Or use empty milk jugs filled with enough water to make them the right weight for you.

The following are only guidelines. You should test the weights before purchasing.

Level One: 1, 2, and/or 3 pounds

Level Two: 3, 5, and/or 8 pounds

Level Three: 5 and 8 or more pounds

It's important to select the right weights to start with—not so light that they're ineffective but not so heavy that you're likely to get injured. You might want to purchase two sets of weights—a light set for now and a heavier one for when you improve. Be aware that some muscle groups (such as quadriceps, buttocks, and back) are typically stronger than others, so you'll be able to start with heavier weights right away for those parts of the body. Select light weights that allow you to do fifteen repetitions of each exercise—not easily but completely and with proper form. Select heavy weights that allow you to do eight repetitions of each exercise—not easily but completely and with proper form.

Note: Some of you will not be able to lift any weight at all, and that's fine. Perhaps you've been ill or are recovering from an injury, or maybe you haven't exercised in so long that you don't want to risk an injury by starting out too aggressively. Or perhaps your doctor has asked you to increase your overall fitness level a little before beginning to strength-train. You will still benefit from doing these exercises without weights. If you find it more comfortable, you can sit in a chair to do them. As soon as you are able and have your doctor's approval, you can begin to add a very light weight such as a roll of pennies to do your exercises.

Strength Training Basics. As always, the focus is on doing the exercises *correctly*. It's crucial to master technique first, not only to get the maximum benefit from these exercises but also to avoid injury. Here are some things to keep in mind:

- Stand with your knees "soft"—neither bent nor hyper-extended. Feet should be hip-width apart unless otherwise noted.

- Keep your back straight, with your shoulders pulled back, and gaze directly forward as though you were meeting your own eyes in a mirror.

- Do your exercises in front of a mirror if possible to ensure that you're doing them correctly.

- Learn to distinguish between the burn of a muscle that's being used and one that's being injured. You should never feel a sharp pain or pull. If you do, stop immediately. When you feel better and the pain is no longer present, try the movement again with a lighter weight. Check your form carefully.

- Control the weight as you return it to the starting position as well as when you extend the muscle. If you can't control the dumbbell in both directions, choose a lighter weight.

- Keep your hands, wrists, and forearms in a straight line. Don't bend your wrist to help move the weight. This can cause a repetitive stress injury.

- Remember to breathe!

The Essential Strengtheners: The First Four. Before we begin, let's define our terms:

An **exercise** is the specific activity to strengthen a particular muscle or muscle group—a bicep curl, for instance.

A **repetition** (also called a rep) is one instance of doing a particular exercise. If you do an exercise 15 times without stopping, you've done 15 repetitions.

A **set** is one complete group of repetitions. The 15 repetitions above would make one set.

You'll do the strength training exercises described next three times this week. You will use light weights for the two arm exercises (unless otherwise indicated), meaning that you are comfortable doing 15 repetitions with this weight. Although you will still "feel the burn," concentrate on learning the exercises and doing them correctly. In later weeks you will advance to heavier weights, though you should not do so until you can complete three sets of 15 reps with the lighter weights.

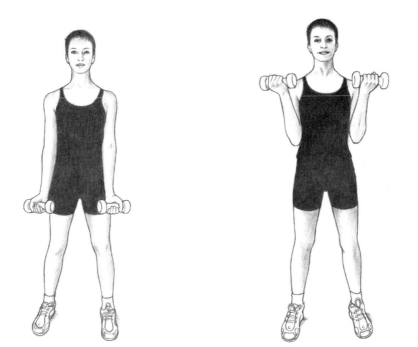

BICEPS CURL

For biceps (front of the upper arm) and posterior deltoids (back of shoulder).

1. Stand or sit with your arms by your sides, dumbbells in hand, palms forward (facing the mirror).

2. As you exhale, slowly begin to pull the weights up toward your shoulder. Your elbows and upper arms should not move.

3. Inhale as you slowly return the weights to your sides.

Number of Reps All Levels: ten
Number of Sets
Level One: one
  Levels Two and Three: two

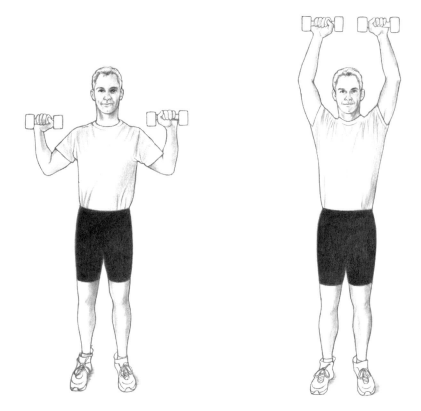

OVERHEAD PRESS

For triceps (back of the upper arm), anterior deltoid (front of the shoulder), and trapezius (upper back and neck).

1. Stand or sit with your arms by your sides, dumbbells in hand, palms facing your sides.

2. Bring the weights up beside your head, level with your shoulders, and rotate the arms so that palms are facing forward.

3. Exhale as you push the weights above your head with a slow, smooth, controlled movement.

4. Inhale as you slowly return the weights to the starting position.

Number of Reps All Levels: ten
Number of Sets
  Level One: one
  Levels Two and Three: two

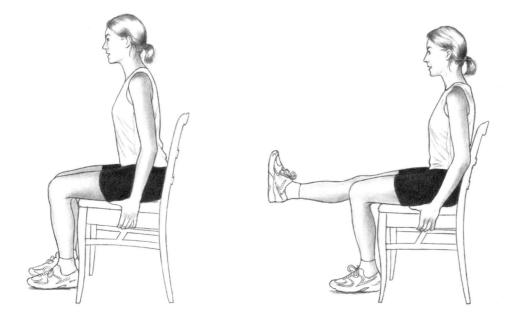

SITTING KNEE EXTENSION

For quadriceps (the big muscles on the fronts of the thighs).

1. Sit on a chair with both feet flat on the floor in front of you.

2. Extend one leg straight and lift it so that it's in line with your hips. Hold for three seconds. Return to start position.

3. Repeat with other leg.

Number of Reps All Levels: ten (five on each leg)
Number of Sets
    Level One: one
    Levels Two and Three: two

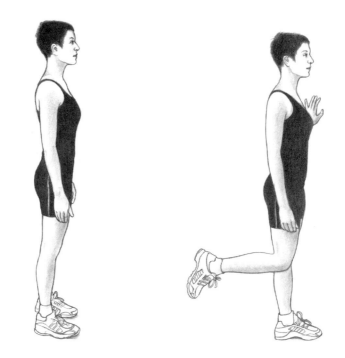

STANDING LEG LIFT

For hamstrings (the big muscles at the backs of the thighs).

1. Holding on to a wall or chair for support, maintain a straight back as you bend one leg at the knee and lift that foot off the floor until your shin is parallel with the floor. (Even if you are unable to raise your foot more than a few inches, you'll still benefit.) Hold for three seconds.

2. Repeat with the other leg.

Number of Reps All Levels: ten (five on each leg)
Number of Sets
    Level One: one
    Levels Two and Three: two

ADVANTAGE CHECKPOINT: END OF WEEK THREE

Weigh and measure yourself. Enter the results in your Atkins Advantage Journal and compare the results with those of last week. To determine whether you are pleased with your results, ask yourself these questions:

Are you free of the signs and symptoms of unstable blood sugar?

Are you continuing to lose pounds and/or inches (albeit perhaps more slowly if you have moved to OWL)?

Are your clothes continuing to feel looser?

Do you feel good overall?

If you answer yes to these questions, then you are to be congratulated. Keep building on the momentum you're developing as you go forward. As long as you continue to lose weight and inches, add 5 grams daily of net carbs to your meal plans if you are in OWL or 10 grams if you are in Pre-Maintenance.

But perhaps you are not entirely happy with your results. Perhaps your weight loss has slowed or stalled and/or symptoms of unstable blood sugar have returned. If you think you might like to experiment with some modifications that could put you on a more accelerated track or if you're simply curious about alternative ways to do the phase you're in, see Customizing OWL (page 106) or Customizing Pre-Maintenance (page 205).

Another possibility is that you gained weight. If so, and if you have not been faithful to Induction, continue at 20 grams of net carbs for another week or two. Regardless of which phase of the Atkins you're in, if you gained weight this week, it's time for action.

See page 156 in Week Seven for strategies if you have experienced a weight gain, slowdown, stall, or plateau in the phase you're in. However, if you have been in OWL for only one week and gained weight, don't assume that Atkins doesn't work for you or that you should return to Induction. It's important to complete two full weeks on OWL before adopting a course correction. One week simply isn't enough time to know if what you're seeing signifies a normal fluctuation or is a bigger issue. For that reason, complete two weeks in OWL before adopting any variations and do the following:

- Stay at your current carbohydrate level for one more week; your metabolism might simply need a little time to adjust.

- Check the rules of OWL (see page 86) to make sure that you're following the plan correctly.

- Enter everything you eat in your Atkins Advantage Journal.

- Be sure to read labels and avoid any products with unacceptable ingredients.

- If you have not yet begun the exercise component, do so now.

EIGHT

WEEK FOUR: FREE SPEED

When a cyclist puts on sleek Lycra pants instead of heavy, wind-catching sweatpants, he can cut down significantly on wind resistance. Likewise, when a skier bends forward into a tuck, she goes faster without expending any extra energy. Athletes call this advantage "free speed."

Whether or not you realize it, you're already taking advantage of free speed. By changing your metabolism, you're making it easier to lose weight and keep it off, and you're making the most of your efforts. You get more free speed every time you sit down to satisfying meals. As you will see, planning ahead plays an important role in helping you pick up even more free speed and gain momentum toward achieving your goals.

NUTRITION: THE HEART OF THE MATTER

In the fourth week of the program, you're shedding pounds and inches and feeling great! For many of you this will mark your second week of Ongoing Weight Loss (OWL). If you are staying at 25 grams daily of net carbs, repeat the meal plans that start on page 278, making some of the modifications we have suggested or your own.

Otherwise, move on to 30 grams of net carbs, referring to the meal plans that begin on page 285.

If you're continuing with Induction (meaning you still have a fair amount of weight to lose), continue to use the Induction meal plans starting on page 264.

If you began Atkins in OWL or Pre-Maintenance, find the meal plans appropriate for your daily net carb intake by referring to the listings beginning on page 278.

Continue to take a good multivitamin, essential fatty acids, and a fiber supplement.

IT'S YOUR PROGRAM

Ongoing Weight Loss is a balancing act between adding variety to your meals and maintaining your weight loss progress. Fortunately, it's not an either/or proposition. You can work the program to suit your preferences.

Do you opt to savor a myriad of textures and tastes even if greater variety means slowing the rate of your weight loss a tad? If you get bored easily and variety will help you comply with the Program long-term, adding carbs back more quickly is probably the right choice for you—as long as your weight loss continues, albeit more slowly. On the other hand, if you'd gladly trade culinary variety for inches lost at your next Advantage Checkpoint, then you might prefer to climb the Carb Ladder more slowly.

As you proceed through OWL, you'll learn how to tailor this phase to your advantage. Pay attention to your body's signals; they'll tell you if you are moving at the right pace. If your weight loss stalls during OWL, you're probably adding back carbs too quickly. Stay put for a couple of weeks instead of adding another 5 grams. (See Customizing OWL below for more on how to keep those inches and pounds falling off.) Conversely, if your weight loss is steady but you crave some new taste sensations, we'll show you how to add back foods from two new food groups each week.

> ### CHOOSING YOUR BERRIES
>
> Unlike nuts or vegetables, in which carb content generally does not vary greatly in portions of the same size, berries and other fruits have a wider range. In Induction you can eat tomatoes, olives, and avocados, which botanically are fruits. Once you are in OWL, we recommend that you start with strawberries, which have one of the lowest carb contents of any fruit. Wait several days before trying a different type of berry. That way, if you have difficulty, you will know which fruit is the culprit. Fruit is a common trigger food for many people, so proceed cautiously.

WATCH FOR TRIGGER FOODS

As you add new carbohydrate foods to your meals and snacks, pay attention to how they make you feel. The reasons for a return to overeating or eating the wrong foods may vary from the physiological (the impact they have on your blood sugar) to the psychological (how certain foods make you feel and the associations they create in your mind).

For some people cheese is a trigger food—meaning they cannot stop with a small portion; for others it is wine and alcohol. For still others it's nuts or berries. Your trigger food may be something else entirely. Here's how to tell if you've added back a trigger food:

- It's hard to control your portions of the food.

- You have become preoccupied with the food.

- You find that eating it makes you crave other higher-carbohydrate foods.

- Eating it stimulates your appetite.

If a particular food is the culprit, get it out of the house and replace it with something else. Likewise, if you're bingeing on a number of high-carb foods, toss them as well. If you have been bingeing for more than a day or two or can't seem to get back in control, go back to Induction to restart fat burning and restabilize your blood sugar as quickly as you can. If you are in control, simply go back to the way you were eating before the binge. Be sure to have the correct foods readily available in case you are tempted again. If you've gained weight, once you're back in control, move through the levels of carb intake until you reach your CCLL.

Keeping a food journal can help you isolate the foods that are causing a problem. When you've identified the culprits, you have a few options:

- Eat these carb foods in combination with fat and/or protein, as you should be doing anyway. Have your berries with a dollop of whipped cream or a handful of almonds on the side.

- If that doesn't work, stay away from the food for a few weeks, then reintroduce it slowly by limiting the number of times you eat it to once or twice a week.

- If you find that a food is still causing problems, you may have to stop eating it for a longer period of time. When you try to reintroduce the food, if symptoms recur, you may have to avoid it indefinitely.

- If you discover that you're really sensitive to a food, don't "cheat" with it. Find something else to say yes to.

The best way to achieve weight loss goals is to personalize each phase of the nutritional program to suit your individual needs and preferences. That way you'll be able to maintain these new habits for a lifetime. The standard rule of OWL, which states that you should add 5 grams daily of net carbs every week, *as long as you continue to lose weight*, can be modified to suit your particular needs.

These variations are intended to keep your motivation high, either by expanding the range of foods you can eat or by accelerating your progress. You'll remain securely within the parameters of OWL; they simply give you more freedom to do it your way.

Please remember that you're not supposed to lose weight as quickly in OWL as you did in Induction and that even if the scale holds steady, as long as you're still losing inches, you're doing fine.

Reminder: It's important to complete two full weeks on OWL before starting to individualize this program because one week isn't enough time to know how your body is responding to this phase.

WHO SHOULD CONSIDER CUSTOMIZING OWL?

Our experience has shown us that the following types do best if they do OWL a little differently:

1. You are a "slow burner." If it is difficult for you to lose weight, even when you strictly adhere to the rules of a weight loss program, then you might be metabolically resistant. The good news is that you will typically get better results by adding carbs a little more slowly and giving your metabolism a chance to catch up. In addition to following the variations below, it is important for you to follow through on the fitness wheel of the program. Exercise is your best chance to rev up your metabolism.

2. You have more than 30 pounds to lose as you enter OWL. If being overweight poses a health risk or you're on medications that slow weight loss, you might want to speed the rate at which you lose in OWL. If adding 5 grams daily of net carbs each week is retarding your weight loss, then exercise and the variations below should help you pick up your pace.

   If you are one of these types, one of these variations should help:

   Slow Climb Variation: Add your carbs back in increments of 5 grams of net carbs, but stay at *each level for two or three weeks* instead of just one. Slowing down the pace at which carbs are reintroduced may allow you to speed up your rate of weight loss. Remember that this isn't a race; there is nothing wrong with adding your carbs slowly. You're still climbing by intervals of 5 grams daily of net carbs. You'll simply be changing the frequency of the intervals in order to give your body a bit more time to catch up.

Alternate Day Variation: Instead of adding back 5 grams daily of net carbs *every* day of the week, add back that extra 5 *every other day*. Let's say you are currently at 25 grams but find your weight loss slower than you'd like. Instead of staying with 25 every day of the week, alternate between 25 and 20 grams: 25 grams on Monday, 20 grams on Tuesday, 25 on Wednesday, and so on. If your weight loss picks up with this pattern of alternating days, stick with it!

3. You are impatient. You miss eating a broad array of foods and know you will be better able to stick with the program if you can vary your menus.

Two-at-a-Time Variation: Add carbs from two food groups at a time, alternating days. For example, when you go from 25 to 30 grams, you might use that extra 5 grams to enjoy tasty nuts on Monday, strawberries on Tuesday, nuts again on Wednesday, and so forth. The daily number of carb grams remains constant, but you can pick from a broader array of carbohydrate foods.

> ## CHROMIUM HELPS CONTROL BLOOD SUGAR
>
> Chromium has been billed as a magic fat-burner and muscle-builder. While some of those claims are exaggerated, this essential trace mineral can help you control your blood sugar and insulin levels as well as your weight. Found in small amounts in many foods, including beef, cheese, dark green leafy vegetables, mushrooms, some shellfish, and barley, chromium must be taken in supplement form to get enough to see results. Taking a chromium supplement may help improve insulin resistance. Doctors and researchers aren't exactly sure how this mineral works to assist insulin, but they believe your body needs it to make one of the compounds used to lower blood sugar and control the appetite. This makes chromium an especially good choice for people who are trying to slim down or who have the metabolic syndrome (page 12), pre-diabetes, or diabetes. It also helps people control their cravings for sugary foods.
>
> There is good evidence that taking a minimum of 200 micrograms of chromium a day in the form of chromium picolinate or chromium polynicotinate is safe and can help control your blood sugar levels. More is not necessarily better, so do not exceed 800 micrograms a day.

EAT BETTER BY PLANNING AHEAD

One way to get some free speed is with advance preparation, and that certainly applies to mealtimes. Planning ahead makes doing Atkins easier, and it can prevent you from going off the program because you won't be caught unprepared when hunger strikes. If you anticipate your meal and snack needs, you won't find yourself hungry without healthy food choices within reach when you're at your most vulnerable.

A well-provisioned pantry saves you time by reducing the number of trips you need to make to the market. If you buy on sale and in bulk, you can save money as well. When you're doing Atkins, it also means that you're never without something suitable to eat. Fresh whole foods are the best choices, and they're the heart of doing Atkins. But what are you going to do on those nights when you have to finish one last thing at work and miss getting to the store? Having nothing fresh in the house should not interfere with your commitment to eat low carb.

Stock your shelves with this list of nonspoilable staples so that you can always put together a healthy, satisfying meal or snack even when the fridge is empty.

- Canned fish, such as tuna, salmon, and sardines, can be the heart of many simple, delicious menu choices.

- Anchovies and anchovy paste are a sophisticated addition to vegetable dishes, sauces, and salad dressings. Look for resealable glass jars that can be kept in the refrigerator.

- Jars of artichoke hearts and hearts of palm are great when added to main-dish salads. Read the label to make sure the artichokes aren't packed in hydrogenated oils.

- Jarred roasted red peppers can be pureed with cream cheese or sour cream to make a dip. They can also be chopped for use in salads or as a flavorful and colorful garnish for vegetable dishes.

- Low-carb soup mixes have a long shelf life and are quick to prepare.

- Sugar-free gelatin and pudding can be used to make satisfying low-carb treats.

- If your daily carb level permits these foods, many grains (such as quinoa) and legumes (such as lentils) can be stored for long periods of time and don't need to be soaked overnight or cooked for a very long time.

Have the following available in the freezer:

- Frozen vegetables such as spinach, broccoli, cauliflower, edamame (soybeans), and green beans are good in a pinch or when the fresh variety is out of season.

- Frozen beef, turkey, or soy burgers defrost quickly for a speedy protein-rich meal.

- Frozen nuts stay fresh for months and can be used in recipes or eaten right out of the freezer. Pack them in small, single-serving ziplock bags that are ready to go when you are.

- Frozen berries without added sugar allow for a quick smoothie or dessert.

IT'S 6:00 P.M. DO YOU KNOW WHAT YOUR DINNER IS?

It's no wonder that a television chef can put together a three-course meal in half an hour, minus commercials: Behind-the-scenes assistants handle the time-consuming prep work. That's one reason that gourmet dining on a weeknight isn't a reality for the vast majority of us. Indeed, research indicates that 70 percent of Americans don't even know what they're eating for dinner until 4:00 in the afternoon. Foraging when you're famished isn't the optimal way to stick with Atkins, but we know it's hard to get a healthy dinner on the table when you're working late and/or picking up two kids from different after-school activities. Because life isn't going to slow down, it's time for some free speed.

Make a menu. Know what you're eating and where. How many dinners will you eat at home this week? What will they be? Draw up a grocery list as you go so you can save time by shopping just once.

> ### MAKE MORE THAN YOU NEED AND FREEZE
>
> When you're making a main dish such as meatloaf, pork tenderloin, or chicken breast for dinner, prepare more than you need and put the unused portions into ziplock freezer bags. Label the items clearly and date them. Frozen raw ground meats should be eaten within one to three months; whole raw pieces, such as chicken breasts, chops, or a roast may be kept for up to six months.
>
> There is nothing better than a steaming bowl of hearty homemade soup. It's no bother to make twice the amount and then freeze half of it in single portions. A delicious, almost-instant meal is never farther away than the defrost setting on the microwave.

Do the prep. You still have to do some slicing and dicing, but it's much less onerous when done other than at mealtime on a weeknight. Do some basic groundwork on the weekend or at another less hectic time—maybe even right after you get back from the grocery store. Here is what you can do in advance:

- Wash and trim greens and herbs. Tear lettuce and other leaves rather than cut them when possible. Pat lettuce greens with a dish towel or paper towel to absorb excess moisture, or just spin dry in a salad spinner. Store in the fridge. Wrap washed herbs in damp paper towels to preserve them.

- Make salad dressing in a jar (for recipes see www.atkins.com), cover, and refrigerate until needed.

- Wash, peel, cut, or chop vegetables and then put them in a ziplock bag overnight or up to three days.

- Trim and season pork, beef, or poultry a day or two before you plan to serve it so that it is ready to be tossed into a heated pan. (Note: Fish should be eaten fairly soon after purchase and not prepared in advance.)

- Marinate meat and poultry in the refrigerator up to 24 hours to deepen the flavor.

Have fun. Enlist some helpers: cooking with older kids can be a great way to bond. Or put a friend on speakerphone and chat while you work. Listen to music, catch up on the news, or keep an eye on your favorite sitcom (just watch your fingers!).

Prepping one or two meals a week in advance will make a big difference. What would have been a real drag on a harried Wednesday night feels quite creative on a lazy Sunday afternoon, and cooking on that harried Wednesday goes from a dreaded chore to a pleasure: Simply open the fridge, drop your prepped veggies into the steamer, toss the salad fixings into a bowl, put the meat, fish, or poultry under the broiler, and presto! Dinner is ready before the table's set—just like a cooking show.

> **ATKINS ADVANTAGE TIP**
> Drinking hot tea or broth before eating a meal can help decrease hunger.

If you are really enjoying this free speed, see if you can't put together Thursday's lunch while you're putting away the leftovers on Wednesday night instead of waiting until you're running out the door the next morning.

SNACKING MADE SIMPLE

Between-meal noshing is fine when you do Atkins. You should eat whenever you're hungry so that your appetite stays under control and you're able to make healthy food choices at mealtime.

Convenience is key: Having snacks at the ready in the fridge or freezer makes reaching for them as easy as grabbing for a bag of chips.

Leftovers: Don't toss "too small for a meal" leftovers or eat them up to avoid the leftover issue. Bag the small portion remaining—a piece of chicken breast, a slice or two of roast beef, or a small cup of stew—for tomorrow's snack.

Snacks in bulk: Make snacks in bulk ahead of time so that there is always something great to grab when your stomach growls. Turkey and cheese roll-ups, for instance, can be prefolded and left in a storage container for a few days until you need them.

Snack packs: Make single-serving snack packs so you won't get carried away reaching into a big container when you're starving. Make a bunch of snack packs filled with nonperishables such as a serving of nuts or homemade, low-carb trail mix in a ziplock bag. Keep a few packs wherever you're likely to be. Pack extra when you know your day is going to involve complications such as a long wait, travel, or back-to-back meetings at work.

Our Favorite Snacks. With snacks like these at the ready, you should be able to avoid high-carb temptations.

- Hard-boiled eggs in the shell will keep in the refrigerator for seven days. If you're inspired, prepare delicious deviled eggs with a little mayo and paprika, or perhaps a little curry powder.

- String cheese or individual packaged cheese slices, rounds, or triangles travel well. (Be sure to avoid processed cheese foods, which can contain added carbs.)

- Turkey, nitrate-free ham, roast beef, and cheese roll-ups are tasty when made with mayonnaise and mustard. For variety and crunch, instead of cheese, wrap meats around a steamed stalk of asparagus or a dill pickle spear or in a lettuce leaf.

- Different types of olives satisfy a salt craving.

- Celery sticks can be filled with cream cheese or natural peanut butter or other nut butters.

- Low-carb soup mixes are a lifesaver. They are inexpensive, highly portable, ready in seconds, and super-easy to prepare—just boil water!

- Add a little excitement to nuts by roasting them in a pan with olive oil and a spice mixture—curry powder and cayenne if you like it hot; ginger, tamari, and sesame oil for an Asian flavor; cinnamon and sucralose for a sweet treat.

- When you make your own trail mix, you can add ingredients as you progress through the phases of Atkins. Start with sesame seeds, soy nuts, or real nuts in OWL, and as your carb threshold increases, low-sugar cereal, unsweetened dried cranberries, popcorn, or sugar-free chocolate chips become options.

- Make nachos with low-carb soy chips. For added texture and color, throw some blanched broccoli florets and red pepper strips on top before you add salsa and melt the cheese.

- Beef or turkey jerky is a fine snack, but be sure to avoid those with nitrates and added sugars.

- Make your own cheese balls by marinating mozzarella in olive oil with a fresh herb such as basil or thyme.

- Cream goat cheese or another spreadable cheese with herbs or olives for a dip with crudités.

- Combine grated cheddar or Swiss cheese with your favorite spices and some pine nuts. Roll them around until they are the size of golf balls, and pack individually as a snack.

- Sausage makes a great appetizer or snack. Experiment with different types, but beware of nitrates and sulfites. Pair them with crunchy cucumber slices and other fresh vegetables. Match with a variety of homemade dips: ketchup, aioli, herbed mayonnaises, and homemade relishes and chutneys.

- Berries with heavy cream make a tasty treat.

- Sugar-free gelatin with whipped cream is easy and refreshing.

- Sugar-free pudding made with cream and water or a reduced-carb dairy beverage instead of milk can be satisfying.

- Try low-carb yogurt or shakes.

MOTIVATION: THE WINNER'S EDGE

In weight loss efforts as in life, thinking ahead is the surest way to get ahead. If you are prepared for temptation, you'll always enjoy the upper hand. Consider these tips from Atkins Achievers to help you stay on course:

Don't leave it to chance. If you have an early meeting where a platter of muffins and bagels is likely to tempt you, pack a low-carb breakfast burrito the night before or that morning. There may be a low-carb option (in which case you can have the burrito for lunch), but if there isn't, you must either go hungry or eat something you shouldn't.

Eat in advance. Eat a snack or meal that is low-carb, high-protein, high-fiber before going off to that cocktail party, and you'll be far less likely to snack on crackers and high-carb hors d'oeuvres. Meet your date *before* the movie for dinner; after a great protein and vegetable meal, you're far less likely to crave the popcorn or sweets at the concession. Or bring a serving of nuts as a substitute if the smell of popcorn becomes too enticing.

Join the fun—the Atkins way. Meet your buddies at your local hangout just as you always have—but with a low-carb strategy in place. Make sure your friends know you're doing Atkins, and if you find yourself hungry when they're ordering nachos, go for the spicy chicken wings and light beer instead.

Call ahead. You won't be the first diner to call a restaurant to ask about the options on the menu. Many restaurants now feature their menus on their Web sites, so you can make judicious choices about what you're going to order before you arrive.

"Hold the rolls." The basket of bread arrives when you're at your hungriest. Don't let it come to roost on your table at all. Tell the server that you're fine without one when you're seated. If your dining companions prefer to have it, push it to the other end of the table and ask for some olives or celery sticks so you can nibble on something, too.

Substitution, please. You can say, "May I have double vegetables instead of potatoes?" and "Please put that chicken on top of salad greens instead of rice pilaf" and "May I have that cheese steak in a bowl?" More and more restaurants now include items such as "naked hamburgers" on the menu to accommodate customers following a low-carb regimen.

> ### SPOTLIGHT ON BROCCOLI
>
> Broccoli—and its close relatives—is a powerhouse of antioxidants, minerals, and phytochemicals. They include lutein and zeaxanthin, two carotenoids that protect vision from age-related macular degeneration; beta-carotene, which the body uses to manufacture vitamin A; indoles, which are compounds that may protect against various cancers; monoterpenes, which are antioxidants that increase immunity; sulforaphane, which boosts the production of cancer-fighting enzymes; and phenethyl isothiocyanate, which is thought to protect against lung cancer. Broccoli is also rich in folate, vitamin A, calcium, iron, and riboflavin, and has more vitamin C than an equal-size portion of oranges. One-half cup of cooked broccoli provides 1.7 grams of net carbs.
>
> Broccolini and broccoli rabe are related to broccoli and have many of the same nutritional benefits. Broccolini is a hybrid of broccoli and Chinese kale, with long stems and buds that look like small heads of broccoli.
>
> Broccoli is frequently maligned because it is so often poorly prepared. There is no question that overcooked, odiferous, khaki-color broccoli is yucky. Instead, steam it for five to seven minutes and see if you don't feel differently.

Bring an entrée. Atkins cookbooks and www.atkins.com offer recipes for every occasion or holiday. If you are dining at someone else's home, offer to bring a special dish; the hostess will appreciate your effort, and there will be at least one healthy choice for you.

Avoid triggers. If planning ahead doesn't work, you may need to make other changes. If you can't go to the movies without beating a path to the popcorn and candy, then invite your friends over for DVDs and low-carb snacks until you feel in complete control of your new lifestyle.

If you are anxious about facing down temptation, this exercise can help you prepare—practically and emotionally—for the challenge. Practice with it now, and then use it when you find yourself nervously anticipating an upcoming event such as a holiday dinner, cocktail party, or wedding.

Find a quiet place, make yourself comfortable, and close your eyes. Imagine yourself in the tempting situation. Perhaps you are sitting down to a Thanksgiving table groaning with platters. Maybe you are all dressed up and watching the candlelight reflect off the heavy silverware at a fine restaurant, or you are draping a red-checkered tablecloth over the picnic table at a summer barbeque.

Envision the scenario in as much detail as possible. If you're at a restaurant, imagine the elegant calligraphy of the menu as you peruse your options. Hear the background music and the murmur of other diners conversing. Smell the aroma of charcoal-grilled meat as you feel the sun on your skin at a barbecue on the beach.

Once you have set the scene, select the food you'll be eating at this meal. If you are envisioning Thanksgiving dinner with your extended family, you decline your sister's famous cornbread stuffing in favor of another slice of perfectly browned turkey and roasted asparagus.

If it is a barbecue you're attending, see yourself sliding the cheeseburger off the bun and taking a helping of salad or the sugar-free coleslaw you brought. Envision yourself making the perfect plate, whether it's colored plastic or the very best china. Reflect on how fortunate you are to be able to eat this way and lose weight at the same time. Chew every bite thoroughly, enjoying the meal completely with no guilt or bad feelings. You are doing the very best thing for your body by choosing these foods. Finally, imagine how good you are going to feel tomorrow when your clothes still fit comfortably.

This visualization activity reinforces your ability to make the healthiest choices. It can be a very useful planning tool, one that will relax and bolster you before you venture into the precarious zone of temptation.

Fitness: The Best You

FOCUS FOR THE WEEK: YOU'LL BUILD ON YOUR EARLIER WEEK'S WORK WITH WALKS THAT WILL PREPARE YOU FOR CARDIO IN FUTURE WEEKS. DON'T FORGET TO PLAY AS MUCH AS POSSIBLE!

Walking ➜ 25–35 minutes ➜ 3 times
Stretching ➜ 30 minutes ➜ 2 times
Strength training ➜ 3 times at a pace that is comfortable for you.

Do your stretches at a pace that is comfortable for you. These stretches may take you longer than 30 minutes.

We'll continue with the four Essential Strengtheners exercises introduced last week, and you'll learn another four. By the end of this week you will likely start noticing a difference in how your body feels as you go about your daily tasks, whether it's lifting grocery bags or a briefcase. You're getting stronger! We're also going to add some light walking to the program so that you begin to rev up your heart and lungs.

EXERTION: HOW HARD SHOULD YOU WORK?

It's important to understand that it's not a matter of putting in the time that makes exercise effective but what you do with that time.

You can do one hundred stretches, but unless you push yourself a bit further with each stretch, your flexibility won't increase. You can lift weights until the cows come home, but unless you increase the amount of weight you use and/or the number of times you lift them, your muscles won't get stronger. The same is true for your heart. You can walk thousands of miles, but unless you gradually increase your pace so that you're working a little harder, you won't maximize the cardiovascular or health benefits.

Working with a weight that is too heavy to lift enough times to benefit from the exercise is pointless; likewise, overexertion with cardiovascular exercises (also known as aerobics) can hinder your efforts. Your goal should be to find the level that produces real results while avoiding the kind of intensity that increases your risks. By gradually building your strength and endurance, you reduce the likelihood of injury. When you choose the right exertion, you get much greater benefit in much less time—and that's free speed!

In fitness as in nutrition, you can do better than a one-size-fits-all approach. The chart below gives you parameters to ensure that you are always getting the best workout for you—whether you are someone with strong fitness fundamentals in place or someone who is just beginning to exercise.

Use this chart to determine how hard you should be working in both the aerobic (cardio) and the strength training components of the program to come. Compare your exertion to the description, and tailor your efforts (in the aerobic portion) or the amount of weight (in the strength training portion) to fit your desired level of exertion.

EXERTION CHART

EXERTION	TYPE OF AEROBICS	TYPE OF STRENGTH TRAINING
LOW: You won't see results, and if an activity is too easy, you'll get bored before you get tired.	Can do all day without getting out of breath; examples are drying dishes, sewing, folding laundry, and playing pool.	Can lift a given weight 15 times without undue effort.
MEDIUM: Your endurance will improve. You are making a noticeable effort, but your strength will not necessarily increase.	You will feel exertion but will not become overtired or work up a sweat; examples are general house cleaning, washing the car, cleaning windows, and raking leaves.	Can lift a given weight 10 times.
HIGH: You'll be challenged, and your muscular and cardiovascular development will increase along with your endurance.	Your heart will be pumping, and you'll sweat but won't be exhausted.	Can lift a given weight 8 times with some effort.
SUPERHIGH: You push yourself beyond your limits.	Activities that leave you breathless and noticeably sore while you are engaging in them.	Cannot lift a given weight more than one to three times.

Next week you will begin cardiovascular exercise, which will strengthen your heart and lungs so they can perform more efficiently. In the spirit of planning ahead, we would like you to spend part of your fitness time this week getting ready by doing some light walking.

The goal is to take three walks of at least 25 minutes each this week. Walk at an easy, comfortable pace (your exertion level should match Low in the Exertion Chart). This is the only time Low is right, so enjoy it! (Of course, if you are already a regular walker, you can certainly pick up the pace.) Your muscles need time to recover from the strength training you've been doing, so alternate between walking one day and strength training the next. Try to take two days off from all exercise during the week, although these should not be consecutive days.

If you have a lot of weight to lose and/or aren't sufficiently conditioned, you don't need to walk for 25 minutes. Break it up into two ten-minute periods of walking separated by a three- to five-minute rest, with the goal of increasing your walking time to two fifteen-minute sessions separated by a three- to five-minute rest. Do this three times a week.

If you already have a cardiovascular fitness routine, by all means, continue! As long as it is at least 25 minutes long and you do it at least three days a week, it satisfies this part of the program.

STRETCHING EXERCISES

Use the same stretching exercises you learned in Weeks One and Two. Do each exercise three times.

Shoulder Hug, page 62

Head Up, Chest Out, page 63

Cat and Dog, page 64

Butterfly, page 65

Quad Stretch, page 77

Press Up, page 78

Low Back and Hamstring Combo Stretch, page 79

Follow Your Hand, page 80

STRENGTH TRAINING

You'll strength-train three times this week, using all eight Essential Strengtheners. With the weight that you can lift fifteen times, first do the four exercises you learned last week:

Biceps Curl, page 97

Overhead Press, page 98

Sitting Knee Extension, page 99

Standing Leg Lift, page 100

Number of Reps All Levels: ten
Number of Sets
   Level One: two
   Level Two: three
   Level Three: three

The Essential Strengtheners: The Final Four. Whether you are Level One, Two, or Three, you will increase the amount of weight you use this week so that your workout is of Medium exertion level. Use weights with which you feel comfortable, completing ten controlled repetitions with effort.

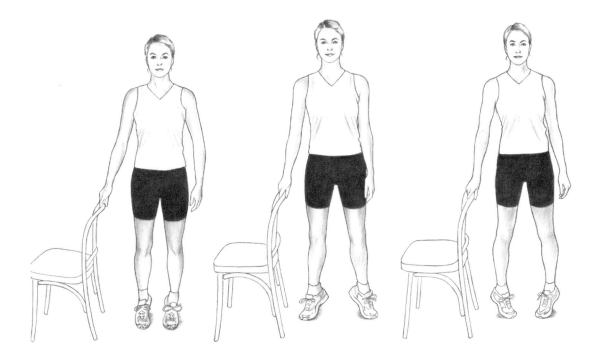

CALF LIFT

For the back of lower legs.

1. Stand, holding on to a chair with one hand for balance if needed.

2. With legs shoulder-width apart and feet parallel, lift yourself slowly onto the balls of your feet.

3. Slowly lower yourself down.

Number of Reps All Levels: ten

Number of Sets

    Level One: One

    Levels Two and Three: One set as above, followed by one set with toes pointed outward and one with toes pointed inward (see diagrams).

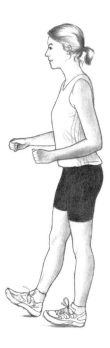

HEEL WALKING

For ankles and lower legs. Perform this exercise on a flat surface at a reasonably slow pace to aid in balance.

1. Walk with short, choppy steps, keeping your weight on your heels and your toes off the ground.

2. Resting either one or both hands on a rolling chair can provide additional support for balance.

Number of Sets

Level One: 10 seconds; aim for two to three sets if possible

Level Two: 20 seconds; aim for three sets with one-minute rest intervals

Level Three: 30 seconds; aim for three sets with one-minute rest intervals

As you become fitter, increase the amount of time per set, first doubling and then tripling your duration.

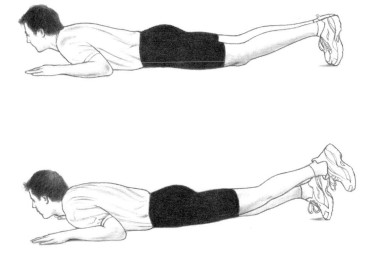

BACK LIFT
For lower back.

1. Lie on your stomach on a thick towel or mat.

2. Keeping both hips pressed against the floor as evenly as possible, lift one leg 6 inches from the floor and hold it for three seconds.

3. Repeat with the other leg.

Number of Reps All Levels: ten, five for each leg
Number of Sets
    Level One: one
    Level Two: two
    Level Three: three

As you become fitter, increase the number of repetitions to 20 per set, ten for each leg.

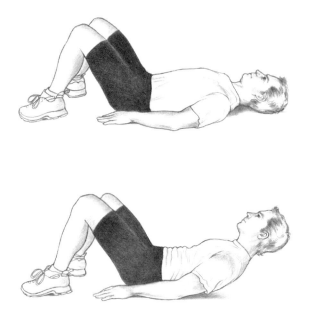

AB LIFT

For strengthening upper abdominals.

1. Lie on your back on a thick towel or mat, with your arms by your sides.

2. Slowly raise your head and shoulders 3 to 5 inches off the floor. Look straight ahead, without craning or putting undue strain on your neck. Hold for three seconds.

Number of Reps All Levels: ten

Number of Sets

    Level One: one

    Level Two: two

    Level Three: three

Modification: For Levels Two and Three, gradually build up to ten reps. Once you are able to perform the appropriate number of sets, cross your arms on your chest instead of placing them by your sides and raise your head and shoulders without using your hands for support.

ADVANTAGE CHECKPOINT: END OF WEEK FOUR

Weigh and measure yourself. Enter the results in your Atkins Advantage Journal and compare the results with those of last week.

If you are still in Induction, consider the following:

If you are pleased with your results and are continuing Induction, fine, but remember that you should eventually cycle through all four phases. Do not remain in Induction until you reach your goal weight.

If you have not been faithful to Induction, continue at 20 grams of net carbs for another week or two.

If you are not entirely happy with your results, see Are You Ready to Leave Induction? on page 82 to review strategies for success in Induction.

If you are ready to move to OWL, see Welcome to OWL on page 86.

If you are in Ongoing Weight Loss, consider the following:

If you are continuing OWL and are pleased with your results, next week add 5 grams of net carbs to your daily menus.

If this is your first week in OWL and you have not lost weight or inches, understand that it is important to complete two full weeks on OWL before adopting a course correction. Stay at your current carbohydrate level for one more week. Your metabolism might simply need a little time to adjust.

If you are beyond your second week of OWL and your weight loss has slowed or stalled and/or symptoms of unstable blood sugar have returned, see Customizing OWL: Do It Your Way on page 106. If you would like to experiment with some modifications that could put you on a more accelerated track or if you are simply curious about alternative ways to do OWL, you can also review this section.

If you're within 5 to 10 pounds of your goal weight, it is time to move to Pre-Maintenance. See The Rules of Pre-Maintenance on page 188.

If you are in Pre-Maintenance, consider the following:

If you are pleased with your results, next week add 10 grams daily of net carbs to your meal plans.

If this is your first week in Pre-Maintenance and you have not lost weight or inches, stay at your current carbohydrate level for one more week. If you have not lost weight by the end of the second week, cut back by 5 or 10 grams daily of net carbs next week.

If you are beyond the first week of Pre-Maintenance and your weight loss has stalled and/or symptoms of blood sugar have returned, see Customizing Pre-Maintenance on page 205. If you would like to experiment with some modifications that could put you on a more accelerated track or if you are simply curious about alternative ways to customize Pre-Maintenance, you can also review this section.

If you have not lost any pounds or inches after four weeks on Pre-Maintenance and are not yet at your goal weight, you may have prematurely found your Atkins Carbohydrate Equilibrium, or ACE (page 25). Cut back by 5 or 10 grams until slow weight loss resumes.

Regardless of what phase of the ANA you are in, if you gained weight this week, it's time to take action. See page 155 in Week Seven for troubleshooting strategies for your appropriate phase.

NINE

WEEK FIVE: GET MOVING!

A s any athletic coach will tell you, *heart* is what wins the game. That is why that vital organ is the theme this week in our Fitness component. We'll be strengthening the heart by slightly intensifying the cardiovascular portion of the Program. We'll also address the larger meaning of the heart as the seat of passion and motivation.

Knowing what gets your juices flowing is important for sustaining high performance. What motivates you? What can you do to beat back boredom? What gets you energized? What makes you put more heart and soul into the things that you do, and how can that motivation become a resource to help you go the distance?

NUTRITION: THE HEART OF THE MATTER

To find meal plans appropriate for your daily net carb level, see the lists beginning on page 278. Remember that if you are staying at the same level of net carb grams for a second or third week, you can modify the meal plans with our suggestions or make your own modifications.

Continue to take a good multivitamin, essential fatty acids, and a fiber supplement.

Before you can get energized, you need to eliminate the old patterns that weigh you down. For many that includes habitually overeating.

Although research confirms that you can eat more calories while losing more weight when you do Atkins than on a low-fat or calorie-restricted program (this is called the metabolic advantage), the ceiling isn't limitless. If you eat excessive amounts of food—even protein—some of it naturally converts to blood sugar and interferes with your weight loss progress. But going too low in calories is counterproductive; your metabolism will slow, impeding weight loss. If you have to cut calories, most men can lose at 1,800 calories a day and women at 1,500. Under no circumstances go below 1,200 calories a day.

> **ATKINS ADVANTAGE TIP**
> Limit all artificial sweeteners to three packets per day and count each packet as 1 gram of net carbs. Although the label will say it contains no carbohydrates, sweeteners can have up to 0.9 gram of carbs without having to declare it.

If you are still having trouble controlling your insulin and blood sugar levels—in other words, you are still experiencing dips in energy and cravings for carbohydrate foods—or if the pace of your weight loss is very slow, you may want to consider taking an additional supplement.

BREAKING THE OVEREATING HABIT

Fortunately, one of the advantages of doing Atkins is that you'll automatically be less hungry and less likely to overeat because the foods you're eating are satisfying and contain slow-burning fuels. You can break the habit of overeating even if you've been doing it for a lifetime. These tips can help:

Concentrate on every bite to battle unconscious eating. It's all too easy to lose track of how much you're consuming if you're doing something else at the same time. Don't eat lunch in front of the computer, don't eat dinner in front of the television, and don't snack while on the phone or reading. Try eating an entire meal without distractions to see how different it feels to focus exclusively on your food.

Slow down. If you eat very rapidly, put your silverware down after every bite and don't pick it up again until you have chewed and swallowed. It will probably feel artificial, but it is a good way to remind yourself to slow down when you catch yourself gobbling.

> **ATKINS ADVANTAGE TIP**
> If you are still on Induction and are getting bored, regardless of how much weight you still have to lose, it's time to move on to OWL.

Chew, chew, chew. In 1903, Horace Fletcher wrote a book advocating that dieters chew every mouthful 32 times, a craze that became known as Fletcherizing. That's a little extreme, but if you're a gulper, try to chew every bite of food at least ten times and give your stomach the chance to tell your brain that it's had enough before your plate is clean.

Eyes bigger than your stomach? Our culture is obsessed with oversized portions. Witness the servings at popular chain restaurants or the super-sized popcorn and soda containers at the movies. If you often feel uncomfortably full after a meal, you are probably in the habit of taking more than you need to feel satisfied. Try this trick: Take your normal portion of protein and vegetables, and divide each selection in half. Put one half out of sight. Enjoy what is left, knowing that there is always the extra portion you've put aside if you're still hungry—but wait twenty minutes after completing your first helping before reaching for the second. This tactic allows your brain to catch up with your stomach. Chances are very good that you won't be hungry anymore. If you are, take from that second half only what you really need to eat to feel satisfied.

Live with leftovers. If frugality is your excuse for eating that extra pork chop or little bit of green beans as you clean up after a meal, stop immediately. Have the chop with eggs for breakfast tomorrow or toss the beans in a salad. There is no reason to be a human garbage pail.

You don't need to leave the table hungry. That's the old way. Now that you are doing Atkins, eat the amount of food you need to feel comfortably full. That's all you need to feel good. Much of stuffing yourself is simply habit. Once you slow down and eat in a more deliberate fashion, you will begin to feel the signals that you've had enough.

REVVING UP YOUR MEALS

One of the surest success spoilers—a challenge as mighty as temptation and perhaps even more insidious—is boredom. It is hard to keep your heart in the program if you feel as though you're stuck in a rut. Boredom happens to everyone—even Atkins Achievers—so it is a good idea to have strategies for coping with it when it strikes.

These tips should help you add a little sparkle to your meals and battle boredom:

SPOTLIGHT ON BLUEBERRIES

Berries have the lowest glycemic impact of all fruits. Nothing says summer like plump, juicy blueberries, but blueberries from southern climes have become increasingly available year round, as is the frozen variety (check to make sure there's no added sugar). A quarter cup of fresh blueberries contains 4 grams of net carbs.

Blueberries offer a bonanza of antioxidants. An excellent source of vitamin C, they are also high in anthocyanins, which are three to four times more potent. Some studies show that anthocyanins may also help improve eyesight and may reduce health problems related to aging.

To select fresh blueberries, check the bottom of a clear container to make sure the berries aren't moldy or squashed. Shaking an opaque package can tell you if they're stuck together. All berries have a short lifespan, although blueberries are hardier than some others. Pop them in the fridge as soon as you get home, and rinse them under cold running water just before eating. (Rinse them earlier, and you'll speed spoilage.)

When snacking, eat blueberries with nuts, cream, or a slice of cheese to ensure that you're getting some fat and protein. This is not necessary when you're having them as dessert because you'll have just consumed plenty of protein.

Eat a wide variety of foods. You don't have to eat chicken every night. Vary your protein choices. You'll be less likely to get bored, and it's the best way to ensure that you'll get the widest range of nutrients. There are hundreds of mouthwatering recipes on www.atkins.com and in *Atkins for Life Low-Carb Cookbook* and numerous other Atkins cookbooks.

Play with texture. Sometimes all it takes to freshen up an old favorite is a little texture. A crispy coating of nuts makes that ho-hum chicken breast something special. Toasted pumpkin seeds or some pomegranate seeds make a simple tossed salad come alive.

Indulge yourself. Have a cheese omelet or real whipped cream on your sugar-free gelatin, or splurge on shrimp for dinner. Such treats will remind you why you love doing Atkins.

Share! Cook for your buddy as Atkins Achiever Laura Herndon did: "I used to swap lunch-making duties with a friend who was also doing Atkins. She'd make lunch for a week, and then I would. There's always that day when you don't feel like making lunch, and that's when you cheat and get a slice of pizza, but if you're accountable to someone else, you stick to it."

MOTIVATION: THE WINNER'S EDGE

A technique for increasing motivation is to turn the things that light your fire into take-away motivational packs that you can break out whenever you need a little extra push to meet your goals.

Choose your Atkins Advantage anthem. If you watched the 2004 summer Olympics, you saw six-time gold medalist swimmer Michael Phelps listening to his headphones until the moment he climbed onto the blocks. Like other athletes, Phelps listens to a fight song to pump himself up just before he competes. Hollywood knows well the inspirational power of a soaring soundtrack rising in the background. When you hear "Gonna Fly Now," don't you think about Rocky sweating his way up those iconic steps?

It's time for you to cash in on some of that inspiration by choosing a fight song of your own: your All-New Atkins Advantage anthem.

Your inspirational anthem should make your heart throb and your energy soar. What tunes do you crank up the volume on when you're alone in the house or in the car? What gets your toes tapping and your fingers snapping when you hear it at a wedding? That's your fight song, the soundtrack to your personal success story.

You can maximize the power your Atkins Advantage anthem has on you by choosing to listen to it at times when your energy level is already high—as you leave for a walk on a beautiful day or on your way out to see friends in the evening or as part of a great workout—so that it becomes loaded with positive associations. Eventually, simply hearing it will restore you to "fight" mode even if you're in the doldrums, meaning you can always pull it out when you need to pump yourself up.

Find your slogan. Just do it. Nothing is impossible. I have a dream. The future begins now. Hang in there. Begin with the end in mind. Attitude is everything. One day at a time.

There is a reason that sports teams, political candidates, and billion-dollar products all have slogans, and now that you've mounted a campaign to realize your fullest potential, you deserve a slogan of your own.

Whether it is one from the list above or one of your own devising, it's time to create your slogan and incorporate it into your life. If you find your slogan inspiring, get creative about it. Say it to yourself often. Have your local copy shop screen it onto a T-shirt. Write it on the soles of your sneakers. Engrave it on a bracelet. Put it on your bulletin board or refrigerator or the visor of your car. Post it on the bathroom mirror.

Sing your praises. You have chosen an anthem, a fight song to inspire you to your very best performance. But your anthem isn't the only thing we want you to sing this week. How about singing your own praises for a change?

If you have been faithful to the program, you've made significant gains toward better health by this point. You are doubtlessly looking and feeling better as you begin to reap the benefits of the good habits you've instituted—habits that will last a lifetime. You have plenty to be proud of, and it's time now to get a little external validation for the hard work you've done.

Call someone—a friend, a family member, or your Atkins buddy—and tell that person about the changes you've made, the results you're seeing, and your goals for the future. Take a moment to bask in their praise and to really feel good about what you've accomplished. It may not be easy to say, "I'm proud of myself," and may even be out of character. But articulating that sentiment and making it public is very empowering—and you'll be surprised at how good the feedback you get makes you feel.

Fitness: The Best You

FOCUS FOR THE WEEK: YOU WILL BE ADDING A CARDIOVASCULAR COMPONENT TO YOUR WORKOUT. AS ALWAYS, DON'T FORGET TO PLAY!

Cardio → 30 minutes → 3 times
Stretching → 20 minutes → 2 times
Strength training → 2 times at a pace that is comfortable for you

Do your stretches at a pace that is comfortable for you. These stretches may take you longer than 20 minutes.

Regular physical activity to increase cardiovascular fitness is, quite simply, one of the best things you can do to improve your appearance, how you feel, and how your body works. As you get more fit, you will

- increase your body's ability to use oxygen efficiently so that your heart doesn't have to work as hard to do the same work.

- increase circulation to your arms and legs.

- be able to work out at a higher intensity so that you burn more calories during your workout—which means that you burn more carbs and more fat!

- help maintain the natural elasticity of the heart and blood vessels, enabling your blood pressure to stay in the normal range.

DOING CARDIO FITNESS

If it has been a long time since you've done any physical activity or if you have quite a bit of weight to lose, you might be feeling some anxiety about beginning cardiovascular exercise. Like every aspect of the Atkins Advantage Program, however, this, too, is individualized. The tools we will introduce in this chapter and in the weeks to come are designed to deliver the optimal workout for you. As long as your doctor has said that it's okay to exercise, you will be able to do so comfortably and safely. The first step is to determine your cardiovascular fitness level.

DETERMINE YOUR CARDIO FITNESS LEVEL

LEVEL ONE

I can't walk continuously for more that 15–20 minutes.

I get winded after a few minutes when doing housework such as sweeping or yardwork such as raking.

I don't have a regular fitness program.

LEVEL TWO

I can walk more than 20 minutes comfortably, but I can't run for more than five or ten minutes.

I don't get winded doing ordinary activities of daily lifting but might during more vigorous activities such as pushing a rotary lawn mower, cleaning windows, and climbing stairs while carrying groceries.

I enjoy occasional physical activity.

LEVEL THREE

I can run 15–20 minutes.

I don't get winded during ordinary or even heavy-duty household activities but might during more heavy-duty activities such as moving furniture.

I participate in regular physical activity.

Once you have ascertained the level that best describes you, follow the recommendations for that level. If, as you progress, you feel that you can do a little more, you can always reevaluate yourself.

THE BENEFITS OF INTERVAL TRAINING

Interval training is a trick used by high-level athletes to optimize their workouts. If you alternate periods of hard work with periods of lighter work, you can work longer than you would be able to otherwise. You also make those periods of lighter work count more because your heart and lungs are still recovering from the period of harder work. Talk about how to pump up the volume!

Let's look at an example using the fitness assignment for Level Two this week where you will alternate intervals of brisk walking with periods of easy walking. The rest periods allow you to work more without becoming overtired; you are also spreading the benefit of the more intense periods of exercise over the more relaxing segments. This is a terrific training strategy not only to maximize the results you get but also to prevent boredom.

How Hard Should You Work? A modification of last week's Exertion Chart (page 116) will help you determine how hard to work. One of the informal ways that exercise physiologists measure how hard their patients are working is by seeing how easy it is for them to carry on a conversation while they're working out. We have modified this technique so you can use it as well.

Low: You can easily hold a conversation.

Medium: You can hold a conversation.

High: Conversation requires effort but is possible.

Superhigh: Conversation is labored or impossible.

CARDIO

You will be walking or running three times this week as you build the cardio routine that will form the foundation for your personal fitness pyramid.

Note: The definition of easy walking below depends on the level you're in.

Level One

Your goal is 20 minutes of continuous walking. This week you will increase the duration of your walk, not the intensity.

Level Two

5 minutes of easy walking (Low) as warm-up

10 minutes of brisk walking (Medium)

5 minutes of easy walking (Low)

10 minutes of brisk walking (Medium)

5 minutes of easy walking (Low) as cooldown

Level Three

5 minutes of easy walking (Medium) as warm-up

10 minutes of brisk walking or jogging (High)

5 minutes of easy walking (Medium)

10 minutes of brisk walking or jogging (High)

5 minutes of easy walking (Medium) as cooldown

For those of you who are already jogging or who feel ready to include light jogging as your new challenge, see Figure 18 for proper running form. Your arms should swing forward and back smoothly at about hip height. Your hands should pass slightly inward in front of your body. Your upper torso should have a slight forward lean, remaining relaxed.

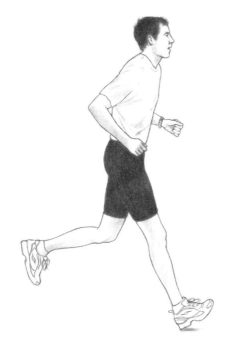

FUEL YOUR ENGINE

Now that you are more active, enjoying increased energy and buoyed spirits, you may also experience an increase in appetite. This is a good sign and is not to be confused with the out-of-control hunger and cravings that plagued you before you got your metabolism back in balance. This hunger won't be as intense, and it won't make you feel out of control. It is more like the healthy appetite you feel after hiking in the country air all day.

When you feel hungry, eat! Don't miss meals and don't get caught without low-carb snacks (keep some in your gym bag or locker) so you can eat whenever you are hungry. Your body will adjust in a week or two, and your appetite will probably decrease.

You may enjoy doing your basic stretches before and after your cardio workout. Perform the stretches twice this week, either after your walk or run or after a five-minute warm-up if it is a nonaerobic day. Remember, if you stretch before your workout, be sure to warm up for five to ten minutes first.

Use the same exercises you learned in previous weeks. Do three sets of ten repetitions of each exercise.

Shoulder Hug, page 62

Head Up, Chest Out, page 63

Cat and Dog, page 64

Butterfly, page 65

Quad Stretch, page 77

Press Up, page 78

Low Back and Hamstring Combo Stretch, page 79

Follow Your Hand, page 80

STRENGTH TRAINING

Strength training continues for all levels. Use the weight at which you can complete two sets of ten controlled repetitions with effort.

Repeat the eight Essential Strengtheners you learned in Weeks Three and Four:

Biceps Curl, page 97

Overhead Press, page 98

Sitting Knee Extension, page 99

Standing Leg Lift, page 100

Calf Lift, page 119

Heel Walking, page 120

Back Lift, page 121

Ab Lift, page 122

Bear in mind as you progress through the Program that for the Essential Strengtheners you should always do at least one set of ten. Once you work up to three sets of ten, build to three sets of 15 before increasing weight.

VISUALIZATION ACTIVITY: OH, SAY CAN YOU SEE?

You have been making momentous changes, both inside and out, for the past four weeks. You may be discovering that one of the hardest things to change is not the way you look or the way others see you but the way you think of yourself.

If you have a negative self-image, it has a negative influence on your life. The way we think about our self can turn into a self-fulfilling prophesy. As you're getting healthier, slimmer, and stronger, it's important to make sure your self-image has caught up to the new you.

By doing Atkins successfully you're already a winner, and it's important that you start seeing yourself that way (no matter how many more pounds you have to lose or how much fitter you'd like to be). One way to do this is to imagine yourself winning. We watch athletes for recreation, but they can also be a source of inspiration, especially now that you're starting a cardio program that will get your heart and lungs in terrific shape.

In this visualization you'll imagine yourself as a star athlete. You'll "see" for yourself what it feels like to make a tremendous effort and to be richly rewarded for it.

Close your eyes and choose the most inspiring scenario for you, whether that means you execute a perfect, splashless dive or hit the serve that aces the tennis match or throw the touchdown that decides the Super Bowl or hit the home run that wins the World Series.

Whatever the event, imagine that last superhuman expenditure of effort that pulls you ahead and brings you the gold. Dedicate yourself, mind, body, and soul, to one last push and then feel the yellow jersey slide over your head as you're proclaimed leader of the Tour de France. Feel the ribbon break across your bursting chest as your burning legs take you across the finish line in a marathon. Hear the national anthem as you bow your head to accept your gold medal. Feel the elation as your teammates rush you off your feet and onto their shoulders for a victory lap.

You can tailor your fantasy however you like. You might feel more comfortable with something a little more realistic, such as shooting the winning basket at a neighborhood pickup game. The only thing you have to do is imagine yourself winning.

Do this visualization, leaving your limitations behind, and know that this tremendous feeling of triumph can be yours every time you achieve a personal victory in the form of one of your personal goals.

ADVANTAGE CHECKPOINT: END OF WEEK FIVE

Weigh and measure yourself. Enter the results in your Atkins Advantage Journal and compare the results with last week's. See page 123 for further guidance about how to evaluate your progress and decide how to proceed.

TEN

WEEK SIX: LOOK AT YOU!

Congratulations! The end of this week will mark the halfway point of your All-New Atkins Advantage Program. This is the perfect time to look back with pride at the ground you've already covered, and it is an ideal vantage point for viewing the path unfolding before you. Let this milestone provide you with the opportunity to celebrate your progress and a chance to refine your goals for the journey ahead.

As you check in with yourself and your progress this week, we'll bring balance, one of the central underpinnings of the Atkins Advantage Program, to the forefront. That inner harmony and focus will help you stay the course in the weeks to come. You have already rebalanced your metabolism by eating in a healthier fashion. Where else do you need to restore balance to your life?

NUTRITION: THE HEART OF THE MATTER

You are midway through the Program and by now have developed a real sense of what is working for you. The beauty of the Atkins Program is that it can be individualized to your needs and you can fine-tune your nutritional needs at any time.

To find meal plans appropriate for your daily net carb intake, see the lists beginning on page 278.

No matter how good your diet, as you add more carbohydrate foods back into your meals, it is important to continue to take the three basic supplements: a multivitamin, essential fatty acids, and fiber to ensure that you are getting a well-balanced diet.

FINDING YOUR CRITICAL CARBOHYDRATE LEVEL FOR LOSING

As long as you still have a substantial number of pounds to lose as determined by your BMI (body mass index), you'll want to stay in Ongoing Weight Loss (OWL), gradually adding back carbohydrates in 5-gram increments. To find your BMI, go to the Web site of the National Institutes of Health (www.nhlbi.nih.gov/guidelines/obesity/bmi_tbl.htm). A BMI between 18.6 and 24.9 is considered normal. A BMI over 30 is generally considered very overweight. As you continue with OWL, you'll eventually approach the threshold known as your Critical Carbohydrate Level for Losing (CCLL), which is the largest number of grams of net carbs you can eat while continuing to lose weight. (Note: If you are still in Induction, continue at 20 grams of net carbs; if you are already in Pre-Maintenance, you are already familiar with this concept.)

> **ATKINS ADVANTAGE TIP**
> By your late twenties you begin to lose muscle mass, so your metabolism slows down, making it harder to manage your weight. The sooner you begin exercising, the better.

Usually, people find their CCLL by overshooting it. At this stage in the Atkins Advantage Program you are determining just how many more carbs you can eat without overtaxing your metabolism and interfering with your weight loss. This level is different for each individual. That is why it is so important to add carbs back gradually and precisely, and monitor your progress. You need to recognize how much is too much and how much is just right for you. If you stop losing pounds and/or inches for a week or two or gain weight, you have probably passed your CCLL.

When this happens, simply cut your carb allowance back by 5 grams; you should then see a return to steady weight loss. For example, if you stopped losing at 50 grams, see if you can resume weight loss at 45. If so, then 45 grams is your personalized CCLL. If you don't see any inches or pounds drop off in a couple of weeks, dial back another 5 grams. (Don't expect the scale to show the same results every week.) After a few more weeks and the loss of more body fat, your metabolism may have speeded up at bit. You can try to reintroduce carbs in 5-gram increments. Be sure to continue to exercise during this time.

Finding your CCLL is part and parcel of the individualization of Atkins. One size most definitely does not fit all. For example, your CCLL may be 55 grams of net carbs; your husband's may be 75. Atkins Achievers have found their CCLLs to be anywhere from 35 to more than 100. Once you locate your personal carb threshold, you'll stay at that level until you are within 5 to 10 pounds of your goal weight, at which point you'll be ready to move on to Pre-Maintenance.

ADJUSTING THE RATIO OF FOODS ON YOUR PLATE

Doing Atkins right isn't an all-you-can-eat cheeseburger fest without the bun. Your body needs a balance of macronutrients. Now that you are eating more carbs in the form of vegetables, nuts, and berries, it's time to adjust slightly the ratio of protein, fat, and carb foods on your plate.

If you want to keep your weight loss progress on track, you must remember that the additions you're making aren't cumulative. You have to compensate for these added carb foods by scaling back a bit on your fat and protein portions. (Of course, many protein foods combine fat and protein to varying degrees.) As you add carbs, if you eat more calories than your body needs, you will gain weight—even on Atkins. Remember that even with the metabolic advantage that Atkins provides, there is a limit to what you can eat without gaining weight.

The rule of thumb for sizing healthy portions is simple: Eat enough food to make you feel comfortably full but not stuffed. Nobody needs five (or even three) cheeseburgers to feel full, especially when the first one is accompanied by a big green salad. If you stop when you're full, you'll do fine. Six ounces (measured uncooked) is the *minimum* amount of protein you should be eating at each of your three meals to keep your blood sugar stable.

> ### SPOTLIGHT ON TOMATOES
>
> Like eggplants, tomatoes are part of the "deadly" nightshade family; for centuries these delicious fruits were thought to be poisonous. Now we know better, of course, and tomatoes are one of the most popular garden "vegetables" even though they are botanically fruits.
>
> Hundreds of varieties are grown and are best in late summer but are available all year round. Tomatoes are rich in vitamins A and C and potassium, and they provide a major source of the antioxidant lycopene, which gives them their color and may provide protection against cancer. One small tomato has 3.2 grams of net carbs; a half cup of canned tomatoes has 2 grams of net carbs. Although tomatoes are acceptable in Induction because they contain a lot of water and therefore cook down considerably, you do have to watch your portions of tomato sauce and other cooked products.

Another way to recognize how much is too much is to follow this simple rule: *Use only one plate.* You'll be eating more types of foods when you leave Induction, but you don't get another plate to accommodate those new foods. Instead, you must make room on the plate you already have for those delicious nutrient-rich carbs.

Most people find that they achieve this balance naturally. In the early stages when carbs were more restricted and you were fueling your body primarily with protein (and fats), you may have needed larger-than-usual portions of meat, fish, and poultry to ensure that you wouldn't go hungry. Now you are adding back the right carbs—those with the fiber content to keep you feeling satisfied and the nutrient content to keep your body working optimally. These carbohydrate foods will keep you satisfied longer because they burn more slowly than the sugar-laden junk carbs you may have eaten before. Learn to listen to your body (rather than be held hostage by your old habits) to tell you how much you really need to be comfortably full.

PREVENT A STALL: ADD ONE GROUP AT A TIME

Many of you will be continuing in OWL this week. For some that will mean being up to 40 grams of net carbs a day. You may have been adding just one new food group a week. If your progress has been smooth, you may have advanced to adding back two food groups each week. If you have been doing the latter, once you approach 40 to 50 grams of net carbs, you should pull back to just one new food group per week. Why? As you get close to 50 grams of net carbs a day, you're less likely to be predominantly burning fat. When you increase your carb intake to this amount, your body naturally begins to burn more carbohydrate as well as fat for energy.

Another reason to slow your introduction of new carb foods is that the greater the variety of foods, the greater the risk of eating a food that ambushes your stable blood sugar or stimulates addictive eating behavior again. Adding food groups back one at a time makes it easier to recognize one that is problematic.

MOTIVATION: THE WINNER'S EDGE

You are almost at the halfway point, which is the perfect spot to check in, make adjustments, and rededicate yourself and your efforts.

JOURNALING ACTIVITY: "BUT NOW" BUSTERS

In Week Two you did a journaling activity called "But Busters" that helped you isolate concerns you might have had about getting started on Atkins. Its purpose was to help you clear potential obstacles *before* they had a chance to interfere with your success. Now you are nearly six successful weeks into the program. You clearly busted those initial *buts*!

Since you have reached this milestone, we'd like you to visit an updated version of that same exercise: "But Now" Busters. The first time around you addressed *potential* obstacles. Now that you've developed a routine and gotten comfortable on the Program, are there any new roadblocks or old "buts" raising their ugly heads to interfere with your continued progress? For example, you might be thinking, "I'm really happy with my results, but now that my kids are out of school for the summer, I'm worried about finding the time to exercise." New hurdles must be dealt with in the same way that you dealt with the old ones.

Motivation is always highest at the beginning of any new endeavor. Sheer optimism can help carry us over occasional bumps in the road. You have been on the program for several weeks, so the novelty of doing Atkins and losing weight may have worn off a little bit. That means it's time to determine whether there are any new worries or dips in motivation that might interfere with continued success.

If everything has gone smoothly and there is no reason to expect anything different in the future, count yourself lucky.

> ## L-GLUTAMINE FOR CONTROLLING CRAVINGS
>
> Another supplement you may find useful in your weight loss efforts is L-glutamine. This versatile amino acid, naturally present in the body, is a major source of energy for cells and plays an important role in supporting the immune system when a person is recovering from illness or injury. L-glutamine helps with wound healing and can improve the nutritional status of people with gastrointestinal problems. It is found in many protein-rich foods, including beef, chicken, beans, and dairy products.
>
> Many Atkins Achievers have found l-glutamine extremely effective at controlling cravings. Although not much research has as yet focused on l-glutamine's role in this regard, a wealth of anecdotal evidence indicates that it may help stop a binge before it happens. To minimize cravings, take 500 to 1,000 milligrams one hour before meals.

Keep this exercise in your back pocket: You can come back to it anytime you find an obstacle in your path. Before you skip it, however, do remember that it is best to address issues before they become full-blown problems. A new job that will require you to travel frequently or an upcoming vacation may not necessarily become problems, but they are things to plan and watch out for. Similarly, a vague feeling of restlessness may be nothing—or a warning sign.

We have all had shoes that rubbed just a little—until there's a painful blister that makes every step excruciating. You have made a lot of changes in your life. Why not take the opportunity to take stock and see how your proverbial new shoes are fitting?

Step One: At the top of a new page in your Atkins Advantage Journal, write the date and the title of this exercise, "But Now" Busters. List all the potential problems or issues, both large and small, that confront you. Do not censor yourself or worry about solutions.

Your original list is a good place to start. Are you still satisfied with the solutions that you came up with to those potential problems? How have your "fixes" stood up? Perhaps your husband, who had agreed to pitch in so you could have time to exercise and dedicate time to the Program, was a good sport about it at first but has gotten lax of late; or perhaps he does the extra chores but takes his resentment out on you. Or maybe your wife initially agreed to cook low-carb meals for you but has fallen back into her traditional cooking habits. Domestic harmony is just as important as success on the Program! If a solution isn't working out or seems to be wearing thin, write it at the top of your list.

Step Two: Think about the road ahead and try to imagine what will produce feelings of anxiety for you. For instance, if you have tried to lose weight using other approaches, you might be concerned that your success on Atkins will be only temporary. Write down anything that occurs to you.

Step Three: Write down every solution you can think of for each item. Aim for at least three solutions—and don't worry if they seem far-fetched or crazy. The key is to think freely and creatively, and to see that there is a wide spectrum of solutions even if they are not ones you can easily implement. Stay open-minded about the range of solutions available to you.

As you begin to find workable solutions, bear in mind that you have to address not just the problem itself but whatever is motivating it. In a sense, the logistical problems are the easy ones! Many of the problems that crop up at this stage in the program are emotional ones—if not for you, then for those around you.

For instance, if your spouse has reneged on his or her offer to help, then a conversation is in order to find out why. Is he starting to feel the pinch from all that pinch-hitting? Is there something in her life that is making it more difficult for her to pick up the slack? Maybe he is a little jealous of your new waistline, new energy level, and new enthusiasm. Or she is nervous about how you'll respond to other women who might now find you as attractive as she always has. Whatever the reason for the change, the first step toward a solution is to come up with a few positive suggestions so that you don't arrive at the conversation empty-handed. Having a few ideas in mind will make a world of difference in reaching a positive outcome.

Sometimes when a person undergoes major changes and begins to see himself or herself in a new light, it is so threatening to his or her partner that it shines a harsh light on the relationship. It can be tempting to undermine yourself to preserve a relationship. It may take the form of finding yourself less focused on the Program and more prone to cheat. Try to examine the reasons for your slip-ups, being as honest as you can. Maybe your own success—and the attention it brings—is scaring you a little. One part of you might be enjoying the compliments you're receiving, while another part of you wants to yell, "I'm the same person I've always been!" You don't want to address this by putting the pounds back on but, rather, by coping with the sometimes complex feelings that big changes can bring.

Your own issues and problems may be different, but they are not insurmountable. Don't let them fester until they become roadblocks. Bring them out into the open, no matter what their nature, and be creative about solutions.

JOURNALING ACTIVITY: COUNT YOUR BLESSINGS

You have many new things to be grateful for, thanks to all your hard work, focus, and dedication to improving the quality of your life. Celebrating your triumphs is another way of taking stock and is as crucial to your continued success on the program as the troubleshooting you did in the last activity. You'll give yourself a well-deserved boost, and reviewing this list will certainly give you incentive in the future.

On a new page of your journal, list the things that you truly value. You'll certainly want to count the people in your life: your spouse, kids, and grandkids; your circle of friends; perhaps the one who introduced you to Atkins; the mentor who has always believed in your talents; and even the pleasant guy at the deli who knows just how you like your morning cup of java. You may also want to include some of your "stuff," whether it's your favorite books, an afghan your grandmother crocheted, or your bicycle.

Don't forget to express gratitude for your own contributions—your talents, your sense of humor, and your continued efforts. Thank yourself for the conviction to begin a lifestyle change like this in the first place and for having the perseverance to carry it through. Enjoy a moment of gratitude for the delicious foods you're eating even as you are shedding excess pounds. Say thanks for the release from the cravings that have plagued you in the past, for your new energy and feelings of well-being, and for the compliments you've received over the last few weeks.

Nothing is too trivial, too abstract, or too sentimental for this list. As the list of the things you really care about grows in front of you, you may find yourself reflecting on the current balance of your life. Do you spend as much time with those family members or friends as you would like? Do you have enough time to read? To bicycle? What weighs down the other side of the scale? You don't have to do anything right now but feel grateful. Simply allow your answers to affect the decisions you make in the future.

Counting your blessings is an appropriate activity mid-program and something you might consider incorporating in your life on a regular basis. Making this list is a terrific way to recharge your batteries anytime you feel you need a reminder of why you're doing what you're doing—not just when you are controlling carbohydrates but when you are struggling with traffic during your commute, going the extra mile on a special project at work, increasing your physical strength and endurance, wiping little noses, and all the other things you do.

When you began this program, you made a promise to the Program and to yourself, and you formalized that promise in the form of a contract.

It is time now to unseal the envelope containing that contract. As you read it, remember the way you felt when you wrote it and your hopes for the future. Appreciate how far you've come since you wrote those words: You have rewired your body's basic chemistry, begun a fitness program, and learned skills that will contribute to a lifetime of good health.

With so much already accomplished and with so much to look forward to, it's time now to renew your promise to yourself and to the Program.

Is there a particular commitment or goal that you'd like to add to your letter, to feed your enthusiasm and steadfastness as you go forward? Perhaps you would like to integrate what you've learned over the past six weeks into this new pledge. What have been the big lessons of this program for you? What has made the greatest impact? Have you seen evidence that small and steady steps are the best way to win the race? That pushing off from each small victory is the way to take the gold? Are you committed to picking up "free speed" wherever and whenever you can? Record the specifics that have resonated most profoundly with you. You may also want to incorporate items from your Personal Goals List from Week Two. What on that list are you most looking forward to achieving?

When you have completed these tasks, renew your commitment to the Atkins Advantage Program by signing and sealing your letter again. Think of this document as your "New You" Resolution. Know that you can open it anytime in the weeks and months to come if and when you feel you need a little extra inspiration.

Fitness: The Best You

FOCUS FOR THE WEEK: YOU WILL ADD A CARDIOVASCULAR COMPONENT TO THE PROGRAM. ONCE AGAIN, DON'T FORGET TO PLAY!

Cardio ➔ 25–35 minutes ➔ 2 times
Stretching ➔ 30 minutes ➔ 2 times
Strength training ➔ 2 times at a pace that is comfortable for you

Do your stretches at a pace that is comfortable for you. These stretches may take you longer than 30 minutes.

YOUR TARGET HEART RATE

We introduced the concept of exertion in Week Four. Remember, this means it's not just exercising that counts but how hard you work. In order to build your endurance and strengthen your heart and lungs, you need to work at the right intensity.

Just as Atkins is individualized in terms of what you eat, one size doesn't fit all when it comes to working out. The Exertion Chart on page 116 is a tool to help measure the intensity of the exercise you're doing and the effect it's having on your body.

This week we're introducing a more scientific and slightly more specific tool that tells how hard you are working—too hard, not hard enough, or, hopefully, just right. This tool, the target heart rate zone, will allow you to "take your pulse" both physically and metaphorically. Here is what's so great about using it:

- It is a simple way to make sure you're getting all the benefits of exercise (by working within your zone) without putting yourself at risk (by working above it).

- It is completely portable. All you need are your fingers and a watch with a second hand to check whether you're in your zone. You can do it in a pool, playing catch with your kids, raking leaves, or doing anything else that gets your heart rate up.

- All you have to do when working out is stay in your zone. You'll probably be pleasantly surprised to see how little you have to do to hit the low end of your target heart rate zone, especially if you're working in intervals.

To find your target heart rate zone:

1. Subtract your age from 220. This number is known as your maximum heart rate.

2. Calculate 60 percent of your maximum heart rate. That's the low end of your heart rate zone.

3. Calculate 70 percent of your maximum heart rate. That's the high end of your heart rate zone.

Example for a 31-year-old:

$$220 - 31 = 189$$

$$189 \times .60 = 113.4$$

$$189 \times .70 = 132.3$$

The heart rate zone for a 31-year-old is therefore between 113 and 132 beats a minute.

You can obtain the beats per minute, known as a pulse, in either of two places:

At the wrist: Press the pointer and middle fingers of one hand to the area on the inside of the other wrist, just below the pad of the thumb.

At the neck: Place the pointer and middle fingers over the soft area on one side of the Adam's apple. Do not massage or apply pressure to this spot.

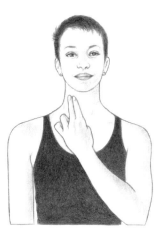

You probably will not want to stop your workout to count out 132 beats as you take your pulse. To ensure that you're in your zone, all you have to do is watch the clock for 10 seconds and multiply your results by six. A 31-year-old needs to count between 19 and 22 beats every ten seconds to know that he is in his zone.

Note: If you have been inactive for some time or if you are more than 50 pounds overweight, you should keep your heart rate in the lower end of your zone. Talk to your doctor to find out how intensely you should work out.

The target heart rate zone is yet another tool you can add to your Atkins Advantage toolbox, one that you can use this week, for the duration of the program, and beyond. As your endurance improves and you become more fit, you may wish to ex-

A SPEEDOMETER FOR YOUR BODY

Consider using an inexpensive heart rate monitor for a real-time look at how hard your heart is working. (Think of the benefit of a speedometer to tell how fast you're going when driving a car.) It's very satisfying to see what your heart can do and is evidence of how you're getting fitter. Basic heart rate sensors and monitors can be purchased online or at a sporting goods or fitness equipment store for about $60 or less. They are extremely user friendly and motivational, providing real-time feedback. Exercise equipment fitted with heart rate monitoring devices are increasingly found in gyms. Although the most accurate readings likely come from chest- or watch-type receivers, these equipment-mounted monitors can also do the job.

ercise at 75 percent of your maximum heart rate, which you can ascertain using the following formula: $220 - (\text{your age}) \times .75$.

CARDIO

Keep your heart rate in the target zone as you do the cardio portion of your fitness program this week.

60–70 percent of your heart rate is considered Medium.

70–75 percent is considered High.

Level One

5 minutes of easy walking

5 minutes of brisk walking (Medium)

Alternate between easy walking and brisk walking for a total of 20 minutes.

5 minutes of easy walking (Low) as cooldown

Levels Two and Three

10 minutes of easy walking

15 minutes of brisk walking (Medium building toward High)

10 minutes of easy walking as cooldown

We're going to add two new exercises to the basic stretches you have been doing so far. Do three sets of ten repetitions of each exercise.

Shoulder Hug, page 62

Head Up, Chest Out, page 63

Cat and Dog, page 64

Butterfly, page 65

Quad Stretch, page 77

Press Up, page 78

Low Back and Hamstring Combo Stretch, page 79

Follow Your Hand, page 80

If you are short on time, you can substitute the new stretches for two of the leg stretches you have already learned. Otherwise, do all ten. Here are the new stretches:

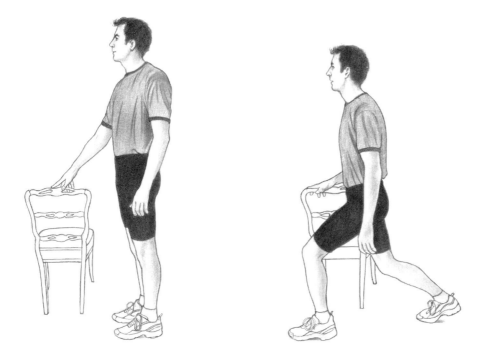

FORWARD LUNGE

The goal with this stretch is to see your front knee bend 90 degrees so that the front of your thigh is as close to parallel with the floor as possible without straining it.

1. Stand with your feet shoulder-width apart and an arm's length away from a chair or wall.

2. Place one palm on the chair or wall and take a large step forward with the opposite leg, bending your front knee and keeping the calf vertical. Your other leg will bend as much as is needed to get the thigh to come as close as possible to being parallel with the floor.

3. Breathe in and hold the stretch for a minimum of ten seconds.

Number of Reps All Levels: three on each leg

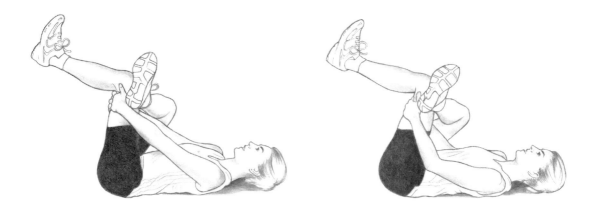

RECLINING ANKLE-TO-KNEE STRETCH

This stretch is particularly good for the piriformis muscle, a common source of pain in hamstrings, buttocks, and the lower back region.

1. Lying on the mat with shoulders flat on the floor, with your left knee bent and the left foot resting flat on ground, bring your right ankle to your left thigh directly above the knee.

2. Reaching forward with both arms extended, grasp the back of the left thigh and interlock your fingers.

3. Pull your left knee and thigh toward your trunk, feeling the stretch in the back of your right thigh, outer hip, buttocks, and lower back.

4. Inhale and hold the stretch for at least ten seconds.

5. Alternate legs and repeat as above.

If the muscles in your lower back and buttocks are extremely tight, begin this stretch sitting back in a chair. Later, as you become more flexible, you should be able to do it comfortably on the floor or a mat.

Number of Reps All Levels: three on each side

Modification: To increase this stretch, lie on your back, making sure that both shoulder blades are in even contact with the floor. As you exhale, gently pull your thigh closer to your torso, easing your hip open. Keep your shoulder blades pressed evenly against the floor and maintain the curve in the small of your back. (Your spine has a slight arch at its base.) Inhale and hold the stretch for a minimum of ten seconds.

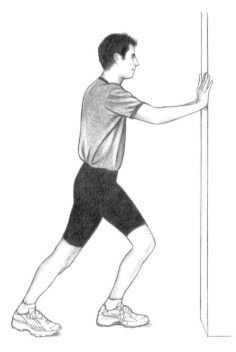

CALF STRETCH

1. Stand with arms extended, using the wall or a sturdy piece of furniture for support.

2. Place one foot approximately 12 inches behind the other, keeping the back knee straight.

3. With your weight on the front foot, slowly move your hips forward, feeling a slight stretch in the upper calf. Build gradually and avoid excessive stretching.

Number of Reps All Levels: three on each side

Now you are going to experiment with adding a cardio component to the Essential Strengtheners. Move through the exercises quickly, without pausing between sets or individual exercises. The goal is to get and keep your heart rate up even if it is into the lower bracket of your target heart rate zone. Use the weight at which you can complete two sets of ten controlled repetitions with effort. Before doing the following exercises, turn to the designated page to review the instructions and illustrations.

Biceps Curl, page 97

Overhead Press, page 98

Sitting Knee Extension, page 99

Standing Leg Lift, page 100

Calf Lift, page 119

Heel Walking, page 120

Back Lift, page 121

Ab Lift, page 122

Note: Speeding up your workout isn't an excuse for getting sloppy. Don't go so quickly that you compromise the integrity of the exercises. That's a sure path to injury. If you become winded, feel exhausted, or are not in full control of the weights, by all means slow down.

YOU CAN DO THE FOLLOWING TO BUILD STRENGTH AND ENDURANCE

Strength training: Build to three sets of ten reps at one weight; then increase the number of reps to 15. Once you reach three sets of 15 repetitions, it's time to increase your weight and build to three sets of ten reps at this weight, increasing to 15 reps and so forth.

Cardio: Your goal is to perform approximately 30 minutes at your target heart rate. As your fitness level increases, increase your speed to keep your target heart rate at the correct level. You can increase the amount of time you spend at that level, add an incline or a treadmill, or walk up hills.

ADVANTAGE CHECKPOINT: END OF WEEK SIX

Weigh and measure yourself. Enter the results in your Atkins Advantage Journal and compare the results with last week's results. See page 123 for further guidance about how to evaluate your progress and decide how to proceed.

RECHECKING YOUR BLOOD WORK

Before you began the Atkins Advantage Program, you saw your doctor and had your blood work done to establish some very important benchmarks. Now it's time to have those tests redone so that you can compare your current cholesterol, including HDL and LDL, triglycerides, blood pressure, glucose, and uric acid levels to those of six weeks ago. These numbers will tell you—as the scale and your measuring tape already have—how well you are responding to the Program.

What you can expect to see: Most people—especially those whose markers were not optimal when they began the Program—should see a marked reduction in their triglycerides, one of the strongest independent markers for heart disease. Many can also expect to see a decrease in their LDL ("bad") cholesterol, along with a welcome increase in their HDL ("good") cholesterol. Eating healthfully is making a difference, and so is being more active. Review the results of the tests with your doctor. If your numbers have improved, you'll have good reason to celebrate.

If your blood work doesn't show improvement, remember that some changes don't appear within the first six weeks. If you had fairly normal results to begin with, you don't have to worry: Your normal results simply stayed normal. (They may very well improve and continue to do so the longer you exercise and eat healthfully.) If you already had high triglycerides or elevated LDL and they haven't shown any improvement or have gotten worse, talk with your doctor. In addition:

1. Ask yourself whether you have rigorously followed the rules of the ANA. In general, people who fail to see an improvement in their blood work have not followed the program to the letter. Unless you faithfully and consistently control carbohydrates, you are not really doing Atkins. As a matter of fact, it could be dangerous to eat liberal amounts of fat during the week and then have a high-carb blowout every weekend. To see the weight and health benefits that make the Atkins program so effective, you must follow it properly.

2. Discuss with your doctor the idea of taking therapeutic levels of supplements to help control your cholesterol. Those covered in this book are chromium (page 107), essential fatty acids such as GLA (borage, primrose, or black-currant

oils), EPA (fish oil), and fiber. For more information about the value of these supplements and others in helping to improve cardiovascular risk factors, see *Dr. Atkins Vita-Nutrient Solution* or www.atkins.com. Note: If you add these nutrients to your program in therapeutic doses (or if your doctor has prescribed any medications after reviewing your laboratory results), be sure to have your lab results rechecked in another six weeks to monitor improvement.

ELEVEN

WEEK SEVEN:
SUCCESS—NO MATTER WHAT

Some days the water is as smooth as glass, the wind is in your sails, and progress is effortless. But there is also the occasional difficult patch when your progress slows or you feel that you're swimming against the current. As frustrating as that might be—and as tempting as it might be to chuck the whole program—choppy seas are a normal part of any journey, and momentary reversals of fortune can only define you if you allow them to. As Henry Ford said, "Obstacles are those frightful things you see when you take your eyes off your goal."

You can overcome any obstacle in your path as long as you have the tools to correct your course.

NUTRITION: THE HEART OF THE MATTER

To find meal plans appropriate for your daily net carb level, see the lists beginning on page 278. Continue to take a multivitamin, essential oils, and a fiber supplement. Chromium (page 107) or L-glutamine (page 141) can be helpful in busting through weight loss slowdowns, stalls, and plateaus.

You are probably still in OWL and will probably continue to add carbohydrates in OWL this week. (If you are still in Induction, that's fine as long as you still have a fair amount of weight to lose. If you are already in Pre-Maintenance, continue to add carbs in 10-gram weekly increments until your weight loss stops. Then back down 5 grams of net carbs, and you should have found your adjusted CCLL.) You can add carbs as long as your weight loss continues to progress and your appetite is under control. If the needle on the scale has been reluctant to move or you are finding that certain foods spark cravings, Customizing OWL: Do It Your Way on page 106 will be useful as you progress.

There is no timetable for when you'll encounter a setback, but one thing we can guarantee: Sooner or later you will experience one. When you do, you can return to this chapter, and you'll benefit from doing these exercises.

If you have lost and regained weight in the past, you may find that you have a tendency to get "stuck" around the same weight over and over again. It's not your imagination! It is natural for your metabolism to settle in a particular range, and it can make it a little harder to jump-start weight loss again. The Plateau Action Plan in this chapter and upping your activity level should help you see renewed weight loss.

SLOWDOWNS, STALLS, PLATEAUS, AND WEIGHT GAINS

If your weight loss slows down, stops entirely, or, worse, you see a gain and you're nowhere near your goal weight, don't panic. A premature rush to action can cause more damage than the problem itself.

Here's what you should do no matter what: Raise your activity level, either by adding another workout session, increasing the amount of time you work out, or upping its intensity. The advice from the Atkins Achievers on this subject is unanimous: exercise, exercise, exercise. This alone may be enough to jog your metabolism into a higher gear.

STEP ONE: ELIMINATE COMMON OBSTACLES

A number of things might be interfering with your weight loss. Ask yourself the following questions:

Have I begun taking a medication? Many medications, both prescription and over the counter, can have metabolic effects that cause a slowdown or a stall in your weight loss progress, including

- diuretics

- blood pressure medication such as beta-blockers

- diabetes medication such as insulin and drugs that stimulate insulin

- birth control medications in any form

- synthetic hormone replacement therapy (HRT)

- nonsteroidal antiinflammatory drugs (NSAIDs), including over-the-counter medications such as ibuprofen and prescription antiinflammatory drugs such as Bextra, Indocin, and Celebrex

- steroids, including prednisone

- antidepressant medications, including serotonin reuptake inhibitors (SSRIs)

- antibiotics

If you are on a short course of medication (two weeks of antibiotics to treat an infection, for instance), your weight loss slowdown or gain will probably resolve itself shortly after you've completed your prescription. Long-term medication is more complicated. You can't go off your meds simply because they're slowing your weight loss progress, but if you suspect that they're the cause of your difficulty, call your doctor. You may be able to take a lower dose or switch to an alternative that won't make you so metabolically resistant.

Note: Never stop or lower the dosage of a medication without consulting your physician.

Have I changed my lifestyle? Subtle changes in our routines can have a big impact on our waistlines. If your spouse has gone back to working the night shift, you might be snacking more heavily in the evening out of loneliness. Wooing a new client might mean dining out a couple of times a week. Take a close look at recent changes in your life, to see what answers lie there.

Am I under a great deal of stress? Many of us overeat as a response to stress; unfortunately, it's a strategy that backfires. Stress is a response to feeling out of control, and nothing makes you feel more out-of-control than overeating. Furthermore, when you get back on the blood sugar roller coaster, your body responds by producing stress hormones, so eating inappropriately actually puts additional stress on your body.

If this is a pattern you tend to fall into, you need to use strategies to cope with stress before you gain back the weight you've worked so hard to lose. If you can remove the stressful element from your life, make that your first priority. If you can't escape the stress altogether, perhaps you can focus on finding constructive ways to relieve the pressure it puts on you.

Time spent doing yoga, meditating, playing with your kids, taking a bubble bath, or venting to a friend is much better than overeating. Make sure you have both the time and the outlets to help you cope. In addition to meditation and breathing techniques, movement is a proven stress-buster, so take a brisk walk to let off some steam.

Am I progressing up the Carb Ladder in the correct order? When you reintroduce carbs in the order in which they are presented in the Atkins Carb Ladder, you first add foods with the least impact on blood sugar. At your present weight your metabolism may not be ready for foods with a higher glycemic impact. This might explain a setback. (Later, you should be able to handle most of these foods in moderate portions.)

Am I eating hidden carbs? You are probably eating a broader array of foods than you were when you first started the Program, as you should be. Make sure that the foods you're choosing really are low carb, especially when you're not preparing them yourself. Is there a sweet glaze on the salmon you eat once or twice a week at your favorite neighborhood restaurant? Were the chicken pieces in your Chinese food dipped in cornstarch before they were sautéed? Sniff out these unwanted extras and eliminate them; the little things can add up.

> **ATKINS ADVANTAGE TIP**
> Just because a product is called low-carb doesn't mean that it is a nutritious choice. Look for products that do not contain manufactured trans fats, high levels of sugar alcohols, or bleached white flour.

Don't get casual about reading labels: Starches and added sugars often lurk in prepackaged foods. Don't allow your carbohydrate portion sizes to creep up, either, and if you find that you're using a quarter cup of lemon juice on your salad instead of two tablespoons, make sure you're counting those extra carbs.

Am I suffering from carb creep? The road back to the size you used to be is littered with "just one bites." Ironically, people who are very successful at losing weight are most at risk for giving in to temptation: Achieving great results can make you get sloppy or feel invulnerable. Keeping a food journal—recording every bite—may increase your accountability and help you get back on track. Cheating every once in a while isn't necessarily the end of the world, but you have to do it carefully and with control. For more information about this, see "Cheating" Smart, page 191. If you remain committed to the Program but are having trouble sticking to it, take your behavior as a sign that you need to adjust the way you are doing it.

Am I adjusting the ratio of foods on my plate? As you add higher-carb foods, you need to decrease the amount of fat you eat and the size of your protein portions, but continue to eat at least 6 ounces (uncooked weight) of protein at every meal (see page 139).

Have I been letting the fitness portion of the Program slip? Besides controlling your carbs, continuing to exercise is the single most important thing you can do to ensure successful weight loss.

STEP TWO: MAKE THE CORRECT DIAGNOSIS

If any of the explanations cited above fit your situation, you need to respond to them first. If you are sure none of the explanations is the reason for your stalled progress, you should pursue another course of action. An essential part of managing a bump in the road is making sure you have identified the problem accurately. Is the snag a normal fluctuation in your weight (remember, your weight can vary by as much as several pounds in a single day), or is it a sign of something that requires action? Because the course correction or treatment needs to be tailored to the problem; a correct diagnosis is crucial. The following three conditions are distinctly different:

Slowdown is a slowing of the pace at which you're losing while remaining at the same level of carb intake. It is not the natural slowdown in weight loss that occurs when you move from Induction to OWL and again from OWL to Pre-Maintenance.

> ### LOW-CARB PRODUCTS
>
> Natural, whole foods are the cornerstone of the Atkins style of healthy eating, and they are especially important during a setback. Reduce your consumption of low-carb products for a while and see if that improves your results. If not, you may have to eliminate them until you start losing again. Make sure you are not overeating low-carb products simply because you like the taste or have gotten in the habit of, say, having a sugar-free chocolate bar after dinner.
>
> Some people can't tolerate certain sugar alcohols (or high levels) found in some sugar-free products. Others find that sweets—even the low-carb versions—stimulate their cravings for "the real thing." See pages 26 and 30 for a refresher course in what to look for in low-carb products.

Stall occurs when there is no measurable loss of pounds or inches for two consecutive weeks.

Plateau exists when you experience no weight loss or inch loss for more than four weeks despite corrective measures.

STEP THREE: TAKE ACTION

You'll want to shift gears before your metabolism gets too far out of whack. It cannot be stressed too strongly again that everyone, no matter what the diagnosis, should increase his or her activity level.

Note: You'll find additional troubleshooting tips for Lifetime Maintenance in Week Twelve.

Action Plan for Slowdown. If you are experiencing a slowdown and are on Induction, make sure you've been following the rules to the letter. Since this is the most rigorous part of the Program, it is the most common time for mistakes. If you have cut back on cheese, olives, avocados, and low-carb products and are still not losing, you'll need to look extra hard at hidden carbs. Perhaps you are eating deli meats that have starchy fillers. Carefully read the ingredients lists on food labels to ferret out any hidden sources of sugar or starches. Also make sure that you are following the fitness part of the Program.

> **ATKINS ADVANTAGE TIP**
>
> As you reintroduce carbohydrates to your diet, pay attention to any reoccurrence of symptoms such as cravings, dips in energy, sleepiness after a meal, or spaciness that disappeared when you first began Atkins. You may be adding too many or too quickly.

If you're in OWL or Pre-Maintenance, it's possible that you have increased your carb level too quickly. If that's the case, cutting back should solve the problem. It doesn't mean that your journey is imperiled but simply that you have to change gears. Review the details of customizing OWL and Pre-Maintenance on pages 106 and 205, respectively.

Action Plan for Stall. If you have hit a stall, do nothing at all for a week. Don't add any more carbs to your daily level, and don't add any new foods or food groups. Your metabolism may need to get used to the current level of carbs (and the type of carbs) in your diet. Be patient and give it the time and space to do so. (During this wait-and-see week, it's important to stick rigorously to the rules of the phase you're in.) If this is simply a natural fluctuation, such as before your period (if you are a woman), then you will probably lose pounds or inches again by the end of the second week without doing anything.

If you see no loss of pounds or inches for two consecutive weeks, you must start keeping a food journal (if you have not already). It can help you identify foods and behavior patterns that may be adversely affecting your progress. Perhaps you are sensitive to one of the foods you've added back in the last few weeks. (See page 104 for help in determining trigger foods.) If you suspect a food is giving you problems, drop it from your repertoire for a week or two and see if that makes a difference. Make a note to pay close attention when you next try to add it back.

If you are in Induction, continue to follow the rules faithfully. Watch cream and cheese portions carefully, and consider cutting back on higher-calorie foods such as avocados and olives. Be sure that your quantities of food are appropriate to assuage hunger but that you're not overeating simply out of habit. Be sure you are eating only low-carb foods suitable for Induction and not eating more than two low-carb products a day.

If you are in OWL or Pre-Maintenance, follow the action plan for slowdown described above. If you begin losing weight again after cutting back, stay at that level for a few weeks and then try to continue adding an additional 5 grams of net carbs (if you're in OWL) or 10 (if you're in Pre-Maintenance).

If you encounter problems again, you may have passed your CCLL, the number of grams of carbs you can eat daily and still continue to lose weight. If you fail to lose weight or inches again at this higher level, reduce by 5 (or 10) grams again, and stay at that number. If you're in OWL, once weight loss resumes, stay there until you're 5 to 10 pounds away from your goal weight and ready to begin Pre-Maintenance. If you're already in Pre-Maintenance, stay at your revised CCLL until you reach your goal weight.

> ### SPOTLIGHT ON RICOTTA CHEESE
>
> There is much to love about ricotta, a soft Italian cheese, but first on the list is versatility. Because of its light, creamy texture and mild, slightly sweet flavor, it works as well as a base for desserts as it does in savory dishes.
>
> It's ironic that a cheese so strongly associated with carb-laden dishes like lasagna should be a staple in the low-carb kitchen. Ricotta is relatively low in carbs—a 3½-ounce serving has 3 grams of net carbs—which makes it appropriate for every phase of the ANA. Like most cheese, ricotta is also a source of calcium, phosphorus, zinc, riboflavin, and vitamins A and B$_{12}$.

Action Plan for Plateau. You have hit a plateau when you've lost neither pounds nor inches for four consecutive weeks and have tried the advice given above for a stall without any resolution.

Almost everyone, including the Atkins Achievers, has experienced a plateau over the course of their weight loss journey. It can be very frustrating, especially if you're doing everything right. But please don't get discouraged! You're not alone, and even though you're stuck right now, chances are you won't be stuck forever.

If you're in Induction and have stuck to the rules and followed our suggestions for a slowdown, take a closer look at your portion sizes. Atkins is not based on calorie counting, and you should feel free to eat protein foods until you're comfortably full. If you are eating very large portions, however, you may be taking in more than your body can comfortably handle—even with the metabolic advantage (see page 126). Try decreasing your intake of protein foods, but be sure not to fall below 6 ounces (measured uncooked) of protein at every meal.

If you are in OWL or Pre-Maintenance, return to the last level of carb intake at which you lost weight or inches. If that doesn't do the trick, continue reducing the number of carbs you're eating in 5-gram increments until you start losing weight again. You may have to return to Induction for a few days to engage your fat-burning metabolism again, but do so only as a last resort.

Be patient. As long as you are not experiencing cravings and an out-of-control appetite, then you are doing fine even if progress is imperceptible on the scale. Stay with the program, increasing your exercise time and/or intensity, and you will see progress.

Action Plan for Weight Gain. The only thing more distressing than hitting a plateau is seeing pounds and inches increase. Again, it's important not to panic. Setbacks are to be expected—which is not to say they are acceptable. If you gain weight at any point in the program, you must act immediately.

Follow the Action Plan for Plateau above and begin reducing your carb intake immediately. When you begin losing weight again, stay at that carb level for three or four weeks before attempting to add carbs.

MOTIVATION: THE WINNER'S EDGE

Everyone—including Olympic athletes, Oscar-winning actors, and high-powered CEOs—feels pressure and anxiety when he hits an obstacle. According to cognitive behavioral therapy, the methodology from which sports psychology (and a host of other popular behavior modification techniques) springs, what distinguishes winners in sports, business, and life, is not the absence of self-doubt but the skills that help them perform even when the stakes and the pressure are at their highest.

TRASHING TRASH TALK

"I can't believe I just said something so stupid."

"I'm too fat to wear this."

"I always choke under pressure."

Sound familiar?

According to one study, up to 80 percent of the 66,000 thoughts an average person has on any given day are negative. This negative "self-talk" creates emotional undertow and has a direct and very negative impact on how we perform in life. Learning to eliminate it can help you accomplish those things you most want.

The first step is to notice negative self-talk. You may be surprised at how incessant and relentless the stream of disapproval is, especially if you're facing a setback. Make a mental note every time you hear yourself talking yourself down, whether you make that comment out loud ("Sorry, Fred, I'm brain-dead today") or to yourself ("I have got to get my life together. I'm such a mess"). We forget that our lives are all works in progress! There is always more left to do.

One way to quiet this hostile soundtrack is to put it into perspective: Imagine yourself saying that horrible comment out loud—not to yourself but to someone you care about. Picture the look on that person's face as you deliver that castigating remark and the way he'd feel after hearing it. Imagine the way *you'd* feel hearing it come out of your mouth. Envision what you'd have to do to mend that person's hurt feelings and to repair the relationship. This tends to be a somewhat shocking fantasy, and that's precisely the point. Now you can see exactly what you're doing to yourself many times a day. Why are you so hard on yourself?

Clearly, the next step is to get rid of these disparagements. Pick one of your favorite self-criticisms (ideally, the one that plays over and over in your head) and imagine writing it in thick magic marker on a large pad of paper. Now see yourself in your mind's eye ripping that piece of paper off the pad, screwing it up into a tiny ball, and tossing it into a large black garbage bag. The next time that thought floats into your brain, remind yourself that you've thrown it into the trash. Do this when you can over the course of the day. When your invisible garbage bag is full of self-hating commentary, tie the top, carry it out to the curb, and leave it there. Or write the words on a piece of paper, rip it up, and throw it away, burn it, whatever. Then write the positive "antidote" and put it someplace prominent as a visible reminder of your new positive self-talk.

FOCUS ON THE MOMENT

I remember quickly learning as a young surgeon that in order to perform the important steps in any surgical procedure, I needed to remain focused on the moment rather than become intimidated by the entirety of the surgical procedure. I have certainly found this to be true when I'm competing in an Ironman event. If I thought about the 112-mile bike race waiting for me during my swim or about the 26-mile run after that, you'd see bubbles as I sunk to the bottom of the ocean, overcome by the anxiety produced by these two looming challenges. Staying focused on the swim when I'm swimming helps me concentrate and continue to swim rather than drown in my own fear. The technical term for this is compartmentalization, but I've come to think of it as "draping the elephant." The massive animal is still there, but you've covered him with a curtain so that he doesn't distract you when it counts the most.

—Stuart L. Trager, M.D.

It may not be possible to eliminate self-criticism from our lives entirely, but it is certainly possible to replace some of those negative thoughts with more gentle encouragements. Stay attentive to your tendency to "trash talk," and whenever you can, especially when you're having a tough time, praise yourself for your myriad accomplishments instead.

One of the real secrets to winning out over adversity is to focus exclusively on the small steps and the moment at hand so that you're not distracted by the white noise of your own insecurities or the overwhelming nature of the big picture.

Think of a mountain climber who needs to focus on the placement of each foot, hand, and piton to achieve success. If he loses concentration by thinking about the risks associated with a fall, he runs the risk of serious injury and even death. In order to keep himself safe, he needs to stay completely focused on each individual move.

How does draping the elephant relate to your success with the Atkins Advantage Program? You must keep an eye on your long-term goals, of course, including better health and your goal weight, but when confronting an obstacle—whether it's a temptation we feel we can't stare down, the results of a serious slipup, or an inexplicable plateau—it can be easy to let anxiety take over and obscure our focus. All we hear is the elephant yelling, "Have a cookie! You're not losing weight anyway!"

Throw a blanket over that elephant and concentrate—on this meal, on your next food choice, on the next bite that goes into your mouth. Keep your head down and focus all your attention and resources on the moment and the task at hand. Perhaps you can use what some dieters call a "secret technique" for avoiding high-carb foods: Put it off. Tell yourself that maybe you'll have some later. Every time you're tempted, say, "We'll see." Eat what you know is healthy for you instead. The next thing you know, it will be time to leave or go to bed or the item is gone because someone else ate it. Voilá! Temptation avoided!

In general, your big-picture goals will provide you with incentive. But when the going gets tough, allow yourself the luxury of concentrating exclusively on putting one foot in front of the other until you're out of danger. Like the massive elephant, your bigger goals will still be there when you can afford to look up from the immediate challenge.

Fitness: The Best You

FOCUS FOR THE WEEK: KEEP YOUR METABOLISM REVVED TO CONTINUE YOUR WEIGHT LOSS. PLAY AS OFTEN AS YOU ARE ABLE.

Cardio → 25–35 minutes → 3 times
Stretching → 30 minutes → 2–3 times
Strength training → 2 times at a pace that is comfortable for you

Do your stretches at a pace that is comfortable for you. These stretches may take you longer than 30 minutes.

Remember, changing your life, like so many things, happens slowly at first and then seemingly all at once. Awkward as it may seem at first, once play becomes part of your daily routine, it will eventually take on a life of its own, drawing you in.

As this chapter makes crystal clear, exercise is the number one prescription to get you out of a slowdown, a stall, or a plateau. Atkins Achievers tell us over and over again how instrumental exercise was in seeing weight loss resume or accelerate. Some of them are actually grateful that they hit a weight loss wall because it gave them the incentive they needed to start exercising.

There is no question that exercise has a revving effect on the metabolism, and its mood-elevating benefits can help you cope with stress, whether from temporary frustrations with your progress or other reasons. Exercising is certainly a healthier response than chowing down on the high-carb comfort foods you relied on in the past. Enjoy exercise this week with the knowledge that it is yet another tool at your disposal if you hit stormy weather.

DEDICATE YOUR PRACTICE

One of the tricks that yoga students and competitive athletes use to meet higher challenges or simply boost their performance to the next level is to dedicate their practice, race, or workout to someone or something else.

While losing weight and getting fit for someone else is a losing proposition (because you need to understand that you are making these changes for yourself), on a day when it is a little harder to get out of bed to go for a walk, a little harder to pass the doughnut box at the coffee station, or a little harder to do the exercises in this program, consider dedicating that activity to someone else. It could be someone who would be proud of you for completing the activity or who could use a little positive energy flowing their way, or it could be someone who embodies an ideal you admire. Maybe it would help you to dedicate your workout to an even more abstract concept, such as people suffering in the world, the abundance in your life, or the very idea of generosity.

You'll draw added focus and energy just by removing yourself from the equation for a little while and dedicating the activity to someone else. Use this not only when you need help getting out of the door but to inspire you to give it your very best.

Level One

10 minutes of brisk walking (Medium)

5 minutes of easy walking (Low)

5 minutes of brisk walking (Medium)

5 minutes of easy walking (Low)

Levels Two and Three

5 minutes easy walking (Low)

20 minutes of brisk walking or jogging (Medium)

10 minutes of easy walking (Low)

All Levels Number of Reps: three

STRETCHING EXERCISES

You have learned a total of 11 stretches to date, and as with strengthening, the goal is to incorporate at least eight of these into your weekly routine. You can choose those that best address your own particular needs. Note, however, that it is important to include Quad Stretch, Low Back and Hamstring Combo Stretch, and Calf Stretch on the days you also do your cardio workout.

Do three sets of ten repetitions of each of the following exercises:

Shoulder Hug, page 62

Head Up, Chest Out, page 63

Cat and Dog, page 64

Butterfly, page 65

Quad Stretch, page 77

Press Up, page 78

Low Back and Hamstring Combo Stretch, page 79

Follow Your Hand, page 80

Do one set of three repetitions of the following exercises:

Forward Lunge, page 149

Reclining Ankle-to-Knee Stretch, page 150

Calf Stretch, page 151

STRENGTH TRAINING
Strength training continues for all three levels. Do three sets of 15 repetitions of each exercise.

Biceps Curl, page 97

Overhead Press, page 98

Sitting Knee Extension, page 99

Standing Leg Lift, page 100

Calf Lift, page 119

Heel Walking, page 120

Back Lift, page 121

Ab Lift, page 122

This week you're going to add two new leg exercises to increase the conditioning you're getting in the lower half of your body. If you are short on time, you can substitute these two exercises for two other leg exercises (Sitting Knee Extension, Standing Leg Lift, Calf Lift, or Heel Walking) at one of your workouts this week.

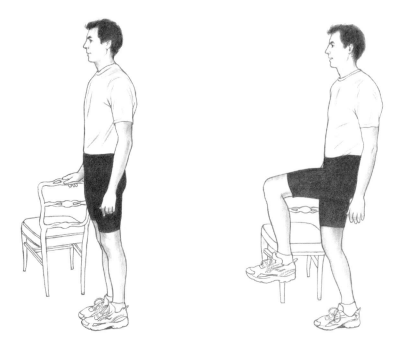

STANDING KNEE LIFTS

For quadriceps (large muscles in the fronts of the thighs)

1. Stand with your feet shoulder-width apart, supporting yourself with your hand on a chair or wall next to you. Inhale.

2. Exhaling, bend your knee and raise your right leg in front of you until your thigh is parallel to the floor. Return your toe to the floor. Pause momentarily and repeat.

3. Without changing the position of your torso, quickly raise and lower your leg ten times, exhaling each time you raise your leg.

4. Repeat with the other leg.

Number of Reps
    Level One: ten for each leg
    Levels Two and Three: ten to start, increasing to 15
Number of Sets
    Level One: one increasing to two and then three if possible
    Levels Two and Three: two, moving to three

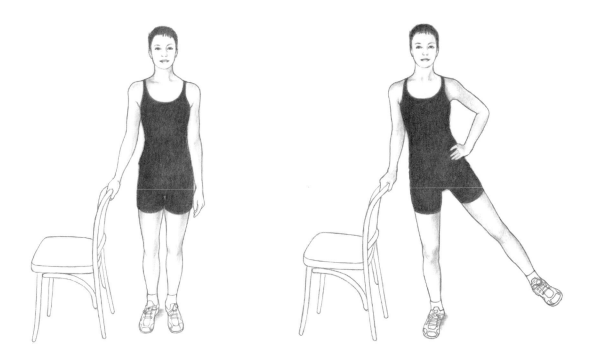

STANDING SIDE LEG RAISES
For outer thighs

1. Stand with feet shoulder-width apart, supporting yourself with your hand on a chair or wall next to you.

2. Without leaning or moving your body, raise your right leg slowly to the side as high as you can comfortably maintain. Control the movement as you slowly raise and lower your leg.

3. Repeat with your left leg.

Number of Reps
    Level One: ten for each leg
    Levels Two and Three: ten on each side, increasing to 15 as tolerated
Number of Sets
    Level One: one, increasing to two and then three if possible
    Levels Two and Three: two, building to three
Modification: As you become more comfortable with this exercise, raise your leg increasingly higher and hold it in this position longer.

ADVANTAGE CHECKPOINT: END OF WEEK SEVEN

Weigh and measure yourself. Enter the results in your Atkins Advantage Journal. See page 123 for further guidance about how to evaluate your progress and decide how to proceed.

TWELVE

WEEK EIGHT: CHALLENGE YOURSELF!

I f it took a leap of faith in yourself and in Atkins for you to begin this journey, something new now propels you forward: the knowledge and confidence that you can do it. Your goal weight may still be some distance away, but the impressive trail you have already forged is evidence that you can achieve your goals one small step at a time.

Last week gave you the knowledge and confidence to get away from danger when it presents itself. This week you'll see that you can give yourself that same boost—in weight loss and elsewhere—even when the going is smooth. The theme of this week is challenging yourself to your full power, to raise the bar in your fitness sessions, your food choices, your work, your play, and even the relationships in your life.

Only by testing your own limits can you find out what your "best" is really like. If you push yourself to give a little extra, your accomplishments will exceed your expectations.

NUTRITION: THE HEART OF THE MATTER

As you advance through the phases, refer again to the Carbohydrate Ladder (page 14) to guide your choices as you reintroduce food groups to your meals. If you are a salad lover, you may elect to use an extra 5 or 10 grams of net carbs on low-glycemic vegetables as you start OWL. For some of you it's time to reintroduce some of the starchy vegetables such as sweet potatoes. Legumes are inexpensive, full of fiber, and add variety to chili, soups, and salads. Remember to pay attention to net carbs and portion size. If you have already added back berries without incident and are ready to advance to higher glycemic fruits, the best way to eat them is after a meal or with protein and/or fat as a snack. To find meal plans appropriate for your daily net carb gram count, see the lists beginning on page 278.

> **ATKINS ADVANTAGE TIP**
>
> If you are experiencing mood swings and dips in energy, it may mean that your blood sugar is unstable as a result of going too long without eating. Have a meal or a low-carb snack with some fat or protein.

Continue to take your multivitamin, essential oils, and fiber supplement.

Take a moment to appreciate how far you've come and what you've done to get here. Pat yourself on the back for all your little victories, day in and day out—at the supermarket, in the kitchen, around the dining table, and when you eat out. You face hundreds of real challenges every day, one with every choice you make, and you deserve recognition for every one you conquer with flying colors. I tip my hat to you, not just for the weight you've lost but for making the individual choices that have brought you to this point in your journey.

A CULINARY CHALLENGE

We tend to stick with the things we know, and nowhere is that truer than in the supermarket, kitchen, or restaurant where we purchase, cook, or order the same things day after day.

This week will include a culinary challenge. For one meal this week, you will be asked to push yourself to do a little more than you think you're capable of. If you're not a cook, you may be surprised by what you can do by opening a cookbook, picking a recipe, and following the instructions.

If you know your way around the kitchen, try one of these ideas:

- Give a favorite oldie a new spin. Take a dish you've prepared countless times or an ingredient you use often, and do something a little more sophisticated with it. Instead of your usual chicken salad, make it with paprika, cumin, cayenne pepper, ground cloves, and ground cinnamon for a Moroccan accent, for instance.

- Convert one of your pre-Atkins favorites into something deliciously low-carb, such as French toast made with low-carb bread and sugar-free syrup.

- Try a new-to-you vegetable; eggplant, jicama, bok choy, and tomatillos are just a few options.

- Try an unfamiliar cooking method. Braising, for instance, is a long, slow method of cooking, perfect for most vegetables or wintry stews. Braise some asparagus instead of steaming them.

- Learn to cook a new-to-you source of protein, such as duck or tofu. If you love fish but fish cookery intimidates you, try an easy recipe such as shrimp sautéed with garlic.

- If you are already an accomplished cook, delve into a recipe a little more complicated than you would ordinarily attempt.

If you enjoy learning new recipes and kitchen skills, make this a weekly ritual. The best way to stay engaged with the Program is to discover how rich and varied you can make it. There is another benefit: Food you have created with enthusiasm and joy satisfies the soul as well as the body. Interestingly enough, that often means you don't need to eat as much of it.

THANKS, BUT NO THANKS
"Come on, you'll love it."
"I spent hours making it especially for you."
"A single bite won't hurt you."
While doing Atkins you can say yes to a lot of the foods traditionally forbidden to someone trying to drop excess pounds, but you do have to say no to some foods—the ones loaded with sugars and other refined carbs. Sometimes finding tactful ways to avoid these unacceptable foods is almost harder than resisting the temptation.

While it can be awkward to turn down your aunt's homemade dessert, you don't want to say yes because it seems impolite not to. Take some advice from Atkins Achiever Tricia Clarke, who has lost 115 pounds. When offered a food that does not fit her new lifestyle, she simply says, "I'd love to, but it's not on my list of appropriate foods." Go ahead—blame it on Atkins!

Having a plan can be a lifesaver at social gatherings, especially if your hosts, friends, colleagues, and family members seem to have trouble accepting your choices. It may help you to rehearse these polite refusals in advance:

"It looks delicious, but I'm doing Atkins."

"Thanks so much for thinking of me! I've brought my lunch today."

"My health doesn't permit me to indulge, but it looks wonderful."

"Sorry, doctor's orders!"

"Everything was delicious; I couldn't eat another bite."

If you sense that someone is genuinely interested in why you're saying no, by all means tell the person why you've eliminated bleached white flour and white sugars from your diet, and about your terrific results thus far. Explain that it can throw your blood sugar out of whack or trigger cravings for more or other unacceptable foods.

SPOTLIGHT ON CARROTS

Inexpensive, available year-round, and high in fiber, carrots are also nutrient powerhouses. They contain vitamins C and B_6, thiamine, folic acid, and magnesium, and they are one of the best sources of carotene, a precursor to vitamin A, which is an important nutrient for healthy eyesight. Beta-carotene is an antioxidant with powerful cancer-fighting potential.

A medium carrot contains 5 grams of net carbs. As a root vegetable, carrots have a higher index ranking than leafy greens and are therefore on rung seven of the Atkins Carbohydrate Ladder (see page 14). You may want to wait to reintroduce carrots until you're in Pre-Maintenance, but a little grated carrot on a salad is not going to interfere with weight loss once you are in Ongoing Weight Loss.

NO NEED FOR A FAT WALLET

It may seem that eating meat and preparing your own meals can get expensive, but you can do Atkins without breaking the bank. While the ANA puts a premium on quality, there are plenty of ways to ensure that you're getting what you need without paying a premium. Once you stop filling your grocery cart with chips, crackers, cereals, and junk food, you can devote your food budget to healthful foods instead. When you pass up the drive-through for a plate filled with fresh vegetables and broiled chicken, you're making an investment in your health and the health of your family. But more than that, Atkins doesn't require eating steak and lobster. Eating the Atkins way means selecting a variety of protein alternatives, and many of them are not expensive. You also eat fresh vegetables and eventually fruit, but that doesn't mean they have to be brought in from Holland, Chile, or Hawaii that morning.

One of your challenges this week is to see how you can get the most bang for your buck. Here's how:

- Instead of paying more for imports, buy vegetables in season when they're plentiful and less expensive, and likely to be local.

- Buy frozen vegetables when the fresh ones are too pricey. Typically, if it is just the vegetable itself, you'll be okay. Steer clear of anything with sauce.

- Cheaper cuts of meat are classic budget stretchers. Often tastier and more tender than their high-ticket relatives, they lend themselves well to long-cooking soups and stews. Hanger steaks are relatively inexpensive, as are chicken legs and thighs, but they are actually more flavorful than flank steak or chicken breasts.

- Eggs aren't just for breakfast! An omelet or frittata is a nutritious and affordable way to incorporate small quantities of leftovers.

- Canned fish, such as tuna and salmon, can often substitute for fresh fish in casseroles, croquettes, and salads.

- Tofu is an inexpensive form of protein that takes well to seasoning and can be enjoyed in Induction. In the Maintenance phases you can use moderate portions of beans to expand a casserole.

- Buy meat in bulk, either from a wholesaler or when it's on sale at the supermarket, and freeze the extra.

- Check out your supermarket's weekly flyer for the best buys.

MOTIVATION: THE WINNER'S EDGE

This week you'll push yourself beyond your already impressive accomplishments to uncover your as-yet-untapped power.

JOURNALING ACTIVITY: MOVE A MOUNTAIN

You already know that wasted motion is anathema to the Atkins credo and that this program requires doing what it takes to make the most of your efforts. So although this next task may feel impossible, it's designed to show you what you're really capable of doing.

This week you're going to challenge yourself to complete a nagging obligation or chore (everyone has at least one) that you've been putting off for weeks, months, or possibly years. It might be a long-unwritten thank-you note; apologizing to a friend for a misunderstanding; or cleaning out the garage or a closet, drawer, or file cabinet.

The mere thought of this task likely unleashes an unpleasant blend of guilt, shame, irritation, and an unending stream of rationalizations to explain why there hasn't yet been a good time to tackle it.

Even the most disciplined and organized among us procrastinates, probably not realizing how much energy these undone tasks actually suck up. As unpleasant as the task may be, the collateral damage you incur by avoiding them is worse: long-postponed chores. The flip side is also true: When you've completed something you've been putting off, you will feel empowered and wonder why you had made such a big deal of it.

You've probably tried to climb this particular mountain before, but this time it will be different. Remember how you felt before you took control of your weight? Compare that feeling to how much better you feel doing something about it. Thanks to the Atkins Advantage, you have finally taken control of your weight by following the nutritional approach that's right for you. Now it's time to take control of something else that has been a burden.

On a blank page of your Atkins Advantage Journal write the name of your much-avoided task and today's date. Commit to spending a minimum of 15 minutes on this task *tomorrow*. No excuses, no reprieves. You don't have to complete the task; simply spend 15 minutes on it.

> **ATKINS ADVANTAGE TIP**
>
> To keep hunger under control until lunchtime, be sure to consume at least 6 ounces of protein at breakfast.

If you are not willing or able to follow through tomorrow, stop reading this exercise and return to it only when you are prepared to take this second step. If you know right now that you absolutely cannot commit to those 15 minutes—because you're leaving town or your day is already overscheduled—you'll have to come back to it later in the week when you know you'll be able to commit to it the following day.

Once you do commit, you must put in your minimum 15 minutes the following day—not the day after or the day after that or after the long weekend, but the day after you write down the task! Get out your calendar and mark it down, assigning a specific start time. Don't leave the time undetermined or loose. "Sometime tomorrow afternoon" doesn't cut it. Determine exactly when you're going to begin, and block out at least 15 minutes.

Tomorrow, when you begin, you can draw on the skills you learned in Creating an Action Plan of Small Steps in Week Three. How much you get done on this first day is not important. Getting a toehold—and discovering how much worse the anticipation of this task is than the execution—is. If you choose to go over your 15 minutes and have the time, that's fine. This is frequently the case. But if there's anything left to be done after your session, remember that you are not finished with your day's work until you have committed specific dates and times in the future—at least another 15 minutes, at least once a week—to completing the task.

Rest assured that in this way you will successfully conquer this long-postponed chore. That weight on your shoulders might have seemed permanent, but you had the power to lift it off all the time. The truth is that by giving it such importance, you also made it even more burdensome.

Note: If you don't return to this exercise by the end of the week, it might be a sign that you're stuck. In this event you might benefit from some additional assistance and support. When you get to a more comfortable place, we hope that you'll come back to this exercise and use it to open some of the doors that have been stuck shut for too long.

JUST SAY NO

One of life's biggest challenges is learning to say no to others so that you can say yes to yourself.

Too many of us give ourselves short shrift. We take care of other people's needs—those of our kids, our spouses, our in-laws, and our bosses—and then find that there's nothing left for us. It is natural and commendable to be agreeable, and saying no when someone asks you for something can be difficult. But when doing for others takes up so much of your resources, time, and energy that you aren't doing enough for you, it has gone too far.

Realizing your own personal dreams and goals requires that you draw some boundaries and put as much stock in your needs as those of the ones you care for. If you don't make yourself a priority by making room on your to-do list for your own goals and dreams, they will always take a backseat to someone else's pressing concerns. So this week we issue this challenge: to say no to any and all requests that you don't have the time, energy, or resources to honor. Instead, do the following:

Make a date with yourself. Figure out exactly what you need or want to do for yourself this week. Your list may include something as luxurious as a massage or as utilitarian as making a long-postponed dentist's appointment, buying a pair of jeans in a smaller size, getting a haircut, or simply setting aside the time to exercise. Make dates with yourself for those activities. Consider them written in stone, as binding as your child's pediatrician's appointment or your next work shift.

Think before you say yes. The next time you find yourself in the hot seat, when you've been asked to do something you don't have time to do, take a moment (and at least one breath) before agreeing. If you can, postpone the answer by asking if you can get back to the person after you have checked your calendar. Then think honestly about your week. Where would this new task fit in? Many of us use taking care of others as an excuse for neglecting ourselves: "I can't work out today. I have to pick the kids up from soccer practice/make something for the bake sale/do this report for my boss." Make sure that you're not falling into the trap of blaming excess weight (and the inability to take it off) on family obligations.

Say no. Many of us say yes partly because we don't know how to say no gracefully. Here are some places to start:

- Be gracious. Instead of saying no, say, "No, but thank you for asking." Thank the person for the opportunity to help.

- If you'd like to be kept in mind for a project at a later date or for something similar, ask the person to keep thinking of you. If you're not at all interested, don't misrepresent yourself. You'll only put yourself in the position of having to say no twice.

- Don't let flattery turn your head and don't let the person's need distract you.

- Don't lie.

- Don't offer a hundred excuses. You don't have to defend your priorities to anyone else. Instead, say you have to check your calendar and will get back to the person either way. If the idea of saying no makes you uncomfortable, try some of these strategies out with a friend, family member, or spouse—or simply visualize yourself saying them. In this way you'll be prepared when the occasion comes up.

This resolution to say no is not a recipe for becoming more self-centered. The only way to be truly generous to others is to be generous to yourself as well. Taking care of your own health and emotional welfare isn't selfish; it's an act of personal responsibility. Making time for yourself won't close your heart; rather, it can open it more fully to others. When you take better care of yourself, both physically and emotionally, you function better in the long run, meaning you have more energy and incentive to give of yourself. The real goal is not just learning to say no but learning when to say no and when to say yes. You may decide to fit something important into your schedule by eliminating something else that is less important.

Obviously, saying no won't work in every scenario; we all face pressing family and work commitments that can't be gracefully declined. But many people find that respecting their own boundaries and taking their commitments to themselves seriously makes other people more likely to respect those commitments as well.

Fitness: The Best You

FOCUS FOR THE WEEK: TO ADD VARIETY AND INCREASED ENDURANCE, ONE DAY OF YOUR ROUTINE WILL INCLUDE A FITNESS CHALLENGE. TO KEEP THINGS INTERESTING, LOOK FOR EVEN MORE WAYS TO INCORPORATE PLAY INTO YOUR LIFE.

Cardio ➜ 35–45 minutes ➜ 2 times
Stretching ➜ 30 minutes ➜ 2–3 times
Strength training ➜ 2–3 times at a pace that is comfortable for you
Fitness challenge ➜ 1 time

The most satisfying aspect of any challenge is proving yourself wrong. "I can't do it," you think in desperation, but then you tap a previously hidden reservoir of unspent strength and, lo and behold, you can do it.

We all need to push our boundaries and limitations a little beyond what we think we can do. The following exercise will allow you to experience that immensely rewarding feeling through a safe physical challenge. It will resonate for you the next time you think, "I can't!"

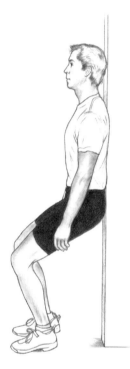

FEEL THE BURN

1. Stand with your back against a wall. Inhale.

2. Keeping the soles of your feet flat on the ground, exhale as you slide down the wall, bending your knees until they are halfway between standing and sitting. You'll feel the "burn" in your thighs.

3. Hold that position for as long as you think you possibly can, and then hold it even longer. Remember to keep breathing.

Modification: As you continue to get in better shape, bend your knees further— to the point where your thighs are parallel to the floor. Going any lower could damage your knees.

Sitting on air is more challenging than you might think; in fact, your thighs will probably begin to shake from the effort. Ignore them and hang in there. Although this is a great leg exercise, particularly for the quadriceps muscles, how long you can hold the position isn't really the point. Passing your threshold—whatever that might be—and staying with the exercise beyond it is the real goal.

When your muscles are screaming and you find yourself thinking, "I can't possibly do this another second," realize that you *can*. Push past that voice in your head and find the one that says, "Okay, maybe one second more." What resources do you have to help you silence that negative voice in your head? Does it help to breathe deeply and concentrate on the sound of your breath as it slowly enters and leaves your body? Does it help to envision a competition where all you have to do to triumph is hold on for three seconds more? Distract yourself by thinking about a winning pop fly or your loved one's face. Use your slogan, hum your anthem, imagine a field filled with cheerleaders shouting your name as they jump up and down.

It is an amazing feeling to press past the point you thought was your limit. Winning feels terrific, doesn't it? As you go through your week, take notice of how many times you limit yourself with the words "I can't" and see if you can't use the techniques that helped you push past that naysaying voice to challenge yourself in a myriad of ways. It is incredibly empowering to meet and master a challenge. Prove yourself wrong over and over again—and love every minute of it!

CARDIO

This week you will walk briskly or run for 20 minutes on two days. You will also participate in a special fitness challenge (see page 186) that counts as your third cardio workout. Keep your heart rate within your target zone the entire time. (For a refresher course on how to do this, see page 145.)

Level One

10 minutes easy walking (Low)

20 minutes brisk walking (Medium)

5–10 minutes easy walking as cooldown (Low)

Levels Two and Three

10 minutes easy walking (Low)

25 minutes walking or running (High or target heart rate [see page 145])

5–10 minutes easy walking as cooldown (Low)

STRENGTH TRAINING: ADVANCED CORE STRENGTHENING

This week you'll concentrate on a particularly challenging body part: your core, comprised of the muscles of your lower back, abdomen, and pelvis.

Everybody wants a flatter, more defined tummy, but did you know that every movement you make actually starts your core? Strengthening this group of muscles not only makes you look and feel more fit, but it also helps you walk, lift objects, sit up straight, and perform countless other everyday tasks. Strengthening the core is also a good way to help relieve back pain.

As always, do at least eight strengthening exercises. Feel free to substitute the new, more advanced core exercises below for the ones you already learned in the Essential Strengtheners (Back Lift on page 121 and Ab Lift on page 122).

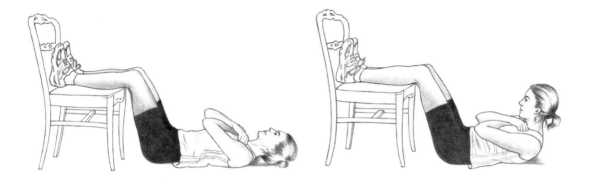

CHAIR AB LIFT

This is a great way to strengthen your entire abdominal region.

1. Lie on your back on a thick towel or mat, with your arms crossed over your chest.

2. Place your lower legs on the seat of a chair. Your thighs should be at approximately a 90-degree angle with the floor (depending on the height of the chair).

3. Inhale at the starting position and then slowly exhale as you raise your head and shoulders 3 to 5 inches off the floor.

4. Look straight ahead without craning or putting undue strain on your neck. Hold for three seconds as you inhale and exhale.

5. Slowly return your head and shoulders to the floor as you exhale.

Number of Reps
   Level One: five
   Level Two and Three: ten
Number of Sets All Levels: one, increasing to three as you get stronger
Modification: For Levels Two and Three, instead of resting your legs on a chair, keep them in the air. Keep your head and shoulders raised for up to five seconds.

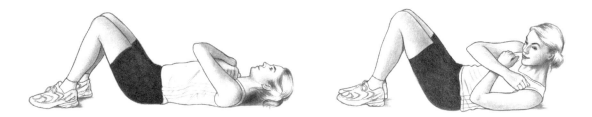

OBLIQUE AB LIFT

This exercise will tone the sides of your torso.

1. Lie on your back on a thick towel or mat, with your arms crossed over your chest, knees bent, and feet flat on the floor.

2. After inhaling, slowly exhale as you raise your head and shoulders while leaning to your left until your left shoulder is 3 to 5 inches off the floor. Your torso should move in one piece.

3. Look toward your left without craning or putting undue strain on the neck. Hold for three seconds.

4. Slowly return to the starting position.

5. Switch sides and repeat.

Number of Reps
  Level One: five on each side
  Levels Two and Three: ten on each side
Number of Sets All Levels: one, increasing to three as you get stronger
Modification: Do this exercise with your feet on a chair and then hold them in midair. If this becomes too easy, hold the flexed position for five seconds.

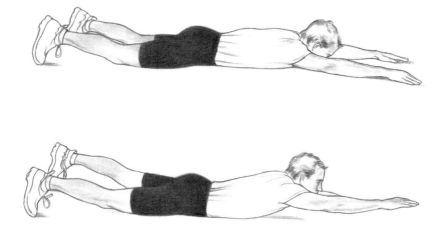

ADVANCED BACK LIFT

1. Lying prone on a mat or thick carpet, raise your entire leg several inches or more from the mat while simultaneously raising your opposite arm. Keep your head and neck relaxed.

2. Alternate your right arm and left leg with your left arm and right leg.

Number of Reps All Levels: ten
Number of Sets All Levels: one, increasing to three as you get stronger

FITNESS CHALLENGE: HOW FAST CAN YOU WALK A MILE?

You are doing only two days of cardio this week. You'll be using your third day to issue yourself another fitness challenge: seeing how long it takes you to walk a mile. To determine how far you have to walk, use a runner's track (the one behind your public school is probably empty in the early morning or evening) or measure a stretch of your neighborhood with your car's odometer. Stretch, walk five minutes to warm up your muscles, and then walk or run the mile as fast as you comfortably can. Note: Do not overtax yourself—especially if you are running! You should be able to speak the entire time and should never feel pain or true shortness of breath.

Record your time in your Atkins Advantage Journal. This is more than just a record of the progress you've made so far, it is a benchmark for the future. This will be the time to beat the next time you issue yourself this challenge. You may want to do this once a month or even more often because it is yet another way to monitor your progress. You can try to shave off minutes with every attempt.

There is an even better reason to reduce your time in the mile: Studies that look at the health benefits of exercise have shown that simply increasing your fitness level translates into a measurable improvement in longevity. In fact, this test is derived from a pivotal study which showed that you can significantly impact your chances of living longer *simply by exercising*. The more fit the people who participated in the study were, the less risk they had for coronary artery disease and heart attack, and the fitter they got, the more the risk decreased. They saw an 8 to 18 percent reduction in coronary artery disease and cardiovascular events, and an 8 to 12 percent reduction in mortality with every minute of oxygen-burning exercise capacity.

The next time you hit the track, think about this: Shaving one minute off your results will make you approximately 8 percent less likely to die of a heart attack if you maintain this level of fitness. Will that help you move a little faster?

ADVANTAGE CHECKPOINT: END OF WEEK EIGHT

Weigh and measure yourself. Enter the results in your Atkins Advantage Journal and compare the results with last week's. See page 123 for other important instructions.

THIRTEEN

WEEK NINE:
THE PRE-MAINTENANCE PHASE

Avoiding "empty" carbs is an essential first step to doing Atkins, but doing it right means learning how to choose the very best carbohydrate foods. The ANA is not just a numbers game: There's a world of difference between the quality of carbs in a slice of white bread and a side of asparagus, between a slice of pizza and a chef's salad, between a plate of pasta and a bowl of old-fashioned oatmeal.

When you take better care of yourself one good result builds on the next. It starts with controlling carbs and losing weight, but eventually this impulse to seek the best choices seeps into every area of your life.

NUTRITION: THE HEART OF THE MATTER

To find meal plans that are appropriate for your daily net carb gram count, see the listings that begin on page 278.

Regardless of which phase you are in, continue to take your multivitamin, essential oils, and fiber supplement.

A CLOSER LOOK AT PRE-MAINTENANCE

If you are within 5 to 10 pounds of your goal weight, it is time for you to move from Phase 2: Ongoing Weight Loss (OWL) to Phase 3: Pre-Maintenance. If your BMI is between 25 and 29.9, you can move to Pre-Maintenance when you have just 5 more pounds to lose. On the other hand, if your BMI is 30 or more, advance to Pre-Maintenance when you have 10 pounds left to lose.

In the Pre-Maintenance phase you can eat more carbs and a broader array of them than you did in the earlier phases. As you increase the amount of carbs you eat, your body will increasingly rely on them for energy rather than using primarily fat. Pre-Maintenance is designed to help you bridge the gap between losing the last of that excess fat and maintaining your goal weight. Although you'll still be dropping pounds at the start of Pre-Maintenance, the driving question should not be how quickly they'll disappear but how you'll be able to stay at your goal weight for good. You already know how to eat for weight loss; Pre-Maintenance teaches you how to eat for life.

THE RULES OF PRE-MAINTENANCE

- Begin Pre-Maintenance when you are 5 to 10 pounds from your goal weight.

- Increase the number of daily grams of net carbs you add back each week in 10-gram increments as long as you continue to lose weight and/or inches with no return of cravings, "pre-Atkins" symptoms, or out-of-control hunger.

- Continue to climb the rungs of the Atkins Carbohydrate Ladder (page 14), adding foods from only one rung each week.

- Add foods within the rung one by one.

- Adjust the ratio of foods on your plate to allow for the increased amount of carbohydrate foods you're eating by reducing the amount of fat and protein. (Most protein foods also contain fat.)

- If you fail to lose weight or you gain weight, see the Advantage Checkpoint on page 123 for help.

In Pre-Maintenance you'll continue to prioritize whole foods while you add the right carbs and continue to take in sufficient protein and a balance of fats. Use low-carb products judiciously.

Slow and steady progress in Pre-Maintenance is crucial to maintaining permanent weight loss. You should continue to lose weight, but your rate of loss will be slower than it was in OWL. On average, you should be losing no more than half a pound a week, which means it could take you some time to lose those last few pounds. Be patient. It's natural to want to rush ahead when the end is in sight, but there's still important work to do: You're retraining your metabolism and learning to make the food choices that will allow you to maintain your goal weight.

Many people experience an increase in appetite as they enter Pre-Maintenance. Fat-burning suppresses appetite, and although you're still burning fat in Pre-Maintenance, you're burning less fat and more carbohydrate in the form of glucose. Actually, your metabolism switches back and forth between the two forms of energy. If you find yourself hungrier than usual, be especially conscientious about having your pantry stocked with low-carb foods and healthy snacks so they are available at all times.

Don't skip meals under any circumstances, and don't allow yourself to get too hungry between meals. Even if dinnertime is on the horizon, a mini-snack such as a cup of broth can help you eat slowly and enjoy your food when it's ready instead of wolfing it down and running the risk of overeating. Don't be afraid if you experience an increase in hunger. As long as you stay within your CCLL and have low-carb snacks when you need them—and as long as you're not stuffing yourself—you should be able to deal with this transition.

Just as you did in OWL, you add daily net carbs (this time in increments of 10 grams) until you come to a point at which you stop losing (you may even gain a pound or two). If you overshoot, which is perfectly normal, reduce your net carbs first by 5 grams and, if necessary, by 10 grams until gradual weight loss resumes.

Because of their higher carb content, nutrient- and fiber-rich carbs such as legumes, higher glycemic fruits, starchy vegetables, and whole grains can usually be added in Pre-Maintenance. These foods need to be reintroduced carefully, however, so as not to interfere with gradual weight loss. You'll probably need to experiment until you find your individual tolerance for portion sizes and frequency of consumption. You can also add whole milk and yogurt without added sugar in this phase, but do not add these foods. (If you are lactose intolerant, watch out for symptoms such as gas, bloating, or mucus production.) For

> **ATKINS ADVANTAGE TIP**
> Read labels: if you see any of the following on the ingredients list of a food product, steer clear: trans fats, trans fatty acids, hydrogenated oils, partially hydrogenated oils.

more on the choices most people can make in Pre-Maintenance, Atkins Glycemic Ranking (AGR) charts are available in *Atkins for Life* and at www.atkins.com.

FORGET ALL OR NOTHING

If you want to continue to reap the benefits of eating this way for the rest of your life, you have to stop thinking in binary terms: all or nothing, never or always, success or failure.

Success does not mean you can eat whatever you want. Likewise, one false step does not mean you're headed for disaster. Being too rigid doesn't work any better over the long haul than being sloppy does. Because a slipup can mean that you're standing on the brink of a binge, you must be able to recognize this potential problem in order to vanquish it.

You have the power to stop a downward spiral before it compromises your terrific progress. Here's how to throw every resource you have at stopping a slipup before it turns into something more serious:

Stop the trend. If you have eaten a food that is not part of the Program or is inappropriate for your phase, the most dangerous line of thinking at this point is: "I've blown it already. I might as well eat whatever I want for the rest of the day." Instead, stop the snowball before it becomes an avalanche by recommitting yourself immediately. Count your carbs for the rest of the day, not because you're "making up" for your splurge (you probably won't be able to anyway) but because controlling carbs is how you eat now. Don't starve yourself. Simply go about your business, eating sensible, carb-conscious meals and exercising normally. Remember, the best opportunity you have of taking back control is right now.

Examine why it happened. If you know why you slipped up, you can be on the alert for temptation in the future. In most cases you can address the problem that led to the slipup with controlled-carb solutions. If you were overcome with hunger while running errands and detoured for some fast food, make sure never to leave the house without some on-the-go snacks (see page 111 for suggestions). If you felt that you needed a treat, perhaps now is a good time to make yourself something that is still low carb. If you were bored, what can you do to spice up your weekly menus? (For starters, sneak a peek at Herbs and Spices on page 208 in Week Ten.)

Don't wallow in guilt. Admit you made a mistake and learn from it.

Be extra careful for a while. Start your food journal again if you had stopped. Plan your meals carefully for the next few days. Carry healthy snacks with you at all times. Call your Atkins buddy and ask for his support. This might be a good time to open the letter you wrote yourself in Renew Your "New You" Resolution on page 144 or to do another one of the activities in this book that inspired you. Reading the Success Stories on www.atkins.com might also help you rededicate your efforts.

Don't think that you can cheat with impunity. The most dangerous thing about cheating is that some people get away with it—for a while. If you eat a piece of cake and the numbers on the scale continue to drop, you might think that you can cheat whenever you want, but you may not be so lucky the next time, and you certainly won't continue to get away with it if cheating becomes a habit. Cake is full of empty carbs and will trigger cravings for other foods that aren't good for you. Find something else that is delicious *and* low carb to spoil yourself with.

"CHEATING" SMART

You may occasionally give in to the powerful pull of temptation. It's better for you to find a low-carb alternative, of course, but, realistically, that is not always the choice you'll make.

Thankfully, the ANA is so effective that most people without blood sugar disorders such as diabetes or the metabolic syndrome find there is some room for flexibility within it, which is why it can become a lifestyle. The key to cheating smart is *control*. There's a difference between bingeing and making room in your program for an occasional bite of something you really want. The guidelines below will help you make the distinction for yourself.

Don't cheat during Induction. You must stay on the straight and narrow in order to kick-start your fat-burning metabolism and stabilize blood sugar.

Don't cheat when your weight loss is stalled. Rather than letting your lack of progress lead to a binge, recognize that this is a time to find other outlets for your frustrations such as a long walk, a heart-to-heart with a friend, or a session at the gym. When the road gets bumpy, it's time to hang on tighter.

Plan for it. Your wedding anniversary is at the end of the week, and your daughter-in-law is replicating the cake served at your wedding. Be realistic: You're probably going to have a couple of bites for symbolic and emotional reasons. "Bank" carbs in anticipation by cutting back 5 or 10 grams a day. Even if you don't see it coming until too late, you can still compensate by cutting carbs for a few days after you bend the rules.

No labeling. On the rare occasions when you do have something you'd be better off not eating, don't label yourself as bad. Think of yourself instead as being supple: bending the rules so that you don't "break" by going off the Program entirely.

Choose whole foods. If you simply must have something sweet, choose fruit over a piece of cake. If you feel empty, have another serving of an acceptable food even if it means going over your CCLL.

Don't waste it. Make sure you have plenty of healthy snacks wherever you go, and save your splurges for something delicious that really matters to you.

Have a little. If you want something very badly, try having just one or two bites

"Parsley/Is gharsley." This is Ogden Nash's poem "Further Reflections on Parsley" in its entirety. Thankfully, many wonderful cooks disagree with him. If you relegate parsley to a garnish, pushing it to the side of your plate, or perhaps give it its due only as a breath freshener, think again. Many cultures treat parsley as a full-fledged vegetable and a centerpiece of their cuisine, and it should certainly take an important supporting role in your Atkins lifestyle.

The two most common types of parsley are curly and flat-leaved (Italian). The curly leaves make an attractive garnish, but flat-leaved parsley is more flavorful and most often used for cooking. Parsley is also available in the form of dried flakes, but fresh is preferable. Here are some ideas:

- Enliven a plain green salad with a sprinkle of chopped parsley or trim the stems and leave the leaves whole.

- Combine chopped parsley with cream cheese as a stuffing for celery sticks or endive "spoons."

- Work chopped parsley into softened butter and add a little garlic and lemon juice if you wish to make a delicious topping for meats, fish, and vegetables. Make extra, roll it into a log with waxed paper, slice it into disks, and freeze.

- Sauté chopped parsley quickly in olive oil and garlic for a wonderful Mediterranean-style sauce for fish.

- Combine chopped parsley and mint with bulgur (cracked wheat), chopped tomatoes, lemon juice, olive oil, and scallions for a Middle Eastern salad called tabbouleh, which is suitable for Pre-Maintenance.

Parsley is loaded with vitamins and minerals, particularly vitamins A and C, iron, and folate. It also contains flavonoids, particularly one called luteolin, which may protect against cancer and cardiovascular disease. A half cup of chopped parsley contains less than a gram of net carbs.

and then stop (assuming you have the willpower). You won't feel deprived, but you won't have sent your blood sugar into a complete tailspin, either. Remember to set limits and stick to them!

Know your trigger foods. You may find certain foods hard to handle. You can't control your portions of them, think about them all the time if you allow yourself even a little, and discover that they trigger cravings for other unhealthy foods. Don't bend the program to include these foods; control is *key* to cheating smart, and these foods, by definition, make you out of control. These are foods you should never eat.

Stop yourself immediately if you feel that you're heading for a binge. The cardinal rule of "cheating" on Atkins is to get right back on the Program after you've eaten a food that is not on the program. The danger of a binge is always there when you cheat. If you feel yourself losing your footing on that slippery slope, it is time to reach deep within yourself and take action. If a binge gets out of hand, you'll compromise your weight loss and may even find yourself back on the blood sugar roller coaster. See the tips on page 190 in Forget All or Nothing on how to pull yourself out of a nosedive.

Keep in mind that cheating, especially after you've been on the Program for a long time, can be more trouble than it's worth, especially if you overdo it. The good news is that with tasty low-carb treats and artificial sweeteners appropriate for baking, there is less reason to cheat than ever before. It was very difficult to pass up cake when your alternative was a chicken leg; now that you can have a slice of a sugar-free cheesecake, it is a different story!

MOTIVATION: THE WINNER'S EDGE

Are you so busy waiting for the big day, the perfect opportunity, the right occasion that you're putting off until tomorrow the wonderful times you could be having today? The activities in this section are designed to help you understand how you can make every moment count.

Many of us don't only procrastinate about tasks, we procrastinate about *life.* Sometimes we do this without even realizing it. As the saying goes, life isn't a dress rehearsal. If you live your life in a state of perpetual delayed gratification, waiting for the perfect moment before you make your move, you're going to miss out on a lot of great stuff along the way.

Now that you're armed with more energy and self-confidence, there is no better time to get in the habit of living the big moments of your life instead of putting them off. It's best to start small. This week give yourself permission to do something you've been putting off because you were waiting for the right occasion. Instead of waiting, make that occasion *now.*

Are you still holding on to that bottle of champagne a friend gave you to celebrate your promotion? How long have you been waiting for the right occasion to enjoy it? Months? Years? Find a reason to celebrate—and pop that cork this week! Perhaps your wife would like to lift a glass of bubbly to commemorate your 5,181-Days wedding anniversary or the "pat on the back" e-mail she received this morning from her boss.

As you put this lesson into practice, notice how good it feels to enjoy the special things that make life sparkle a little brighter instead of putting them off for "someday." Doesn't food taste a little better when served on fine china even though it's an ordinary Wednesday night dinner? Don't you feel a little more glamorous after you've spritzed yourself with your "special occasion" perfume for absolutely no reason at all?

If you don't use the gift certificate for a massage that has been languishing under that refrigerator magnet for months, it will expire—and that's a waste. The curtain has risen on your life—what are you waiting for?

Building on success provides motivation for further progress. You are already a very different person from the one who started this program two months ago. So if you have been waiting to reach your goal weight to go after something that is important—whether it's looking for a new job, going out on dates, joining a health club, running for president of the PTA—even though you still have pounds to banish, go for it. Feeling accomplished can only enhance your weight loss progress.

MAKE YOUR LUNCH HOUR COUNT

This week you'll learn techniques for making every moment count, and that means paying attention to everything. Life is made up of ordinary events that are so much a part of our daily routine that we don't even notice them long enough to think about them. But when you "make them count," you can put a shine on even the most pedestrian, workaday aspect of that routine.

Take lunch, for example. For too many of us the lunch hour is a wasted opportunity. We do the same humdrum thing day after day, sleepwalking through the experience, hardly noticing the surroundings or the food. How do you use yours? Do you grab a salad or eat reheated leftovers while flipping through the newspaper? Do you go to the same drab food court with your work friends or sit at the same table in the company cafeteria day after day, week after week? Do you hunch over your computer playing video games or e-shopping? Or do you use the time to run errands?

This week enliven your lunch hour. Here are some suggestions:

- Go to see just one amazing painting at a museum near work.

- Check out a book at the library by an author you've never read before.

- Go out for a special but speedy meal at a restaurant instead of grabbing something from a nearby deli.

- Visit a farmers' market and treat yourself to some berries and wildflowers.

- Make a picnic lunch, bring a blanket to the park (or the scrap of grass outside your workplace), and eat lunch outside.

- Make a date with a friend, your spouse, a family member, or someone you work with.

- Visit a favorite place—a garden, a special spot by the lake, or a stretch where you love to window-shop.

- Check out a tourist attraction in your hometown that you've never been to, whether it's a presidential birthplace, a war memorial, a famous writer's home, or the observatory at the top of the tallest building in town.

Remember, skipping meals isn't an option on Atkins. No matter how far your lunch wandering takes you, make sure you always have a meal and leave yourself the time to eat it!

Make this hour a true hiatus from the rest of your day, a time to do something you'll remember—a real treat. Instead of taking it for granted, make it count.

Fitness: The Best You

FOCUS FOR THE WEEK: YOU'RE GOING TO PICK UP THE PACE A NOTCH AS YOU CONTINUE TO BUILD YOUR ENDURANCE. THE MORE CHALLENGES YOU BRING TO YOUR WORKOUTS, THE BIGGER THE PAYOFF WILL BE. KEEP ON FINDING NEW WAYS TO PLAY.

Cardio → 30 minutes, minimum → 3 times
Stretching → 30 minutes → 2 times
Strength training → 2 times at a pace that is comfortable for you

Do your stretches at a pace that is comfortable for you. These stretches may take you longer than half an hour.

When it comes to fitness, making it count is a state of mind. You've probably seen people at the gym who spend more time chatting with their friends and visiting the water fountain than they do on the machines or in classes. Those people might get some satisfaction from telling themselves that they've been to the gym, but they're not really taking full advantage of their time there. Be sure that what you're doing at the gym is going to get results.

NEGATIVE REPETITIONS

This week you will learn another concept that will help you make the most of the time you dedicate to fitness: negative repetitions.

Every exercise has two parts: the concentric repetition when you shorten or tighten the muscle you're working, and an eccentric repetition when the muscle exerts force as it returns to the starting position. Pick up one of your lighter dumbbells and do a repetition of the simplest exercise you know, let's say the biceps curl. Chances are that you focused almost exclusively on the concentric rep, the part of the exercise where you curl the dumbbell up toward your shoulder and can feel the biceps tightening and working. Most of us do. But you can get twice the benefit from this exercise if you concentrate on the second half as well.

Do the exercise again. This time, instead of letting the weight swing back to your side, return it very slowly, almost as if gravity had been reversed so that it is pushing against the dumbbell. Feel how that works the bicep muscle more intensely. That's a negative repetition. It's a little change, but one with a big impact. In fact, sports science suggests that the greatest gains in strength training actually occur though eccentric exercises.

ANKLE WEIGHTS

When an exercise feels challenging, you're building muscle strength. With time, as you become stronger and the effort is less challenging, you need to add more weight to continue to build strength. You're probably feeling a little more solid and toned, and that's great! But it also means that your body has gotten used to doing these exercises. You may choose to add more resistance in the form of ankle weights.

Ankle weights are a convenient and inexpensive way to add resistance to home strengthening exercises. They can be purchased in any sporting goods store, and be sure to try them on before you buy. Ankle weights start at 2 pounds and can go up to 20 pounds. Most are adjustable in weight. Start small and build slowly to reduce your risk of injury.

Don't assume that one weight will be appropriate for every exercise. Differences in muscle strength and the nature of different exercises will determine where you should begin. This week you can use the ankle weights for both the Sitting Knee Extension (page 99) and the Standing Leg Lift (page 100). Beginning with a light weight, perform repetitions and sets as before. Gradually increase the weight as you become comfortable performing three sets of 15 reps.

Control the weight; don't let your legs swing wildly. Don't run or walk in ankle weights because it places added stress on joints and increases injury risk from muscle strain.

If you are not comfortable adding ankle weights, there are other ways to increase workout effort and intensity. You can increase your speed and/or add hills (or elevation on a treadmill) to your walking or running program.

STRETCHING EXERCISES

You've learned a total of 11 stretching exercises to date, and you'll learn two more this week. Your goal is to incorporate eight of these into your weekly routine. Choose those that target areas where you are less flexible. There is no reason that you can't do all of them if you wish.

Shoulder Hug (to stretch the upper back), page 62

Head Up, Chest Out (to stretch the chest and fronts of the shoulders), page 63

Cat and Dog (to warm up the back), page 64

Butterfly (to stretch the inner thighs and hips), page 65

Quad Stretch (to stretch the fronts of the thighs), page 77

Press Up (to stretch the chest), page 78

Low Back and Hamstring Combo Stretch, page 79

Follow Your Hand (to exercise the spine), page 80

Forward Lunge (to stretch the hip flexors), page 149

Reclining Ankle-to-Knee Stretch (to stretch the outer hip and low back), page 150

Calf Stretch (to stretch the backs of the lower legs), page 151

Following are two more stretches to add to your repertoire.

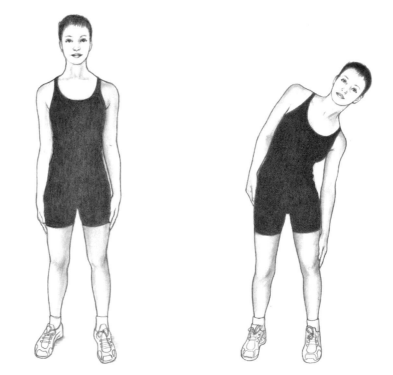

SIDE BENDING

1. Stand with your feet shoulder-width apart and arms relaxed at sides.

2. Lean first to the right, allowing your right hand to slide down the outside of your thigh toward the knee.

3. Slowly return to the starting position and then repeat on the other side.

Number of Repetitions All Levels: ten
Number of Sets All Levels: one, increasing to three as tolerated

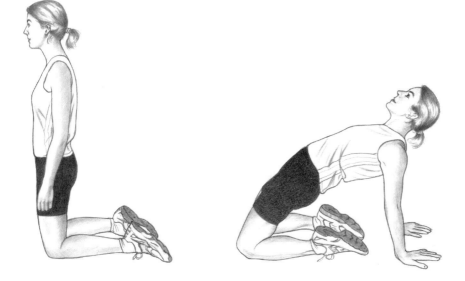

BELLY UP

1. Kneel on a mat or folded towel.

2. Reach both hands behind your feet (fingers pointing backward) while slowly leaning back until you're able to rest your weight on your hands.

3. Extend your back, lifting your abdomen as much as you can.

4. Relax your back, allowing your abdomen to lower while keeping your hands in place.

Number of Reps All Levels: five, increasing to ten as tolerated
Number of Sets All Levels: one, increasing to three as tolerated

STRENGTH TRAINING

This week you should do the following strengthening exercises.

Combined Biceps Curl/Overhead Press, page 201

Sitting Knee Extension (with ankle weights), page 99

Standing Leg Lift (with ankle weights), page 100

Back Lift, page 121

Ab Lift, page 122

Chair Ab Lift, page 183

Oblique Ab Lift, page 184

Advanced Back Lift, page 185

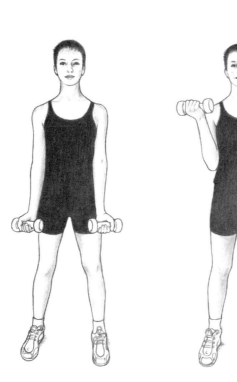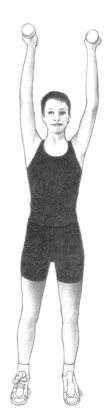

COMBINED BICEPS CURL/OVERHEAD PRESS

You are already familiar with the overhead press and the biceps curl. They are two of the Essential Strengtheners, and you've been doing them a couple of times a week since Week Three. Now let's take them up a notch by combining them into one single exercise.

For the biceps (fronts of the upper arms) and the shoulders. Concentrate first and foremost on proper technique.

1. Stand or sit with your arms by your sides, dumbbells in hand, palms facing forward. Inhale.

2. Exhaling, bend at the elbows and slowly pull the weights up toward your shoulders. Your upper arms should not move.

3. Inhale. As your hands reach shoulder height, turn them so that your palms face toward each other over your head.

4. Push the weights up above your head with a slow, smooth, and controlled movement on an exhale.

5. Inhaling, slowly return the weights to shoulder height.

6. Turn your palms to face your shoulders, and slowly lower your arms to the starting position as you exhale.

Number of Reps All Levels: ten
Number of Sets All Levels: one, increasing to three as tolerated
Modification: Once you can perform three sets of ten, increase to three sets of 15 and then increase the weight again.

FITNESS REWARDS

Your fitness program has taken shape over the past two months, and your body is probably showing the results. Congratulations for sticking with it, and in order to sweeten the pot a little, we'd like to introduce a brand-new concept, one that will change the way you think about fitness and about carbohydrates.

There is unanimous agreement that exercise has numerous health benefits. But despite years of recommendations to exercise to lose weight, it has become apparent that exercise itself isn't the most efficient weight loss tool. When you do Atkins, you lose weight in a way that is much more effective and easier than burning 3,500 calories to lose a single pound. For a 150-pound person, that's about seven hours of tennis, ten hours of walking, and five hours of high-impact step aerobics! No wonder people exercising to lose weight feel daunted by the task.

You don't have to work out like a maniac to eat until you're satisfied on Atkins. You *do* have to control your carbohydrate intake, but working out is a way to increase the amount of carbs you can eat.

Exercise can provide an extra measure of control. As you know, your age, gender, and genes all impact your carb threshold. So does your activity level. Most of those things are out of your control, but when you exercise, you *take* control.

Using the chart below, you'll find the additional grams of net carbs you can introduce on a given day, as a tradeoff for every half hour of workout time at the level described in Determine Your Strength Level on page 94. We call these additional grams Fitness Rewards.

You can double-check the group you're in by using the results of last week's fitness challenge. If it took you more than 20 minutes to walk a mile, you're in Group One; between 16½ and 20 minutes, Group Two; 16 minutes or less, Group Three.

FITNESS REWARDS CHART			
CURRENT BODY WEIGHT (IN POUNDS)	NUMBER OF GRAMS FOR FITNESS GROUPS		
	ONE	TWO	THREE
100–150	2.5	5.0	5.0
151–200	5.0	7.5	10.0
201–250	7.5	10.0	12.5

This is for every half hour of workout time.

Adding carbs is dependent on your weight and what you're doing during your exercise sessions. So, for example, if you're in Group One and you weigh 175 pounds, you get to consume an additional 5 grams of net carbs for each half hour workout or 10 grams for an hour's workout. Larger bodies burn more carbs per unit of time, so someone weighing 225 pounds who is in Group 2 would earn twice as many fitness points: 10 grams of net carbs for each half hour and 20 grams for a full hour. We have deliberately calculated these to stay below the number of carb grams you actually burn so you are not replacing all those you burn. Because there is some level of individuality to all this, you may be able to add back even more. Begin at this level and increase as you become fitter and move up a level.

ADVANTAGE CHECKPOINT: END OF WEEK NINE

Weigh and measure yourself. Enter the results in your Atkins Advantage Journal and compare the results with last week's results. See page 123 for guidance about how to evaluate your progress and decide how to proceed.

FOURTEEN

WEEK TEN: SPICE IT UP

Whether it is your meals, your workouts, or your job, nothing compromises your chances of long-term success more than boredom. You can avoid this trap by making sure there's room for plenty of variety in all aspects of your life.

It's also important to break out of old, self-defeating behavior patterns, the ones that can trip you up again and again in the same ways. It's as important to refresh your self-image periodically as it is to restock your pantry.

It's time to spice things up so that you don't let yourself get stuck. Since you're already undergoing a tremendous process of renewal, what better time to make sure you're adopting a brand-new outlook that can help you make every day better?

NUTRITION: THE HEART OF THE MATTER

To find meal plans appropriate for your daily net carb gram count, see the listings that begin on page 278.

Continue to take a good multivitamin, essential oils, and a fiber supplement. If you are experiencing a return of hunger or cravings, you may want to consider chromium (see page 107) or L-glutamine (page 141).

CUSTOMIZING PRE-MAINTENANCE: DO IT YOUR WAY

As you know by now, Atkins isn't one-size-fits-all. The ability to customize each phase is what makes people successful over the long haul.

In this section you'll find modifications to the standard rule of Pre-Maintenance: You add 10 grams of daily net carbs every week as long as you continue to lose weight. You should lose weight very slowly in Pre-Maintenance so that you learn to make the right choices. These variations keep you within the parameters of the Program while affording you the opportunity to influence the rate at which you lose.

Remember that even if the scale holds steady, as long as you're still losing inches, you're doing fine.

Note: Unless you've gained weight, it's important to complete two full weeks in Pre-Maintenance before starting to customize this program because one week isn't enough time to know how your body is responding to this phase.

Should you consider customizing Pre-Maintenance? As in OWL, we've found that some groups benefit from adapting the rules of Pre-Maintenance:

1. You are metabolically resistant, a "slow burner." If your weight loss pace has been slow throughout the earlier phases, you're probably a slow burner. If you found one of the customized variations of OWL helpful, you may well find variations helpful in this phase as well.

2. You find that hunger, cravings, and other symptoms are recurring. If your body signals you that your blood sugar has become unstable, you're probably over-filling the tank. Red flags aren't apparent only in the form of pounds and inches; sometimes they express themselves in the way we feel long before they show up on the scale or tape measure. Take note of early warning flares such as extreme frustration at the snail's pace of weight loss in Pre-Maintenance or if you're thinking about food more than you have since starting Atkins.

By noting these signs early, you can avert setbacks before they happen. See page 66 to review those symptoms that alert you to the need for an adjustment.

These variations give you the latitude to adapt the rate at which you add carbs to better suit your needs. Think of these variations as tools that allow you even more flexibility as you attempt to create your personalized program.

Slow Climb: In this variation, as long as you are making progress, albeit slow, you'll still add carbs in increments of 10 grams; however, you'll stay at your new level for two or three weeks before making each addition instead of every week. This should help you stay on course as you progress toward your goal.

or

Alternate Days: If you choose this option—and, again, assuming you are not gaining but your progress is very slow—instead of eating an extra 10 grams of net carbs every day of the week, have them only every other day. For example, have 60 grams on Monday, 50 on Tuesday, 60 on Wednesday, and so forth.

THE USES AND ABUSES OF INDUCTION

Induction can be hard to resist. That's why some people don't let themselves advance as far or as quickly as they should. They stay too long in Induction or return whenever the going gets tough. People who find it difficult to add the right carbs in the right amounts without compromising their results sometimes hide in Induction.

Even worse, some people go off the Program entirely until the pounds pile on again, and then they return to Induction.

Induction is a critically important phase of Atkins, and there certainly are times when it is necessary or advisable to return, however briefly, but the promise of lifelong weight control cannot be fulfilled with this phase of the program. When you use Induction as a corrective for overeating or eating the wrong foods, you turn Atkins into just another yo-yo diet. Yo-yo dieting is bad for your immune system and your HDL cholesterol. If you overuse Induction, it may make your metabolism less likely to respond to it.

Everyone who begins in Induction should move eventually to Ongoing Weight Loss and, finally, to Phase 3: Pre-Maintenance and Phase 4: Lifelong Maintenance to ensure long-term success. With Atkins you always have the freedom to speed up or slow down your weight loss, and you can choose the pace that works best for you (see Customizing OWL, page 106, and Customizing Pre-Maintenance, 205). You do not need to return to Induction to achieve that control, and you shouldn't.

Instead, try to follow the rules of the phase you're in. When you are feeling restless, treat yourself to something new on the Acceptable Foods in Induction list (page 26), a new recipe, or some low-carb alternatives to those foods you are especially missing.

If you have already fallen off the wagon and gained a pound or two, you do not need to go back on Induction to get your metabolism burning fat again unless you have experienced unmanageable cravings, an out-of-control appetite, or any of the other symptoms given on page 66. You should be able to regain control by reducing your net carb intake by 5 or 10 grams for a week or two.

On the other hand, you may need to go back to Induction if either of the following has occurred:

1. You've gone off Atkins for more than a few weeks and/or are experiencing symptoms such as hunger, cravings, mood swings, brain fog, and/or you've regained more than 5 pounds. If you stopped doing Atkins altogether and upset your metabolism to some degree, you will probably need Induction to trigger the "reset" button and help calm those cravings and excessive hunger. Unlike a few episodes of cheating or even a binge of a day or two, a complete return to your pre-Atkins eating habits requires serious action. You won't have to stay in Induction very long; it will probably take only a week or two to stabilize your blood sugar and insulin levels: You'll know because you won't feel as hungry, and you'll be liberated from your cravings. You can then begin to add back carbs.

2. You have gained less than 5 pounds but can't correct your course by cutting back. Normally, you can get back on track by reducing your daily carb intake by 5 grams of net carbs (or 10 grams if you're in Pre-Maintenance). If that doesn't work, it may be necessary to go back to Induction to get your metabolism back into balance, but you should use this only as a last resort.

If you have hit a plateau that can't be budged—meaning that you have not lost any pounds or inches—for four consecutive weeks and your attempts at cutting back by increments of 5 grams of net carbs (if you're in OWL) or 10 grams (if you're in Pre-Maintenance) has not worked, then it may be necessary to go back to Induction.

Don't return to Induction unless you absolutely have to, but if you do go back, you must do Induction to the letter. Commit to this phase again wholeheartedly and do everything you did the first time. Doing it halfway isn't how you got results the first time around.

If your behavior has led to a slip, take this opportunity to determine why. What was it that made it hard for you to stick with the program? What triggered your noncompliance? What kinds of feelings were you experiencing when you stopped doing Atkins? Take a look at how you felt physically and how you were feeling about yourself at that time. What can you do, going forward, to prevent another derailment in the future? Because this is a very common pattern for many people, it's vitally important for you to confront this behavior pattern. It will not change unless you commit to changing it.

The goal, of course, is to incorporate Atkins into your life, and that means following the whole program so that it's not a diet but a healthy way of eating based on making smarter choices.

Some people are perfectly content to eat the same things every day, but if you're not one of them, then you risk straying to less wholesome alternatives if you don't keep your urge for variety sated with low-carb options. You can enjoy a perpetually varied and exciting array of foods by eating seasonally and locally.

In another era when families were dependent on their own gardens and those of their neighbors, people had no choice but to eat what was in season. Our forebears ate apples in the fall, berries in the spring, and an abundance of vegetables and fruits in late summer. Now, of course, a cornucopia of choices awaits us at the supermarket: produce grown, packaged, and shipped from all over the world.

That abundance of choice is a mixed blessing. As professional chefs know, foods generally taste better when they're in season. There's a world of difference between the taste of a farm-stand tomato just hours off the vine in late summer and that of a supermarket tomato in the dead of winter. That second tomato is picked long before it's ripe so it can travel a long distance and sit in the market. It's bred to be shiny and round and red; taste is secondary.

There's another boon to eating seasonally: Foods you may not be familiar with at your farmers' market can be a delicious and nutritious way to add variety to your table. If you take a walk through the stalls, you'll likely see melons and eggplants and tomatoes, in a myriad of shapes and colors. Some of these are heirloom varieties, grown from seeds that may be direct descendants of those our ancestors ate! You will also be supporting local growers—a boon to your local economy.

Nature has its own way of ensuring that we vary our diets—by making some of the most delicious foods extremely elusive. Some of the most delectable fruits and vegetables come out to play for only a short period of time each year. Pomegranates are in season only in the late fall. Fiddlehead ferns are available for only a few weeks in the spring. Some other less familiar seasonal taste treats include white peaches, rhubarb, currants, and gooseberries. Nature ensures that our palates need never have a dull moment.

A CURE FOR BOREDOM

Sometimes the only difference between "Chicken again?" and "Wow!" is the judicious use of herbs, spices, and sauces. With creativity (but little expense and effort) you can transform everyday foods into exotic and flavorful meals based on cuisines from around the world.

Herbs and Spices. Each cuisine is defined by certain spices or spice mixtures. For example, curry powder and garam masala in India, five-spice powder in China, and gomasio in Japan all put you a mere shake away from transforming tonight's chicken, shrimp, or beef into a new adventure. Spices and herbs contain a negligible amount of carbs, but do read labels to avoid mixtures that have added sugars. Here are some other flavorful hints:

If you're been relying on dried herbs, experiment with fresh. There's a big difference in taste. Since dried herbs tend to be more pungent, you may want to increase the amount of fresh herbs you use.

Make sure your spices are fresh. Those past their prime lose pungency. Purists recommend buying spices whole and grinding them yourself in a coffee grinder reserved for the purpose. At the very least, purchase spices from a store that has a rapid turnover and buy in small quantities.

Toast your spices. Toasting spices over a very low heat greatly increases the complexity of their flavor. Be careful; they scorch easily.

Experiment with dry spice rubs. Pick and choose from ingredients such as cumin, cayenne, chili powder, garlic powder, lemon pepper, celery salt, paprika, five-spice powder, curry powder, thyme, and sage. Brush chicken, fish, or meat with a little oil before dipping it into your spice mixture.

> ### SPOTLIGHT ON GARLIC
>
> Garlic, "the stinking rose," was so highly valued by the Egyptians that they used it as a form of currency. It is a significant component of many cuisines, and its health benefits are legendary. Raw garlic has an antibacterial effect, which is why it plays a role in many topical home remedies and can be purchased as a supplement as well. Some studies suggest that garlic can help lower cholesterol.
>
> Garlic might not help you against vampires, but it is a natural antibiotic and is known to support the immune system. As you know, antioxidants are a special group of nutrients that protect cells against the damage that can in turn cause signs of age and diseases such as cancer. Garlic has the highest antioxidant power of any vegetable, and a medium clove contains about 1 gram of net carbs.
>
> Eating garlic has other advantages. Well-seasoned food is more satisfying, meaning you are less likely to overeat. Garlic, like onions, appears in many recipes as part of a seasoning mixture to flavor meats, soups, and sauces. Raw pressed garlic is very pungent, while garlic that has cooked for a long time becomes mellow and almost sweet. The bigger the variety—think of the well-named elephant garlic—the less punch it packs.

Marinate! Don't underestimate the power of a simple marinade. Even a modest combination of ingredients—garlic, lemon juice, olive oil, and maybe a sprig of thyme—can dramatically enhance the flavor of meat or other source of protein.

Get Saucy. Herbs and spices aren't the only way to expand your culinary artistry. Sauces are another simple, inexpensive, and inexhaustibly delicious way to enliven mealtime. Try these ideas:

Deglaze the pan. You might associate sauces with fancy French cooking, but a simple sauce is as easy as splashing a little wine or chicken broth into the pan that you just used to cook your entrée. (If you're using wine, turn off the heat while you're pouring.) Cook the mixture until it is reduced, scraping up the delicious brown drippings at the bottom of the pan, and voilá!

Thicken the low-carb way. There are now low-carb alternatives to cornstarch and flour that make delectable sauces without compromising your carb intake. Two products to look for are Thicken Thin not/Starch Thickener and Thick It Up!

Don't get stuck in a protein rut! Chicken, beef, pork, and fish are fine, but also explore lamb, bison, ostrich, and soy products, for example.

MOTIVATION: THE WINNER'S EDGE

This week combat the same-old, same-old by opening your heart and mind to new experiences—and don't be surprised if you discover that what's new is *you*.

Get too comfortable, and complacency and boredom can set in. Your familiar routine may have much to recommend it, but if you allow your vantage point to become too narrow, you'll go stir-crazy. The first exercise this week is designed to encourage you to expand your horizons: Learn something new for each of the next seven days.

THINK BIG

You don't need to pick up astrophysics on the side (although a few phrases in a foreign language might be fun). This activity needn't take a lot of time or energy, but you do have to make an effort to explore one new thing this week.

But this is not necessarily about physical achievements. Instead, the point is to introduce a bit of bravado into your life by challenging yourself to do something new. By declaring your goal out loud or writing it in your Atkins Advantage Journal, you will be stimulated to "think big." The definition of big is relative. What is big for you may not be big for someone else. Your goal should challenge you and your image of yourself. Here are some ideas to consider:

- Offer to coach your daughter's softball team.

- Take a class in a foreign language you have always wanted to learn.

- Explore your heritage by interviewing a relative about his childhood and knowledge of the family's history.

- Volunteer for a project that needs to be done in your community.

- Organize a book club for friends and coworkers.

Think of this assignment as a scavenger hunt of sorts. You may well have to get out of your comfort zone, but you will likely uncover some buried treasure.

THE ONE THAT GOT AWAY

Have you ever found yourself saying, "If I knew then what I know now, I would . . . not have left that job . . . passed up the opportunity to buy that house . . . let that friendship wither," or whatever. If you like the idea of second chances, you'll love this next activity. The assignment itself is very simple: Go back to one of the activities you skipped in this book and do it.

As dedicated as you've been to this program each step of the way, chances are good that you have bypassed—or given short shrift to—at least one of the activities in the motivational wheel of the Program. You may have intended to revisit it later, or you may have started it, gotten interrupted, and never returned to it. Maybe you did it in your head instead of writing it out in your Atkins Advantage Journal. Or you may simply have opted to skip it altogether.

If that's the case, it's probably because something about it didn't quite fit with your ideas about yourself. Maybe you thought, "I can't do that. I'd feel like an idiot." Or "I don't need to do this one. I don't have that problem."

> **ATKINS ADVANTAGE TIP**
>
> Be realistic about your goal weight. Perhaps you're trying to get too low. This is especially true if you have gained a few pounds of muscle mass with exercise or you're trying to get down to the weight you were in your teens. If you haven't rechecked your BMI, do so now. This can help you get a realistic idea of your healthy weight range.

Now is the time to revisit one of the activities you initially resisted. There's a line of thinking that says we avoid the very things we most need to do. As a result, we repeat thought patterns and actions that run counter to our best interests. Coming face-to-face with your resistance to something often offers you the solution you need to break that pattern. Imagine the joy and sense of accomplishment you would experience if you could break habits that have limited you in the past.

This week's theme is to make sure you don't get stuck in a rut, and one of the sinkholes we're likely to fall into is our own perception of ourselves. You've already seen that it's possible to wrestle one of your self-defeating behaviors to the ground by confronting your eating habits and doing the hard work necessary to change them. That's why I urge you to continue that good work by facing down one of the activities you avoided earlier.

If the exercise is truly uncomfortable for you, you may still not be ready for it. If that's the case, take some time to consider what it is about it that causes you such discomfort, and then examine what your resistance can tell you about yourself.

Our perceptions of ourselves tend to get stuck and not change. Nowhere is this more evident than when we're assessing our own limitations and capabilities. "I'm a terrible singer." "I've never been athletic." "I'm right-brain and logical, not creative." Unless we challenge these self-imposed boundaries, they become a prison of our own making.

Have you ever tried a food you thought you hated, only to discover that it wasn't so bad after all? Fresh spinach sautéed with garlic, olive oil, and a sprinkle of sea salt is a far cry from a frozen green block cooked into soggy oblivion. Or maybe it's just that your tastes have changed, and you're not a spinach hater after all.

You are now going to "taste" some supposed truths about yourself to see whether they still exist or if your self-perceptions need to evolve in order to keep up with *you*.

Sit comfortably in a chair in a quiet room where you are unlikely to be interrupted.

Close your eyes. Breathe deeply and slowly, and relax.

As you begin to relax, reflect on the phrases and words you use to describe yourself.

Let the thoughts flit through your brain. There's no need to examine closely what you know about yourself and the veracity of the claims. Simply see how those impressions feel to you. For instance, do you describe yourself as "responsible" or "a caretaker" or "bad about money," "scatterbrained," or "the funny one"? The qualities you focus on don't have to be deep fundamentals. Perhaps you're convinced that you're "a bad singer" because your seventh grade music teacher chided you for being off-key in front of the whole class.

Again, the point is not so much whether the statements are accurate but how they make you *feel*. Some will make you feel proud. Take a moment to appreciate that feeling and the accomplishments that gave rise to it. Others won't sit as comfortably. You may feel irritated. Or the statement may feel oppressive to you or in need of qualification.

Pay special attention to those. The chafing you feel is a sign that you're no longer comfortable with the label you (and possibly others) have assigned to you. Now might be the time to leave that self-perception behind by gently exploring what happens when you challenge the boundaries of your personal box.

You don't have to leap into it. You might not want to think of yourself as "a bad singer" anymore, but that doesn't necessarily mean karaoke at a crowded club. Start by humming a few bars when a song you like comes on the radio even if there's someone else in the car. It's possible that your old teacher was right and that stray cats will answer if you give that song full voice—but who cares? If you can find pleasure in the activity (and nobody's getting hurt), what's the harm?

Remember: You were once a person who had problems controlling what foods you put into your mouth, someone who perhaps feasted on junk foods filled with empty carbs. That's no longer true, is it? If you've been following the program, you've undoubtedly discovered a number of surprises about yourself and your capacities: that you're someone who likes to move—and to sweat; someone who passes up triple-layer fudge cake for a bowl of blueberries; or even someone who can look great in a bathing suit. Now that you know how incredibly powerful you can be and how good change can feel, where else in your life—what other labels—would you like to focus on changing?

Fitness: The Best You

FOCUS FOR THE WEEK: STEP UP YOUR CARDIO WITH FOUR DAYS OF WORKING OUT. KEEP PLAYING!

Cardio → 30 minutes, minimum → 4 times
Stretching → 30 minutes → 2 times
Strength training → 2 times at a pace that is comfortable for you

Do your stretches at a pace that is comfortable for you. These stretches may take you longer than half an hour.

The extra day of cardio will give your heart and lungs an extra workout. Of course, there's nothing wrong with running or walking on the fourth day as long as you enjoy it and it allows you to keep your heart rate up. You could also use this day to try something new. You've accomplished so much and are so much fitter than you were when you first started the program, so it's time to take advantage of your new potential. You can not only do more but do *different* things. As you'll discover, there are many benefits to switching out the components of your workout and introducing new ones. One benefit, of course, is that it's a surefire way to avoid boredom. You're a lot less likely to dread your workout if you kickbox on Monday, run on Tuesday, and take a vigorous vinyasa yoga class on Thursday. The more your workouts engage your mind, the more likely you are to stick with the program.

There are physical benefits as well. The more you exercise in a particular way, the better your body gets at the activity. That's how you know you're getting fit! But you don't want to "outgrow" your workout. If you persist in doing the exact same things as your fitness level improves, your workouts won't continue to offer as many benefits.

As you know from Week Eight, one way to challenge yourself is to increase the intensity of your workout. This week we'll provide you with another option: changing what you do. You'll work different muscles in that yoga class than you do when you're kickboxing. You'll also build different balancing skills, reflexes, and methods of acceleration and deceleration—all of which will contribute to greater fitness in the long run. Of course, you probably won't realize all this is happening, just that you're a little sore (in a good way) the day after your new class because you've done something different.

Here are some ways you can mix up your cardio workouts:

- Are you curious about martial arts? Sign up for a karate, judo, aikido, jujitsu, Krav Maga, or capoeira class.

- If you belong to a health club or gym, investigate the group classes, whether low-impact aerobic exercises or high-impact step classes that use dance choreography, spin classes on stationary bikes, or even classes that incorporate the treadmill. If you're self-conscious at first, ask if there's a beginner class so you can learn the basics, and always proceed at your own pace.

- Styles and types of yoga range from relaxing and meditative to the athletic. All are noncompetitive, and you'll leave class feeling restored in both body and soul. There are yoga studios now in most communities.

- Dance. Take a class at a dance school, join a club, or take a cardio class that incorporates dance—whether hip-hop or Broadway style. Swing dancing is a great way to meet people while you're working up a sweat. Belly dancing is terrific for the core muscles. Ballet, Masala Bhangra, and African and Brazilian dancing are all good workouts and will certainly shake you out of your exercise doldrums.

- Classes that teach Pilates and the Lotte Berk method can do wonders for the all-important core, the system of muscles at the center of the body encompassing your pelvis, lower back, and abs.

- There are Strollercize classes that let new mothers work out while their babies socialize in their strollers. Try Mommy and Me yoga classes, and Mommy and Me Pilates, but remember: Exercise time is *your* time. Make sure baby's not getting a better workout than you are.

- Boot camp programs get you out of bed early for an alfresco military-style workout in a neighborhood park.

- Invest in some home workout equipment, especially if winters make it hard for you to walk or run outside. The classic treadmill, stationary bike, Nordic-Track, or elliptical machine lets you get your cardio workout without leaving home. (You'll often find secondhand machines offered at tag sales, in classified sale ads, and on the Internet.) There are also a number of good machines that will allow you to do a variety of strength training exercises.

- Be aware that the quality of exercise equipment can vary dramatically. You're likely to get what you pay for. Identify the features that are most important to you to prevent buyer's remorse. Any mechanical devices should be sold with a warranty. Equipment should feel smooth and offer significant resistance to provide training benefit with room for progressive gains in strength.

- At-home props don't have to cost a lot of money. You can get a wonderful and fun workout on a mini trampoline or rebounder. What about an exercise ball? A balance trainer? Exertubes or resistance bands? A hula hoop?

- Ask friends for recommendations on workout tapes they've enjoyed using. Trade them back and forth so you don't get bored with the ones you own.

Note: If you discover that a class you've signed up for is hard work for your muscles but is not getting (and keeping) your heart rate in its optimal target zone, substitute that class for one of your strength training sessions and do something else to make up the cardio workout.

STRETCHING EXERCISES

Incorporate eight of the 11 stretching exercises you've learned to date. Choose from the following those that best address your particular needs:

Shoulder Hug, page 62

Head Up, Chest Out, page 63

Cat and Dog, page 64

Butterfly, page 65

Quad Stretch, page 77

Press Up, page 78

Low Back and Hamstring Combo Stretch, page 79

Follow Your Hand, page 80

Forward Lunge, page 149

Reclining Ankle-to-Knee Stretch, page 150

Calf Stretch, page 151

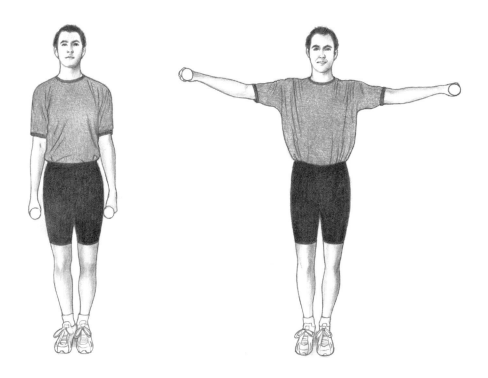

SIDE RAISES FOR ARMS
For deltoids (shoulders)

1. Stand with feet shoulder-width apart and your arms straight against your outer thigh muscles, holding a light dumbbell.

2. Inhale and then exhale as you slowly raise the dumbbells to the sides (abduct to shoulder level), keeping your arms straight.

3. Inhale as you hold each arm parallel to the floor momentarily. Exhaling, slowly lower each dumbbell to the starting position.

Number of Reps All Levels: ten
Number of Sets
    Level One: one, gradually increasing to three if possible
    Levels Two and Three: two, increasing to three sets, then to 15 reps per set before adding more weight

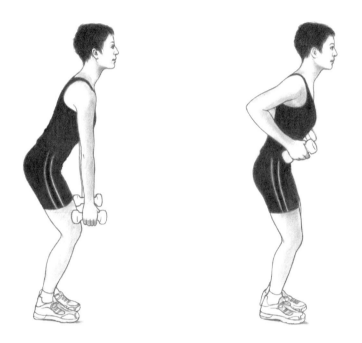

UPRIGHT ROWS

For biceps (fronts of upper arms) and latissimus dorsi (sides of back)

1. Stand with your feet shoulder-width apart and knees slightly bent. Hold a dumbbell in each hand. Bend slightly forward from the waist and let your arms hang down naturally. Your palms should be facing each other.

2. Inhale. Exhale as you pull both arms up and slightly back toward the sides of your chest.

3. Hold for a second as you inhale. Exhaling, slowly lower your arms back to the starting position.

Number of Reps All Levels: ten
Number of Sets
    Level One: one, gradually increasing to three if possible
    Levels Two and Three: two, increasing to three sets and then to 15 reps per set before adding more weight

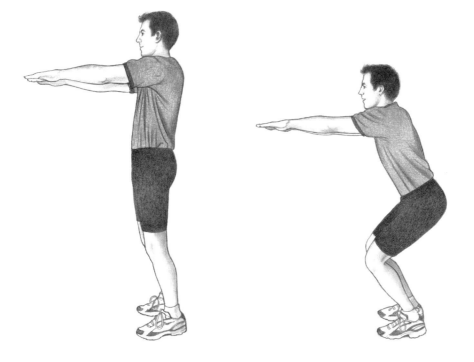

HALF SQUATS

1. Stand with your feet shoulder width apart and your arms extended in front for balance. Inhale.

2. Exhaling, slowly squat halfway down, at a 45-degree angle.

3. Hold to a count of three. Inhaling, fairly quickly raise yourself to the starting position.

Number of Reps All Levels: ten

Number of Sets

   Level One: one, increasing to three as you get stronger

   Levels Two and Three: two, increasing to three sets, and then to 15 reps per set before adding dumbbells

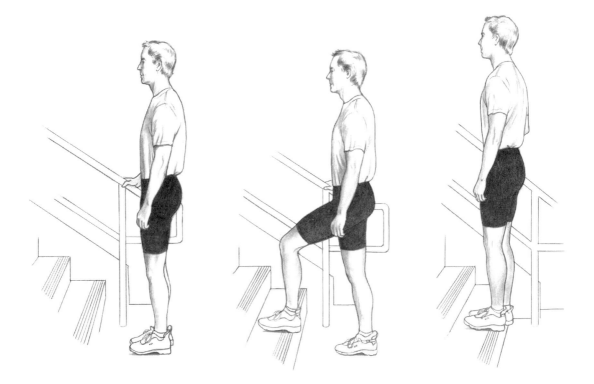

TWO-LEGGED STEP-UPS

1. Stand about 6 inches in front of a step, with feet shoulder-width apart. Hold a side rail if needed.

2. To a count of four, step up with one foot (1), bring your other foot alongside on the step (2), step down with the first foot (3), and step down with the second foot (4).

3. Switch the starting leg and repeat.

Number of Reps All Levels: ten (five reps for each leg)
Number of Sets
    Level One: one, increasing to three as you get stronger
    Levels Two and Three: two, increasing to three sets and then to 15 reps per set before adding dumbbells

ADVANTAGE CHECKPOINT: END OF WEEK TEN

Weigh and measure yourself. Enter the results in your Atkins Advantage Journal and compare the results with last week's results. See page 123 for further guidance about how to evaluate your progress and decide how to proceed.

FIFTEEN

WEEK ELEVEN: ATKINS YOUR WAY

You deserve to be slim, healthy, and able to accomplish all your dreams. With the successful completion of each week, you have acquired valuable tools, each one building on others to help you work the Program—and the rest of your life—to your advantage. With these tools you can build the best program for you, one that will sustain you for the remainder of the time it takes you to reach your goal weight and ultimately maintain that weight for life.

Now it's time to do Atkins *your* way. When you truly master any skill or craft, your performance looks natural. Think of a basketball player's vertical leap, an ice skater's triple axle, or a prima ballerina's perfect series of turns. Physics may explain how such feats happen, but after years of practice, they come naturally. Now it's time to take the skills you've learned and incorporate them naturally into your healthy lifestyle.

NUTRITION: THE HEART OF THE MATTER

Continue to add new foods, following the Atkins Carbohydrate Ladder (see page 14). Gradually, as you create your personalized dietary regimen, you will learn exactly what your body can and cannot handle. Those of you who have been in OWL for a few weeks should already have a good idea of what you can eat without weight gain or return of pre-Atkins symptoms.

If you are already in Pre-Maintenance, legumes such as lentils, baby lima beans, and black beans are among the first foods you can reintroduce, followed by fruits such as kiwi, Granny Smith apples, and melons, and then starchy vegetables such as carrots, sweet potatoes, and acorn squash. The remaining food group is whole grains. Because they are highly concentrated sources of carbs and are foods that many people have difficulty controlling, whole grains are usually added last. In this category are no-added-sugar cereals, brown rice, millet, old-fashioned oats, other unrefined grains, and breads and other baked goods made from them.

To find meal plans appropriate for your daily net carb gram count, see the listings beginning on page 278.

Continue to take a good multivitamin, essential oils, and a fiber supplement. If you are experiencing a return of hunger or cravings, you may want to consider chromium (see page 107) or L-glutamine (page 141).

FOCUS ON QUALITY

Remember that it's not only the quantity of carbs that matters, but the quality as well. You should be focusing on adding back carbohydrate foods high in fiber and nutrients.

You may recall Glycemic Index Versus Glycemic Load (page 13). These are both difficult tools to apply to meal planning, so the Atkins Glycemic Ranking (AGR) combines the two. The AGR lists vegetables, fruits, grains, dairy, nuts, and legumes, recommending which to eat regularly, which to eat in moderation, and which to eat sparingly once you are at or close to your goal weight. Of course, you still must count grams of net carbs and control portion sizes. Based on your individual tolerance, some of you will not be able to eat all these foods. Following is the AGR chart for fruit. (For AGR charts for other carbohydrate food groups, see *Atkins for Life* or www.atkins.com/agr.)

> **ATKINS ADVANTAGE TIP**
> Vegetables that are high in fiber make you feel full longer because they tend to contain more bulk than low-fiber foods and take longer to digest. Use a carb gram counter to choose low-glycemic vegetables with the most fiber.

EAT SPARINGLY

APPLES	APRICOTS	APPLE JUICE
BLACKBERRIES	CRANBERRY JUICE, UNSWEETENED	BANANAS
BLUEBERRIES		DATES
CHERRIES	GRAPEFRUIT JUICE, UNSWEETENED	FRUIT COCKTAIL, CANNED IN JUICE
CRANBERRIES	GRAPES	
GOOSEBERRIES	GUAVAS	GRAPE JUICE
GRAPEFRUIT	KIWI FRUIT	ORANGE JUICE
ORANGES	MANGOS	PRUNES
PEACHES	MELONS	RAISINS
PEARS	NECTARINES	
PLUMS	PAPAYAS	
RASPBERRIES	PINEAPPLES	
STRAWBERRIES	POMEGRANATES	
TANGERINES	WATERMELONS	

DOING ATKINS YOUR WAY

Atkins truly is about declaring independence. Most people who do Atkins say that for the first time in their lives they are no longer obsessed with or controlled by food. The ability to eat the way you can eat on Atkins, while still losing weight, is true freedom. If you can tailor an eating plan that perfectly meets your needs, you'll be able to stick with it happily for the rest of your life.

Make no mistake: Doing Atkins your way doesn't mean doing it any old way. Tearing open a bag of "low-carb" soy chips doesn't mean you're living the low-carb lifestyle. You'll enjoy the flexibility of accommodating your individual needs and preferences, but you must hold fast to a series of principles without which the Program does not work. For example, you know that you have to count carbs and stay within your daily carb allowance—that's a rule. Within those parameters, however, there's freedom. Once you know your carb threshold, you're free to eat from a rich and varied banquet of foods.

Pre-Maintenance is the phase in which all this truly begins. The focus is no longer primarily on losing pounds but on developing an optimal eating plan—as long as those fixed points remain just that. So even while you're doing Atkins *your* way, you'll be doing Atkins *right* if you do the following:

Control carbohydrate intake and stay at or just below your daily threshold. You enjoy considerable latitude in making food choices, but you must always remain true to your CCLL (if you're in Pre-Maintenance) or your ACE (once you're maintaining your weight).

Put quality before quantity. We've said it before, and we'll say it again: It's not just how many grams of carbs you add back but the quality of the carbs that counts. You're not doing Atkins right if you're eating added sugars and added trans fats, bleached white flour, and other refined foods even if you stay within your daily carb limit. Healthy carbs come from whole foods.

Plan ahead. You know what you're going to be eating, especially in situations where you are not in control such as in a restaurant or at a party. You pack healthy snacks and don't allow yourself to get too hungry between meals.

> **ATKINS ADVANTAGE TIP**
> When you're traveling, keep snacks handy so that you won't be tempted to grab a slice of pizza between connections or eat the roll in the airline meal.

Keep products in their place. Is it okay to grab a low-carb nutrition bar for breakfast, if you're running late? Sure. Is it okay to have another one mid-morning, before a lunch consisting of another bar and a shake? Of course not. Low-carb products are convenient, provide variety, and offer alternatives to foods that are off-limits, but overreliance can displace whole foods and interfere with weight management.

Keep an eye on your carb threshold. The number of carbs you can eat—whether you're losing or maintaining—isn't set in stone. If you start exercising more seriously, you may be able to eat slightly more carbs than before. Watch out for anything that may lower your carb threshold, too. Do you have an injury that makes it difficult to exercise? Have you started a new medication? Sometimes people who have kept the weight off successfully for many years begin to gain weight even though they're not eating any differently. The culprit in these cases may simply be the natural metabolic slowdown that comes with age or hormonal changes. As a result, you may need to adjust your carb intake or increase your activity level.

Stay on the Program. If you spend a few days loading up on too many or the wrong kinds of carbs, it's going to take you three or four days just to rebalance your metabolism. If you make this a pattern, alternating periods where you control carbs with ones where you don't, you will not reap the health or weight loss rewards that come from doing Atkins right.

Stay active. Fitness is an essential part of doing Atkins right. It will make you look and feel better, and it will help you lose weight more quickly and avoid (or get off) a plateau—not to mention allowing you to eat more carbs. If you're not exercising, you're not doing Atkins correctly.

Adjust the ratio of foods on your plate. As you eat more carbs, you'll need to reduce the amount of both fat and protein you eat.

Get enough protein. Don't skip meals, and try not to allow yourself to get too hungry between meals. Even though you will be cutting back a bit on protein as you add carbs, don't skimp on it no matter what. Protein is the backbone of a healthy diet, and eating sufficient quantities—at least 6 ounces (weighed before cooking) at each meal—ensures that you will stay satisfied and your blood sugar will be stable.

Eat a healthy mix of fats. Don't create your own fat-restricted version of Atkins. If you avoid natural fat, you'll be hungry and need to eat more often, your food will lack taste, and you'll rob yourself of valuable nutrients.

Cheat smart. You "bank" your carbs in anticipation of a splurge or compensate later. You are satisfied with a small portion and don't squander a splurge on something not worth it. You treat yourself to trigger foods. You remain mindful and under control even when you are choosing to occasionally veer from the Program.

SPOTLIGHT ON LENTILS

Lentils are quick, economical, delicious, and a staple of many cuisines. Unlike many other legumes, you don't have to presoak lentils, and they take only 20 to 30 minutes to cook. You can also buy canned cooked lentils. Lentils are delicious hot or cold, served as a side dish with chicken, fish, or meat. Half a cup of cooked lentils logs in at 12 grams of net carbs, less than most other legumes. You'll find them sold whole or split in half, like split peas. They come in a variety of colors and sizes. The brown and green ones retain their shape when cooked, unlike the red and yellow ones, which take on a creamy consistency, making them perfect for soup and purees.

Lentils are a good source of fiber, which makes them very filling. Although most people wait until they are in Pre-Maintenance to add them back into their meals, their glycemic impact is relatively low because they take a long time to digest. They're a good source of protein as well as folate, vitamin B_6, magnesium, and iron.

Are savvy about your patterns. Be aware of any triggers—foods, environments, and emotions—that pose a threat to your progress. If you know when you're likely to cheat or overeat, you can be proactive when danger looms. Get support during stressful times, stop slipups before they become binges, and don't allow yourself to get too hungry or bored. Use the exercises in this book to make sure you know what's likely to trip you up and have an action plan prepared in advance that will help you troubleshoot those problem spots.

THE PASTA PERFORMANCE CONNECTION

An endurance athlete sitting down to an enormous bowl of pasta the night before a race is one of the enduring clichés of the sports world. Unfortunately, this has sent the misleading message that having an active lifestyle means you have to eat lots of carbs. In fact, many athletes are coming to appreciate the benefits of controlling carbohydrates.

As with nonathletes, doing Atkins can be the right strategy for many competitive athletes. Those engaging in sports who are also trying to manage their weight have found they have more energy and no drops in blood sugar—and peaks and troughs in energy—that come with eating a lot of carbs, especially poor quality ones.

When performance counts, even a few extra pounds can compromise results. Athletes at any skill level can benefit from competing at optimal body weight—not just to move faster but to reduce wear and tear on the body and make participation more enjoyable.

What many recreational athletes don't realize is that when they try to lose weight by restricting calories, they may not be giving their bodies sufficient fuel. In one study, for example, cyclists on a diet comprised of 7 percent carbohydrate have been able to pedal nearly twice as long as those eating a diet comprised of 75 percent carbohydrate.

Another advantage is that when you do Atkins, you get enough protein and calories to prevent the muscle loss that can accompany weight loss on low-calorie diets. Your efforts are spent building new muscle tissue, not trying to make up for what your body has broken down. Another example of free speed!

MOTIVATION: THE WINNER'S EDGE

While Ongoing Weight Loss and Maintenance on Atkins will be easier and more pleasurable than methods you've tried in the past, it will take a little effort and a little finesse. This week we'll show you how you can take what you've learned over the last ten weeks to make a program you can live with for life.

MAKING IT WORK

When faced with a real-life challenge, ask yourself, "How am I going to make this work?"

If your lunch was higher in carbs than it should have been, how can you shift your schedule to get in a little extra exercise to compensate? Or how can you reduce the amount of carbs in tonight's dinner menu?

Making it work means not accepting excuses from that self-defeating inner voice. If you want to find excuses not to work out, control your carbs, or make the extra time to do something special for yourself, you will. Excuses are low-hanging fruit, there for the picking. Most of us are experts at this form of self-delusion. But you can also choose *not* to give those excuses the power to stop you.

This week pay attention to your inner voice. You should hear alarm bells go off every time it attempts to distract you from your goals. "It's so chilly outside. I don't feel like going for my walk tonight," it might say, or "I've had such a terrible day. I really deserve those chocolate chip cookies."

When you hear that bell, you have a mandate: Turn your negative thoughts into positive action. You know how to do the right thing, now do it! Silence that self-defeating inner voice by asking yourself not *whether* you can make it work but *how* you're going to make it happen.

"Not wanting to" is no excuse for not showing up. It's no reason to sacrifice the rewards of achieving the goals you've set for yourself. It's okay not to want to—it's even okay to complain and feel sorry for yourself while you're doing it. The important thing is that you not give up.

You might think that a "no excuses" policy sounds like something you'd hear from a drill sergeant. But you now have the tools to step up to the challenge. We're not asking anything from you that you can't deliver. That "I don't want to" voice sounds hollow in your ears, as well it should. When you take positive action instead of giving in to the excuse, you replace that whine with a strong, steadying voice, an authority whose calm builds your confidence. If you need a little boost, look back to see how far you've already come by reviewing your accomplishments in your Atkins Advantage Journal.

COPING WITH CURVE BALLS

There's a difference between failing to follow through on your evening walk because you "don't want to" and falling off the Program because of real obstacles that life serves up. You might argue that tough talk can get you through a moment of ennui or laziness, but what if the barrier is much more significant than merely feeling sorry for yourself?

Of the people who have slimmed down on Atkins only to gain the weight back later, more often than not they can point to a life-changing event that got them off track: a divorce, the death of a parent, a sick child, a lost job. Still, without exception, every one of these people wished they had stayed on Atkins, and some were able to resume Atkins later and achieve permanent weight loss.

Abandoning Atkins makes things worse, not better. When something devastating happens, you already feel out of control. Relinquishing control over your weight and your health by getting back on the blood sugar roller coaster will only compound your misery.

Atkins isn't a "diet" or something you do only when the sun is shining. It's what you do and how you eat for good. That's really what it means to do Atkins your way: to incorporate it into your life in such a way that it's not negotiable.

It is possible to cope with a major life event without gaining back the weight. We hope you won't have to use these tips, but they'll help if you do:

Avoid the trap of "I have bigger things to worry about than my weight right now." Think about how bad it will feel to lose control of your carb intake—the mood and energy swings, the return of symptoms and cravings, the weight gain. Remember that by eating correctly and exercising, you're helping your body better cope with stress.

Talk about it. Talk about the stresses in your life and about the difficulties you're having in weight loss as well. Enlist a close friend, your Atkins buddy, or a professional to listen.

You matter, too. You might find yourself putting someone else first during a difficult time, and that's to be commended. Remember, however, that you are a better and more able caretaker if you make it a priority to keep yourself in good health.

Do your best. We've talked extensively about how important it is to "make it count," to challenge and push yourself to do your best. Sometimes that means bettering your best, exceeding your expectations, and blazing past your self-imposed limitations. Other times doing your best means asking nothing more of yourself than showing up. Some days, especially during periods of great stress when it's hard to do anything at all, it's enough just to do *something*. You don't have to beat your best time, for example, but do try to go for a 20-minute walk.

Make time to relax. Revisit the relaxation technique on page 54 as often as you need. It can make a big difference in a small amount of time. Taking a short break in the form of meditation or relaxation can be restorative and centering when your life seems to be falling apart.

It isn't only health and weight loss commitments that we're tempted to jettison when under severe stress. It's everything—our personal appearance, our friendships, our family relationships, and even the housekeeping. Doing so only makes the situation worse. We know that it's hard to feel motivated when the rug has been pulled out from under you, but that's when it is all the more important.

You *will* come out on the other side of whatever you're going through. The more you do, the better you'll feel. Whatever victories you can push yourself to achieve when things are tough will buoy you. So don't ask too much of yourself, but don't ask for too little, either.

Fitness: The Best You

FOCUS FOR THE WEEK: YOU WILL FURTHER INDIVIDUALIZE YOUR FITNESS REGIMEN AND CONTINUE TO INCREASE THE INTENSITY OF YOUR WORKOUTS TO KEEP CHALLENGING YOURSELF AS YOU GET MORE FIT.

Cardio → 30 minutes, minimum → 4 times
Stretching → 30 minutes → 3 times
Strength training → 2 times at a pace that is comfortable for you

> **ATKINS ADVANTAGE TIP**
>
> Keep a spare set of sneakers and workout clothes in the trunk of your car or in your office. That way your good intentions won't be derailed when a meeting runs long and you don't have time to run home to get your workout gear. You'll also be prepared to work out if you find yourself with the time and inclination. Clothing layers and foul-weather gear will mean that a change in weather won't spoil your plans.

Do your stretches at a pace that is comfortable for you. These stretches may take you longer than 30 minutes.

One of the most consistent messages we hear from Atkins Achievers is that they became involved with a sport after losing some of their weight, and this, in turn, helped them lose the rest. Whether a sport satisfies your competitive spirit or your need for social contact, or you simply find it fun, here are some ideas for you:

- Play ball! Tossing a baseball, throwing a Frisbee, or kicking a ball in the park with your kids all count as long as your heart rate stays in the target zone.

- Partner up for a racket sport such as tennis, squash, or racquetball.

- Don't forget about winter sports such as skiing (downhill and cross-country), snowshoeing, and ice skating.

- There are lots of adult leagues for team sports such as basketball, volleyball, softball, football, soccer, and even swimming. Check your YMCA, community bulletin board, high school, or local community college.

Reinvestigate an activity you enjoyed as a child but have let fall by the wayside.

CARDIO

Use at least one of your cardio sessions this week to explore a sport or activity as a substitute for one of your workouts. The chart below provides some suggestions at various levels, but first go to page 131 and reevaluate your current cardio fitness level. Based on how much you have increased your endurance and strength, find your fitness level on the chart to see the activities you can substitute for at least one of your cardio sessions. Once you are able to maintain your High cardio effort for 20 minutes, you will add five to ten minutes per session each week until you can maintain this effort for 45 minutes. Be sure to include a five- to ten-minute warm-up and a five- to ten-minute cooldown. As your fitness level improves, increase your speed to maintain the High level.

If you can, move from brisk walking to jogging, beginning with slow jogging lasting for five to ten minutes and alternating with brisk walking. Gradually increase the amount of time spent jogging until you are able to jog continuously. Following this approach, combined with four aerobic sessions as outlined in this chapter, will ensure that you meet the fitness recommendations of the Centers for Disease Control and the American College of Sports Medicine.

ALTERNATIVE CARDIO ACTIVITIES

LEVEL ONE	LEVEL TWO	LEVEL THREE
BOWLING	BADMINTON	BASKETBALL
CANOEING (LIGHT)	SHOOTING BASKETS	HANDBALL
CROQUET	SKATING (ICE, ROLLER)	RACQUETBALL
DANCING (SQUARE, SOCIAL)	SKIING (LIGHT CROSS-COUNTRY)	ROPE SKIPPING
FISHING (WADING)	SKIING (MODERATE DOWNHILL)	SKIING (HEAVY DOWNHILL)
GOLF (USING CART)	SOFTBALL	SKIING (MODERATE CROSS-COUNTRY)
PING-PONG	SWIMMING	SNOWSHOEING
VOLLEYBALL (MODERATE)	TENNIS (MODERATE SKILL)	SOCCER
	WATERSKIING	SQUASH
		TOUCH FOOTBALL

STRETCHING EXERCISES

As a visit to any yoga class will reveal, we're all flexible in different parts of our body. Some people can't grasp their hands behind their backs, while others can do this easily but only dream of the day when they can touch their toes. This week, although you'll do stretching exercises for every part of the body as usual, we'd like to encourage you to focus on learning and addressing your personal trouble spots.

Lie quietly on the floor, perhaps after a workout, and feel where the tension is in your body. Which areas are relaxed, and which are clenched like a fist? When you have your answers, you're going to do another round of stretching this week that concentrates specifically on those tight areas. If you can, do these additional stretches every day. Over the course of the week you will notice how much more flexible you become in these previously locked-down areas.

You have now learned how to stretch from head to toe. As you declare your independence, choose from the information below to meet your individual needs.

LEGS

Calf Stretch, page 151

Quad Stretch, page 77

Low Back and Hamstring Combo Stretch, page 79

Butterfly, page 65

Forward Lunge, page 149

LOWER BACK

Low Back and Hamstring Combo Stretch, page 79

Side Bending, page 198

Press Up, page 78

Cat and Dog, page 64

Reclining Ankle-to-Knee Stretch, page 150

ABS

Press Up, page 78

Belly Up, page 199

Cat and Dog, page 64

ARMS

Shoulder Hug, page 62

Head Up, Chest Out, page 63

STRENGTH TRAINING

This week you'll replace the strength training portions of your workout with the following exercises. They are designed to help you develop muscles and skills that will stand you in good stead no matter what sport you choose.

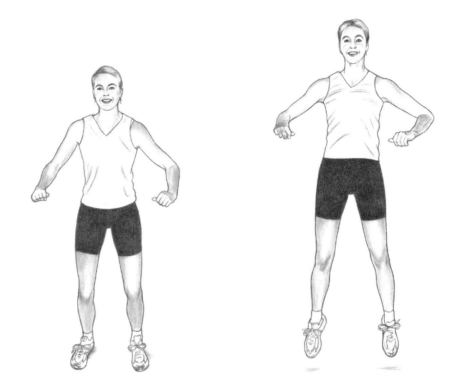

VERTICAL JUMPS

For quadriceps (the big muscles on the front of your thighs). This exercise is designed to build your strength, speed, and bone strength, and enhance your balance. It will also improve your "jump" for sports such as basketball and volleyball. Note: If you're in Level One or have arthritis or other joint problems, you may want to skip this exercise or do it in a swimming pool.

Bending your knees slightly and keeping your feet shoulder-width apart, hold your arms slightly out to each side (ready for action), jump, and try to land in the same spot.

Number of Reps

Level One: five, jumping only high enough to barely lift feet from the ground. With time, jump higher and gradually increase reps to ten per set.

Levels Two and Three: ten, increasing to 20 and gradually jumping higher

Number of Sets All Levels: three

Modification: Instead of jumping in place, jump back and forth across a line on the ground to improve agility and balance, and strengthen additional muscle groups.

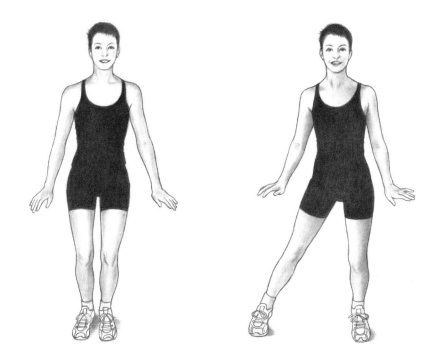

SIDE SHUFFLE

For quadriceps and inner thighs. This exercise will build leg strength, balance, and agility. It's a favorite among basketball and football players.

1. Bend your knees slightly.

2. Shuffle sideways to your left for four steps, without allowing your feet to cross one another.

3. Shuffle sideways to the right for four steps, and shuffle back to the left for four steps.

Number of Reps All Levels: three (repeating all steps three times)

Modification: For Levels Two and Three, hold light weights and shuffle for ten steps if you have enough space. If space does not allow this, perform ten reps without weights.

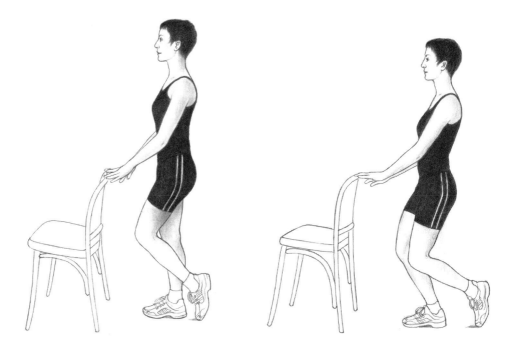

ONE-LEGGED STAND

For building leg strength and overall balance. Balance is useful in all sports, but it is equally important in daily life and can help avoid injury.

1. Stand with your left hand on a support such as a chair, a low bookshelf, or an arm rail, at hip height.

2. Inhale, gazing straight ahead at a fixed point. Slowly exhale, bending your right knee so that you lower yourself about 6 to 8 inches while holding your left heel just off the floor. Do not bend too far, which would put undue stress on the knee joint.

3. Try to hold this position for three seconds as you inhale and exhale evenly, then slowly push up to the starting position.

4. Switch sides and repeat.

Number of Reps All Levels: five

Number of Sets

    Level One: one

    Levels Two and Three: two, increasing to three, and then add reps slowly, building to 15 per set

Modifications: If this is easy for you, try these variations:

- Do the exercise without holding on to the support. (Stay close to it in case you lose your balance.)

- Change the orientation of your gaze. Look first over your right shoulder, then over your left.

- To improve balance, keep your eyes closed instead of focused on a point in front of you.

- For a more advanced version, perform the original exercise while holding dumbbells.

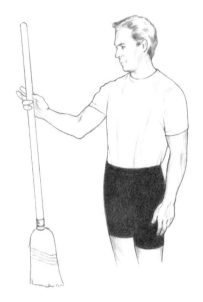

BROOM BUILDER

For building hand and forearm strength, which is particularly useful if you play racket sports.

1. Hold a broom vertical to the floor with your right hand. The bottom of the broom should be a few inches off the floor.

2. Move your fingers down the full length of the broom handle so that you are gradually advancing it upward. Don't move your arm but use your forearm muscles to stabilize your hand while your fingers do the work.

3. Switch hands and repeat.

Number of Reps All Levels: one, increasing to five or more per hand

ADVANTAGE CHECKPOINT: END OF WEEK ELEVEN

Weigh and measure yourself. Enter the results in your Atkins Advantage Journal and compare the results with last week's. See page 123 for further guidance about evaluating your progress and decide how to proceed.

SIXTEEN

WEEK TWELVE: LIFETIME MAINTENANCE, OR THE BEGINNING OF THE REST OF YOUR LIFE

Over the last eleven weeks you have learned that it's possible to control your carbohydrate intake—and, in turn, your weight and your health. You've also learned that when many people realize they have the power to control their weight, they awaken to the fact that they can extend this success to other areas of their lives as well.

If you continue to apply to your own dreams the same focus, commitment, and energy that you brought to the Atkins Advantage Program, there is truly no limit to what you can accomplish. Mastery is a great multiplier. The feeling of empowerment you get from a success like this doesn't fade easily because it's one that provides you with renewable benefits each day. The Atkins Advantage Program was designed to continuously stoke this flame so that it burns brighter with each passing week, lighting your path through the rest of your life. The 12-week program may be drawing to its end, but your own success story is just beginning—and is yours to create.

NUTRITION: THE HEART OF THE MATTER

All the work you've done on the Program thus far has prepared you for this moment: the beginning of the rest of your life. No matter which phase of the Atkins Nutritional Approach you're in, when the Atkins Advantage Program is over, you'll take with you the tools you need to make this new, healthy way of eating a permanent part of your life.

To find meal plans appropriate for your daily net carb gram count, see the lists that begin on page 278.

Continue to take a good multivitamin, essential oils, and a fiber supplement. If you are experiencing a return of hunger or cravings, you may want to consider chromium (page 107) or L-glutamine (page 141).

If you are still in the process of losing weight, you will continue to add back carbs according to the rules of the phase that you're in, moving up the Atkins Carbohydrate Ladder (page 14).

If you are already in Lifetime Maintenance, continue to stay at your Atkins Carbohydrate Equilibrium (ACE).

If you're ready to cross the threshold from Pre-Maintenance to Lifetime Maintenance, it's time to review the rules of this phase that will allow you to maintain your goal weight permanently. Even if you are not there yet, continue reading to learn what's ahead for you.

You are ready to segue to Lifetime Maintenance when you've been able to successfully maintain your goal weight for four consecutive weeks.

This is a subtle but important point: You don't begin Lifetime Maintenance the day you reach your goal weight. Instead, you stay in Pre-Maintenance until you're firmly in control. Only after you have maintained your goal weight for a full month are you officially in Lifetime Maintenance. If you have reached that important milestone, you deserve a round of applause for your tremendous accomplishment.

By committing to this program and seeing it through, you have achieved the first part of your goal: reaching your target weight. Now the most rewarding and challenging work begins: maintaining it for life.

THE RULES OF LIFETIME MAINTENANCE

- Continue to choose from a wide variety of natural, whole, nutrient-rich carbohydrates.

- Continue to eat sufficient protein, fiber-rich veggies, and natural fats to feel comfortably full.

- Continue to count your carbs so that you stay at or just below your ACE, the maximum number of grams of net carbs you can eat without gaining or losing weight.

- Continue with your fitness program.

- Continue with your supplementation program.

- Weigh yourself once a week and never let yourself gain more than 5 pounds without making an immediate course correction.

- Adjust your ACE as necessary if your lifestyle or other changes affect your metabolism.

- Drink plenty of water.

TROUBLESHOOTING LIFETIME MAINTENANCE

Slight fluctuations in your weight—2 or 3 pounds or even more—will occur and are perfectly normal, sometimes even over the course of a day. If you see the numbers on the scale begin to creep up, and you think those pounds reflect more than water weight, hormonal fluctuations, or the big dinner you ate last night, it's time to pay attention. Another indicator of trouble is if your clothes start to feel tight. Inches were as important as pounds when you were taking off weight and they are just as important when it comes to maintaining it. Keep up with your Atkins Advantage Journal to ensure that you're paying attention to your actions and your goals. Make sure that you do not revert to old habits that got you into trouble in the first place.

If straightening up your act gets the needle on the scale back under control, that's great, but remember: If you don't maintain the Atkins lifestyle, you won't maintain your goal weight. If that happens and you begin to approach the crucial 5-pound mark, you must reduce your daily carbs by 5 or 10 grams until you regain control and reestablish your goal weight.

If cutting back on carbs isn't effective, however, or if you experience out-of-control hunger, cravings, energy dips in the afternoon, or any of the other symptoms of unstable blood sugar that you had before you started doing Atkins, you may need to return to Induction to correct your metabolism along with your behavior. Generally a week or two is all that is needed. Then don't leap from Induction back to Lifetime Maintenance; instead, gradually increase your carb intake. You should be able to fairly quickly retrace your progress through the Program back to your goal weight (see page 23).

Circumstances change—and with them your carbohydrate tolerance. Your ACE isn't etched in stone. If you stop your fitness program—due to an injury or because you're traveling more—or there are changes in your health or hormonal status or you start taking certain medications, your ACE may change as a result. Let's say you hurt your knee, and your doctor tells you to stay off it for a while. The 80 grams daily of net carbs you were eating while exercising regularly may now be too much; you will likely have to scale back to avoid weight gain. On the other hand, if you change jobs and start walking to work or stop taking a certain drug, you could experience weight loss, meaning your ACE could move up.

Most injuries are temporary issues; aging isn't. Dr. Atkins used to see patients who had been in control of their weight for years. "I'm not doing anything differently," they'd say, "so why have I gained 5 pounds?" The answer, of course, was that time had done its inevitable work on their metabolism, and their carbohydrate tolerance had lowered as a result. Women and men both go through hormonal changes that make weight management more of a challenge as they age, and taking certain medications (see the list on page 157) may also result in a metabolic slowdown.

Although most people's metabolism does slow with the passage of years, that doesn't mean you're powerless to affect your destiny. By keeping up with your fitness routine and even intensifying it, you can resist the natural tendency for your ACE to drop as you age. That way you can continue to enjoy a wide variety of nutritious foods that will help you maintain your health and vigor.

To make sure you maintain your goal weight, keep an eye on your ACE and make adjustments if you find that you're either losing or gaining weight.

LIFETIME MAINTENANCE *DON'TS*

The difference between diets and Atkins is that this program doesn't end when you reach your target. You want your goal weight to be your *permanent* weight! The difference between Lifetime Maintenance and the three phases that preceded it is that this is not only a phase but a lifestyle. So don't fall into the trap of thinking that reaching your goal is the end of the journey, that you're "done" when you get there. It might be the end of weight loss, but it's only the beginning of the Atkins lifestyle.

Avoiding the following pitfalls guarantees your success for life:

Don't slip back into the way you used to eat. Although you can eat more grams of carbs and a wider variety of carbohydrate foods than you could in the earlier phases of the Program, you must continue to make healthy choices. Sugary sodas, candy, processed foods made with added sugars, bleached white flour, and trans fats are all still out of bounds.

Don't stop reading labels. At this point you have a much better feel for what is an acceptable food and what isn't than you did when you started, but you still need to read labels and check your carb gram counter if there is any question in your mind.

Don't ignore warning signs. Pay attention to your body. If you experience mood swings, energy dips, cravings, or out-of-control hunger, you know that you're in danger of losing control of your metabolism. Be sensitive to these changes and make a course correction by decreasing your carb intake before damage has been done.

ATKINS FOR THE BEST OF LIFE

Over the last 11 weeks you have changed your life. You look and feel better, and you've reduced your risk of heart disease, diabetes, and a host of other diseases and conditions directly linked to carrying too much weight.

To stay focused on the goal of permanent weight control in the weeks, months, and years to come, return to this book whenever you feel it can help. While you've probably internalized the healthy lifestyle choices introduced in this program, it's still a good idea to reinforce those new habits by continuing to use the new techniques you have learned. In particular, your Atkins Advantage Journal is a powerful resource. You can use it to keep track of your victories, setbacks, and challenges. Even if you decide not to use it all the time, you can return to it when confronting a setback.

The activities in this book will come in handy as you set and meet challenges for yourself in the future. An activity that didn't resonate with you when you first read it may have new meaning down the road. Or you may find that you have "all new answers" for an activity you've already done.

SPOTLIGHT ON OATS

Oats, the most nutritious of the cereal grasses, are filled with an abundance of fiber, making them effective at lowering cholesterol levels. Oat bran is an excellent way to add supplementary fiber to your diet without adding carbs that impact blood sugar levels. Oats also contain high concentrations of vitamin B_1 and goodly amounts of vitamins B_2 and E.

Oats come in many different forms. In the United States, rolled oats are the most popular and include old-fashioned oats, quick-cooking oats, and instant oatmeal. Instant oatmeal may be convenient, but it is by far the least nutritious of the bunch. Your best bet is old-fashioned oats, which takes only five minutes to prepare. Equally nutritious are steel-cut oats, sometimes known as Scotch or Irish oatmeal, which has a nutty texture. Instead of being rolled, the whole grain is cut into smaller pieces. It requires longer cooking than rolled varieties, although soaking them overnight cuts cooking time in half.

Oats are part of the final rung on the Carbohydrate Ladder, so most people doing Atkins don't add oats to their meals until they are in Pre-Maintenance. If you have a high metabolism, you may be able to do so earlier. A half cup of uncooked old-fashioned oatmeal contains 27 grams of net carbs. Serve it with a little butter or cream to cut the glycemic impact.

Oats are for more than just oatmeal. Enjoy low-carb granola for breakfast or snacks (see www.atkins.com for a recipe), perhaps with low-carb or no-sugar-added yogurt. Rolled oats are a nutritious replacement for bread crumbs in your favorite meatloaf recipe.

Atkins.com is another invaluable resource at your disposal. Use the carb gram counter to keep track of your daily carb count. Surf the recipes for ideas and use the list to find out what you'll need to make them.

The tools you've acquired, the habits you've adopted, and the healthier lifestyle you've embraced as you have progressed through the 12 weeks of the Atkins Advantage Program are yours for good. You've learned healthy new eating and fitness habits that will stand you in good stead for a lifetime. You've learned how to motivate yourself when the going gets tough. And you now have all the skills you need to get yourself back on track no matter what derails you. These tools are what distinguish Atkins, and they'll make it possible to hold on to this slim new you forever.

MOTIVATION: THE WINNER'S EDGE

The Atkins Advantage Program has acted as your "training wheels." Now that you know how to ride, you're free to make your own course.

If the idea of riding solo has you afraid that you'll lose control or spin off course, rest assured that you've developed the skills and techniques you'll need to reach your goal weight and maintain it for life. Twelve weeks can transform new behaviors into ingrained habits. That's why we know that your successes will only continue to multiply in the weeks, months, and years to come.

In this section you'll acquire motivational tools that you can take with you into Week Thirteen and beyond.

In the same way that you began this program by tossing or giving away every last scrap of processed, refined, starchy, sugary, trans-fat-filled food in your pantry, it's essential this week to jettison your anxieties and self-doubts about the program going forward. Lighten your load by eliminating thoughts that weigh you down and hold you back. Once you banish your unhealthy thoughts, you can go about replacing them with productive, enriching, nourishing ones.

Your first activity this week (and any other time that negative feelings threaten to drag you down) is to eliminate any worries you might have about maintaining your new healthy lifestyle. Worrying doesn't do much to solve your problems. This visualization is surprisingly effective, especially when you're tossing and turning in bed, unable to calm your mind.

UP, UP, AND AWAY

Do this activity with your eyes closed in a quiet spot where you will not be disturbed. Take a few slow, deep breaths. Start at your toes and work your way up your body, willing each muscle group to relax, until you reach the crown of your head.

Once you are completely relaxed, imagine yourself in the middle of an enormous meadow filled with green grass and open space as far as the eye can see. As you look up into the cloudless blue sky, you see a small shape. As it gets closer, you can see that it's a beautiful hot air balloon, making a slow and graceful descent to the meadow. (Or perhaps you prefer a gleaming silvery rocket ship—whatever works for you.)

The balloon lands silently on the grass a few feet away from you. You see that there is a basket at your feet, filled with heavy polished flat stones. Each one of these stones is engraved with the name of one of your worries. One might read "Gaining it all back," for instance, or "Getting stuck" or simply "Macaroni and cheese." There are as many rocks in the basket as there are worries in your mind.

You're going to let those worries go now. Walk over to the hot air balloon and, one by one, take the stones from the basket and load them into the gondola. Read each stone as you hold it in your hands and feel its weight slip from your fingers as you place it into the bottom of the gondola. When you have transferred every one of the stones, untie the rope tethering the balloon to the ground. Stand and watch as it rises, heavier now but still ascending into the blue sky. Watch it until it's only a speck and then finally disappears, carrying your worries with it.

This may sound like an unlikely cure for real anxieties, but if you give it a chance, you'll find that it's a very effective treatment for the worries that stalk you in the dark hours of the night.

Fitness: The Best You

FOCUS FOR THE WEEK: IT'S TIME TO CONSIDER JOINING A GYM OR HEALTH CLUB. YOU WILL MAINTAIN THE SAME FREQUENCY AS LAST WEEK FOR ALL COMPONENTS OF YOUR FITNESS PROGRAM, BUT TAKE ADVANTAGE OF MACHINES TO TAKE YOUR CARDIO AND STRENGTH TRAINING ROUTINES TO A NEW LEVEL.

Cardio → 30 minutes, minimum → 4 times
Stretching → 20–30 minutes → 2–3 times
Strength training → 2 times

Do your stretches and complete the exercises at a pace that is comfortable for you. The stretches may take you longer than 30 minutes.

During the last few weeks you have individualized your fitness program by taking a dance class, picking up a sport, or engaging in other activities. A gym, health club, or fitness center can be another great option for getting the most out of your workouts.

Some people find the energy of other people working out at a gym infectious and enjoy using the available equipment. Others are motivated by having paid for a membership: They show up to get their money's worth—and get fit as part of the bargain!

You may already belong to a club, or you may only now be feeling fit enough to work out with other people. If you find the idea intriguing, then one of your tasks this week is to get a day pass at a local gym or health club to see if you'd be interested in joining. Like all businesses, different gyms have different styles. You'll want to visit before you sign up. Keep in mind that cost can vary a great deal, and you should probably be able to find a place that fits your budget.

Here is some helpful information when choosing a gym or health club:

- Choose a gym close to work or home. You're more likely to go if you don't have to travel far for your workouts.

- Visit at the times you think you're most likely to attend. Most establishments cater to different crowds at different times of the day, and some time periods are much busier than others.

- Some gyms are friendlier to beginners than others. If you're just starting out, look for other beginners and ask the staff if there's someone available to answer questions.

- Make sure there's enough equipment to handle the traffic and that there are sign-up sheets for the machines that are most in demand. You don't want to waste time waiting to use a machine.

- Inspect the facilities to learn whether the space is clean and orderly and that the equipment is well maintained and in good working order. Check locker rooms and bathrooms as well.

- You should feel comfortable with the music they're playing—and the decibel level they're playing it at.

- Find out whether the classes they offer are ones you're interested in and at an appropriate level for you.

Some people feel self-conscious when they're beginning at a gym. If you're just starting out, you certainly have nothing to be embarrassed about. You're doing what it takes to get in great shape. Take heart: In most cases you'll find that the majority of people are there to get a workout and to concentrate on *their* bodies, not yours!

CARDIO

Experiment with the cardio equipment at the gym: stationary bikes, elliptical trainers, rowing machines, stair-climbing machines, treadmills. Try a class or, if available, enjoy the pool or running track. Don't forget about intensity: Take your pulse or use a heart rate monitor to make sure you're working at the right level. If you want to hit the gym for just one of your four cardio days and keep your other three days the same, that's fine. Feel free to divide your program up in the way that suits you best.

STRENGTH TRAINING

Gym equipment is a terrific way to get fit, but you must use it correctly or run the risk of serious injury. If you haven't worked out at a gym, or if it has been a while, you'll definitely want to consider getting some one-on-one training. Some gyms offer an introductory lesson for new members. Ask, and if yours does, don't miss it. A session with a personal trainer is a splurge, but it may be worthwhile if you need a lesson on how to use the machines correctly. As with your cardio workouts, you can enjoy the novelty of the strength training equipment at the gym for as many or as few days as you like.

> **ATKINS ADVANTAGE TIP**
>
> Choosing the right weight takes a bit of trial and error, and it's better to err on the side of too light. Starting too heavy can lead to injury and loud clanging of weights!

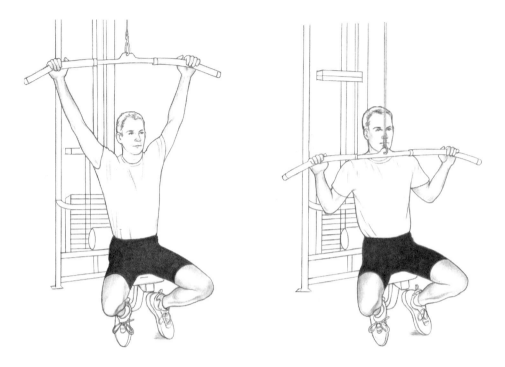

LAT PULL DOWN

For latissimus dorsi and biceps, helping to increase upper back strength and definition.

1. Kneel or sit facing away from the machine. Grab the bar, palms facing outward, with your hands on the bar just beyond the width of your shoulders. Keep your gaze forward and your head and torso in a straight line.

2. Inhaling, bring the bar down to the level of your chin. Do not yank the bar; the movement should be smooth and controlled.

3. Exhaling, return the bar to the starting position, again with control. Don't let it jerk you out of your seat.

Number of Reps All Levels: ten, using the weight at which you can comfortably reach this goal

Number of Sets All Levels: one set of ten, gradually increasing to three sets of ten, before increasing reps to 15. Once at three sets of 15, increase weight by one 5-pound increment.

Modification: You can do a number of variations of this exercise by changing the position of your hands.

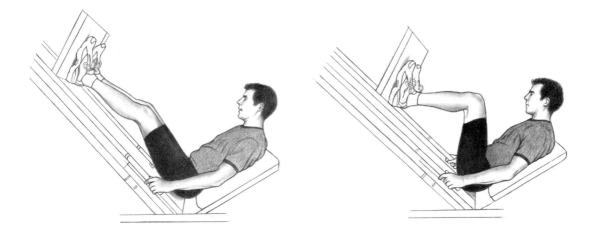

LEG PRESS

For quadriceps, hamstrings, gluteus maximus (butt), leading to greater overall leg strength and power for cycling, jumping, and running.

1. Sit with your back against the padded seat, keeping your abdominal muscles engaged and your knees bent at approximately 90 degrees. With each leg in alignment, place your feet flat on the platform, shoulder-width apart. Your weight should be evenly distributed between the balls of your feet and your heels.

2. Exhaling, press the platform out until your legs are almost straight. Do not lock your knees.

3. Inhaling, return the weight smoothly to the starting position.

Number of Reps All Levels: ten, using a weight at which you can comfortably reach this goal

Number of Sets All Levels: one set of ten, gradually increasing to three sets of ten, before increasing reps to 15. Once at three sets of 15, increase weight by one 5-pound increment.

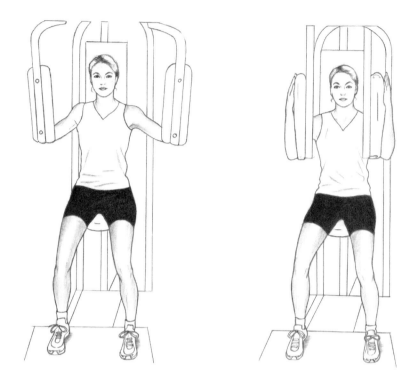

PECTORAL FLY

For pectoralis major and minor (chest muscles) and anterior and lateral deltoids (fronts and backs of shoulders).

1. Sit with your back against the padded seat and your feet on the ground. Hold the handles with both hands.

2. Exhaling, slowly pull the handles toward the center of your chest as you concentrate on squeezing the muscles in your chest.

3. Inhaling, slowly return your hands to the starting position.

Number of Reps All Levels: ten, using a weight at which you can comfortably reach this goal

Number of Sets All Levels: one set of ten, gradually increasing to three sets of ten, before increasing reps to 15. Once at three sets of 15, increase weight by one 5-pound increment.

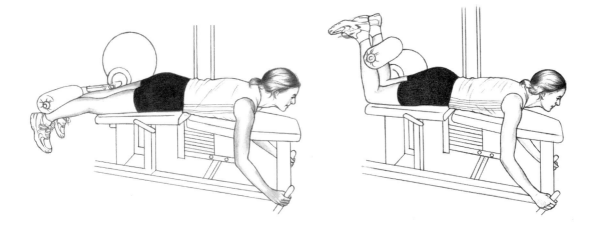

HAMSTRING CURLS

For hamstrings (the large muscles behind the upper leg, used for running, jumping, cycling, and walking).

1. Lie prone on the bench with the pad resting just over your ankles.

2. With your hips and abdomen pressing against the bench or pad, bring your feet toward your buttocks by bending your knees to almost a 90-degree position.

3. Inhaling, release the weight slowly and with control, returning to the starting position and stopping just before your legs are completely straight. (It is worth noting that this is a very common weight-clanging exercise, typically caused by not maintaining full control of the weight as it is lowered.)

Number of Reps All Levels: ten, using a weight at which you can comfortably reach this goal.

Number of Sets All Levels: one set of ten, gradually increasing to three sets of ten, before increasing reps to 15. Once at three sets of 15, increase weight by one 6-pound increment.

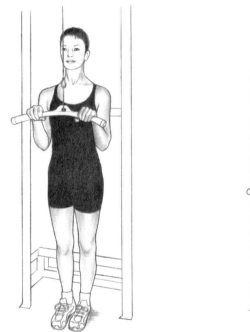
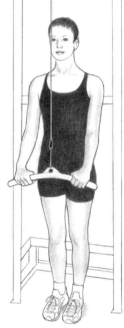

TRICEPS PULL DOWN

To firm and add definition to the upper arms and shoulders.

1. Stand with your back straight and your feet slightly spread apart.

2. Grasp the bar with your hands in a comfortable position (about 12 inches apart).

3. Slowly, keeping your elbows close to your torso, press your hands downward toward your thighs until your elbows are straight.

Number of Reps All Levels: ten
Number of Sets All Levels: one, increasing to three as you get stronger

If you've discovered over the last 12 weeks that you enjoy setting and achieving goals, reaching the end of the Atkins Advantage Program doesn't mean you have to stop.

Many of the Atkins Achievers have signed up for an athletic event as a way of giving themselves a fitness goal. It doesn't have to be a competition, although it can be. One popular choice is a walk or run to benefit a cause, such as those that raise funds for breast cancer and AIDS research. Doing good adds a little incentive.

Even if the event isn't competitive, you'll find that preparing for it changes the focus of your workout. You're not just exercising, you are "in training." Making your fitness goals concrete in the form of an event can be another aid to help you achieve your personal best.

ADVANTAGE CHECKPOINT: END OF WEEK TWELVE

Weigh and measure yourself. Enter the results in your Atkins Advantage Journal and compare the results with those of last week. See page 123 for further guidance about how to evaluate your progress and decide how to proceed.

For those of you who are not yet at your goal weight, the meal plans at progressively higher carb levels will help you as you move forward. Also, be sure to reread each section as you enter a new phase and continue to use your Atkins Advantage Journal to track your progress.

For OWL, see page 86.

For Pre-Maintenance, see page 188.

For Lifetime Maintenance, see page 241.

By now you undoubtedly have your own definition of the Atkins Advantage. Is it the ability to lose weight without deprivation or guilt? Is it the metabolic advantage of being able to consume more calories than you would on a low-fat program? Is it the ability to customize the program to your needs and tastes? Is it the fact that you can keep that lost weight off permanently and painlessly? Is it the "toolbox" of healthy life skills you now possess? Is it the collateral advantage that spills into the rest of your life that comes from knowing that there's nothing beyond your reach?

It's all of those things—and more. It's empowerment. As you leave the Atkins Advantage Program, take with you the incomparable satisfaction of knowing that you are now in control of your life for good! Your new habits and the mindfulness you bring to your choices will be with you not just at the supermarket and dining table but in life. You'll stay on the Advantage path long after this book is finished.

The end of this program is both a finish line and a new beginning. It represents both an incredible accomplishment and a very exciting new opportunity. With that in mind, we'd like to leave you with a final challenge: Now that you've transformed yourself both inside and out, let your dreams be your guide, and empowerment the fuel you use to reach your destination.

PART III

THE MEAL PLANS

SEVENTEEN

TWELVE WEEKS OF MEAL PLANS WITH 20 TO 80 GRAMS OF NET CARBS

These plans were designed to give you a "taste" of how your food choices grow as you increase your intake of carbohydrates. And never fear, even in Induction you will be able to savor an exciting array of foods every day. Just give the two weeks of Induction meal plans the once-over and see for yourself. (We've provided one week's worth of meal plans from 25 to 80 daily grams of net carbs.)

These sample plans are just a guideline—because you should always feel free to eat the foods that best suit your tastes and economic considerations. As you have learned, the Atkins Advantage Program is meant to be customized for you, which will in turn maximize your chances of achieving long-term success.

A few things to keep in mind: To a certain extent the numbers of grams of net carbs are an approximation. Moreover, there is a 10 percent spread in either direction for a given day, but each week averages out to the appropriate level. Therefore, 20-gram meals range from 18 to 22 grams of net carbs a day; 60-gram meals range from 54 to 66 grams a day. Also, when it comes to dressing salad greens, we've assumed 1 tablespoon for 1 cup of greens and 2 tablespoons for 2 to 3 cups. Each tablespoon of dressing is equal to about 1 gram of net carbs. (Of course you will be using your own dressings or low-carb or sugar-free dressings.) It's up to you to measure dressings and condiments to be sure you're not exceeding your carb intake. The same goes for cheeses, which vary slightly in their carb counts. Here we've assumed 1 gram of net carbs for each ounce of cheese, no matter the variety.

Although it is not generally necessary to count calories on Atkins, the meal plans illustrate that as you begin to add more nutrient-rich carbohydrates, you decrease the amount of fat and protein.

INDUCTION GUIDELINES

During the first two weeks of Induction, eating more frequently can ease the transition to fat-burning and stabilizing your blood sugar, which is why we have included a morning and afternoon or evening snack. Many people find that after their blood sugar stabilizes at the end of the first week, they are comfortable and have less need to snack. If this is the case, be sure to continue to eat about 20 grams of net carbs each day. After two weeks on Induction, whether or not you move on to Ongoing Weight Loss, most people find they do not need more than one snack a day, so the meal plans for 25 grams of net carbs and beyond include only one. You can have that single snack whenever it suits you or not at all. Likewise, if you prefer four or five smaller meals, you can modify the meal plans by spreading out the suggested foods as long as you always consume carbs with fat and/or protein. Sweet snacks can also be used as desserts following a meal—and vice versa.

To better absorb fat-soluble nutrients in vegetables, it is important to have them with fat. When a vegetable is listed on a meal plan, feel free to add a pat of butter or a drizzle of olive oil. On the other hand, if you are also having an oil-based salad dressing at that same meal, it is not necessary to use any additional fat or oil.

TYPICAL MENUS

As you look at the Induction meal plans (20 grams of net carbs) and those for the ensuing weeks when carb count is still relatively low, starches such as potatoes, rice, and regular bread are absent. Instead of assuming that dinner must comprise a protein dish, a vegetable or salad, and a starch, your protein dish is typically accompanied by a salad and a cooked veggie dish. (Grains and starchy vegetables will put in an appearance as your net carb count climbs, although portions will generally be smaller than you may have been accustomed to in the past.)

Feel free to substitute your favorite vegetables and sources of protein. If, for example, a meal plan calls for asparagus and you're not a fan or it isn't in season, simply substitute another vegetable, with about the same carb count, such as green beans. Likewise, if a meal plan calls for baked halibut, feel free to substitute another fish or even chicken or tofu.

Follow serving sizes carefully. If you eat larger portions of carbohydrates, your net carb gram counts will be higher. You'll note that we have also included suggested portions for protein foods, starting with 8 ounces at each meal in Induction. You may find you need more, which is fine as long as you are not stuffing yourself. Or you may find you want to eat less. Clearly, a large active man will have different caloric needs and may require more protein than a petite, sedentary woman.

Here are some "portions at a glance":

Protein: 6 ounces of meat, poultry, or fish is the size of two bars of soap.

Cheese: 1 ounce of cheese is the size of four dice.

Butter: 1 serving of butter (1 teaspoon) is the size of a thimble.

Vegetables: 1 cup of salad greens is the size of a clenched fist, and ½ cup of cooked veggies is the size of a scoop of ice cream.

Nuts and seeds: 1 ounce of nuts or seeds is the size of a ping-pong ball.

HIGHER CARB MEAL PLANS

Beginning at 40 grams of net carbs a day, we have reduced the suggested protein portions to 6 ounces to compensate for the additional carbohydrates you are now consuming. If you previously needed more than 8 ounces, you should slowly decrease your portions to find the amount you now need to feel satisfied. To make room for more carb foods without overeating, you also need to cut down on fat (which will happen naturally as you reduce portion sizes of proteins). In cases where the meal contains other protein sources—soybeans or low-carb bread, for example—the meat or fish portions can be further reduced. From 40 grams on, it is also a good idea to cut down the frequency with which you include foods such as cream, cheese, olives, and avocado.

FAVORITE CARBOHYDRATE FOODS

Certain carbohydrate foods are integral to the Atkins Nutritional Approach; among them are olives, avocados, and blueberries. Others such as broccoli and garlic were among Dr. Atkins' favorites because they are high in nutrients and/or fiber. You'll see them frequently in the meal plans that follow. For example, olives and avocados are often used as snacks in the meal plans with lower carb counts. Some carb foods that deserve to play a starring role once you are close to your goal weight—carrots, lentils, and oats, for example—may not have received the recognition they deserve.

The meal plans list most low-carb ingredients generically, so just because a slice of low-carb bread is listed as 5 grams of net carbs does not mean that all so-called low-carb breads are suitable. Some include 12 grams of net carbs per slice! As always, check carb counts on products before you buy them. If they do not comply with the counts provided on the meal plans, you may have to modify that day's plan. In a few cases we have listed an Atkins product by name because carb counts and ingredients can vary so greatly. In these cases the flavors of shakes and bars are just a suggestion; if you use another product or another flavor, make sure the carb count is the same.

CUSTOMIZING MEAL PLANS

Just because you are consuming a certain number of daily grams of net carbs does not mean that every dish or ingredient on a meal plan is suitable for you. For example, if you are at 60 grams of net carbs but have not yet introduced starchy vegetables, avoid recipes with such ingredients until you have reached that rung on the Carbohydrate Ladder. Or if you find that apples, for example, trigger cravings, don't consume a dish made with that fruit.

Go to www.atkins.com for delicious recipes. Keep the following in mind as you select recipes to individualize your meal plans:

Recipes for Phase 1: Induction

- Main dishes generally contain no more than 7 grams of net carbs per serving.

- Side dishes, desserts, snacks, and sauces generally contain no more than 3 grams of net carbs per serving.

- The following ingredients are not included: nuts, seeds, nut or seed butters, fruit, legumes, grains, starchy vegetables, dairy products other than butter, cheese or cream, or low-carb treats such as chocolate. (Nuts and seeds are permissible after the first two weeks of Induction.)

Recipes for Phase 2: Ongoing Weight Loss

- Main dishes generally contain no more than 12 grams of net carbs per serving.

- Side dishes, desserts, snacks, and sauces generally contain no more than 9 grams of net carbs per serving.

- Nuts and seeds, nut and seed butters, and berries are not included.

- Main dishes can contain 18 or more grams of net carbs per serving.

- Side dishes, desserts, snacks, and sauces can contain 10 or more grams of net carbs per serving.

- Ingredients restricted in earlier phases may be included but not bleached white flour or other refined grains or sugar in any form.

COOKING ATKINS STYLE

There are no major differences between regular cooking and controlled-carb cooking. To a large extent, cutting unnecessary carbs is simply a matter of eliminating certain habits. The bigger difference is one of ingredients.

DAY ONE

BREAKFAST

Atkins® Advantage Morning Bar (3)

2 hard-boiled eggs (1)

SUBTOTAL: 4

SNACK

¼ cup ricotta cheese (2) with 1 stalk celery (1)

Ricotta cheese makes a deliciously creamy spread for crudités.

LUNCH

Salmon salad: 8 ounces canned salmon, mixed with 2 tablespoons mayonnaise, 1 table-spoon flat-leaf parsley, and ½ cup sliced cucumber (1)

2 cups mixed greens (2), topped with 4 spears steamed asparagus (2) and vinaigrette (2)

Assume each tablespoon of vinaigrette or low-carb salad dressing contains 1 gram of net carbs.

SUBTOTAL: 7

DINNER

8 ounces grilled chicken breast

½ cup roasted broccoli (1)

1 cup romaine lettuce (1) with 2 ounces Parmesan cheese, shaved (2), 5 olives (1), and Caesar dressing (1)

Grill an extra chicken breast tonight so that making the chicken salad for tomorrow's lunch will be a breeze!

SUBTOTAL: 6

SNACK

½ cup sugar-free strawberry gelatin (1) with 2 tablespoons whipped heavy cream (0.5)

TOTAL: 21.5 GRAMS

DAY TWO

BREAKFAST

Florentine omelet: 2 eggs (1), 2 ounces cheddar cheese, shredded (2), and 1 cup chopped spinach (1)

3 slices Canadian bacon (1)

SUBTOTAL: 5

SNACK

½ Hass avocado (2)

Love avocado? Instead of enjoying it as a snack here, fill the pitted half with 6 ounces of crab salad, season with salt and pepper, and swap it for the chicken salad in today's lunch. Serve with 8 asparagus spears for the same amount of net carbs.

LUNCH

Chicken salad: 8 ounces of chicken mixed with ½ cup sliced cucumber (1), ½ cup chopped cherry tomatoes (2), chopped dill, and 2 tablespoons mayonnaise
2 cups mixed greens (2) with vinaigrette (2)

SUBTOTAL: 7

DINNER

1 cup clear broth (1)

Shrimp scampi: 8 ounces shrimp, sautéed in butter, garlic (1), and chopped parsley

2 cups romaine lettuce (2), 5 black olives (1), and ranch dressing (2)

SUBTOTAL: 7

SNACK

1 ounce Monterey Jack cheese (1)

TOTAL: 21 GRAMS

DAY THREE

BREAKFAST

1 slice rye toast (3) topped with 2 slices lox and 2 tablespoons cream cheese (1)

SUBTOTAL: 4

SNACK

1 deviled egg (0.5)

LUNCH

1 cup chicken broth (1)

Chef salad: 2 slices each thinly sliced ham, turkey, and roast beef, plus 1 chopped hard-boiled egg (0.5), 1 ounce crumbled blue cheese (1), and 2 slices crumbled bacon over 3 cups mixed greens (3) with vinaigrette (2)

SUBTOTAL: 7.5

DINNER

8 ounces grilled skirt steak

½ cup each zucchini (1) and mushrooms (1.5), sautéed

1 cup arugula salad (1), ½ cup sliced cucumber (1) with ranch dressing (1)

SUBTOTAL: 5.5

SNACK

Hot cocoa nip: ½ cup reduced-carb milk dairy beverage (1.5) with 1 tablespoon unsweetened cocoa (1) and ½ packet Splenda (0.5), heated

Looking to jazz up your hot cocoa? Add a teaspoon or two of peppermint or rum extract for no carbs and unique flavor.

TOTAL: 20.5 GRAMS

DAY FOUR

BREAKFAST

2 scrambled eggs (1)

1 slice rye toast (3)

2 slices bacon

SUBTOTAL: 4

SNACK

½ cup raw jicama (2.5) with 1 tablespoon vinaigrette (1)

If you've never had jicama, you're in for a treat! This crunchy root vegetable adds a satisfying nutty flavor to any salad and is an exciting alternative to same-old celery.

LUNCH

8-ounce turkey burger and 1 tablespoon ketchup (1), 2 cups romaine lettuce (2), and 1 ounce crumbled feta cheese (1) with vinaigrette (2)

SUBTOTAL: 6

DINNER

8 ounces grilled tuna

½ cup steamed artichoke hearts (2)

2 cups mixed greens (2) with vinaigrette (2)

Look for canned artichoke hearts in water. Those packed in oil sometimes contain hydrogenated oils.

SUBTOTAL: 6

SNACK

Atkins® Advantage Chocolate Peanut Butter Bar (2)

TOTAL: 21.5 GRAMS

DAY FIVE

BREAKFAST

Spicy turkey-and-egg scramble: 3 ounces browned ground turkey, mixed with 2 scrambled eggs (1) and seasoned with salt, red pepper flakes, and hot pepper sauce

SUBTOTAL: 1

SNACK

1 ounce Swiss cheese (1)

LUNCH

Chicken and mushroom soup: 8 ounces shredded poached chicken and ½ cup sliced mushrooms (1.5), simmered in 1 cup chicken broth (1)

2 cups endive (1), with 5 black olives (1) and vinaigrette (2)

SUBTOTAL: 6.5

DINNER

8 ounces roasted pork tenderloin

3 cups romaine lettuce (3) with 1 ounce blue cheese, crumbled (1), 2 tablespoons sun-dried tomatoes in olive oil (2), and vinaigrette (2)

SUBTOTAL: 8

SNACK

1 stalk celery (1) with 2 tablespoons soy nut butter (2)

While you should wait to introduce nuts and seeds until you're past the first two weeks of Induction, soy nuts and soy nut butter are okay. Add soy nuts to salads and spread the butter on your favorite crunchy vegetable.

TOTAL: 19.5 GRAMS

DAY SIX

BREAKFAST

Atkins® Advantage Peanut Butter Granola Bar (3)

1 hard-boiled egg (0.5)

SUBTOTAL: 4.5

SNACK

1 ounce cheddar cheese (1)

LUNCH

Cobb salad: 6 ounces grilled chicken, 1 slice bacon, crumbled, ½ Hass avocado (2), and 1 ounce blue cheese, crumbled (1), over 3 cups mixed greens (3) with vinaigrette (2)

SUBTOTAL: 8

DINNER

Beef sauté: 8 ounces ground beef sautéed with 5 chopped black olives (1), ¼ cup tomato sauce (3), and 1 cup chopped spinach (1)

Creamy mashed cauliflower: 1 cup steamed cauliflower (2) pureed with 1 tablespoon butter and 2 tablespoons heavy cream (0.5)

When pureed as described cauliflower is magically transformed into a dead ringer for mashed potatoes.

SUBTOTAL: 7.5

SNACK

5 black olives (1)

TOTAL: 22 GRAMS

DAY SEVEN

BREAKFAST
3 waffles (3) made from soya flour pancake and waffle mix with sugar-free pancake syrup

2 turkey sausages (0.5)

SUBTOTAL: 3.5

SNACK
½ Hass avocado (2)

LUNCH
Blue-cheese burger: one 8-ounce hamburger patty topped with 1 ounce melted blue cheese (1) and ½ cup chopped cherry tomatoes (2)

2 cups mixed greens (2) with ranch dressing (2)

SUBTOTAL: 7

DINNER
Chicken "parmigiana": one 8-ounce grilled chicken breast topped with small tomato, chopped (3), and 1 ounce fresh mozzarella cheese, shredded (1)

½ cup broiled eggplant (2)

1 cup mixed greens (1) with vinaigrette (1)

If eggplant is not your thing, have a cup of steamed greens instead for the same amount of net carbs.

SUBTOTAL: 8

SNACK
1 deviled egg (0.5)

TOTAL: 21 GRAMS

DAY ONE

BREAKFAST

Nutty smoothie: 1 tablespoon soy nut butter (1) blended with 1 cup reduced-carb milk dairy beverage (3), 2 scoops whey protein vanilla shake mix (3), and 4 ice cubes

If you don't have controlled-carb dairy beverages on hand, you may substitute water and 2 tablespoons heavy cream.

SUBTOTAL: 7

SNACK

1 hard-boiled egg (0.5)

LUNCH

"Bread-free" Reuben: 4 slices corned beef, 2 slices Swiss cheese (2), and ½ cup sauerkraut (2) over 2 cups spinach, steamed (1), with mustard vinaigrette (2)

SUBTOTAL: 7

DINNER

One 8-ounce grilled salmon steak glazed with 1 tablespoon low-carb teriyaki sauce (1)

2 cups mixed greens (2) drizzled with 1 tablespoon peanut oil and 1 tablespoon unseasoned rice wine vinegar (2)

Be sure to use unseasoned rice wine vinegar.

SUBTOTAL: 5

SNACK

5 black olives (1)

TOTAL: 20.5 GRAMS

DAY TWO

BREAKFAST
1 poached egg (0.5) on 1 slice low-carb multigrain toast (3) with 1 ounce American cheese, melted (1)

½ cup halved cherry tomatoes (2)

SUBTOTAL: 6.5

SNACK
1 Atkins® Advantage Morning Start Bar (2)

LUNCH
1 cup vegetable broth (1)

2 cups baby spinach (1) with 8 ounces roasted turkey, 1 slice bacon, crumbled, and blue cheese dressing (2)

SUBTOTAL: 4

DINNER
8 ounces lamb chops, broiled

1 cup steamed cauliflower (2)

1 cup mixed greens (1) with ranch dressing (1)

SUBTOTAL: 4

SNACK
Classic shrimp cocktail: 6 medium steamed shrimp with cocktail sauce (combine ketchup and jarred horseradish) (3)

TOTAL: 19.5 GRAMS

DAY THREE

BREAKFAST

2 scrambled eggs (1) with 1 ounce Monterey Jack cheese, shredded (1), and 1 tablespoon each green salsa and sour cream (1)

2 turkey sausage links (1)

SUBTOTAL: 4

SNACK

Atkins® Advantage Ready-to-Drink French Vanilla Shake (2)

LUNCH

1 cup chicken broth (1)

One 8-ounce grilled chicken breast half topped with nut-free pesto sauce—combine ¼ cup fresh basil leaves, 2 tablespoons olive oil, and 1 ounce Parmesan cheese, grated (1)

1 cup romaine hearts (1) with vinaigrette (1)

If you're making your own pesto and don't have fresh basil on hand, try substituting flat-leaf parsley.

SUBTOTAL: 4

DINNER

Fish fajita: 8 ounces panfried cod and 1 slice cheddar cheese (1) wrapped in a low-carb tortilla (3) and heated

2 cups mixed greens (2) with ½ cup button mushrooms, chopped (1), and vinaigrette (2)

SUBTOTAL: 9

SNACK

½ Hass avocado (2)

TOTAL: 21 GRAMS

DAY FOUR

BREAKFAST

1 Atkins® Advantage Morning Bar (2)

1 hard-boiled egg (0.5)

SUBTOTAL: 2.5

SNACK

1 celery stalk (1) with herb dip (sour cream with fresh chopped herbs such as dill, basil, or rosemary) (1)

LUNCH

Cream of broccoli soup: ½ cup broccoli, steamed (2) and pureed with ¼ cup cooking liquid and ¼ cup heavy cream; season to taste

½ Hass avocado (2) filled with 8 ounces crab or tuna salad (combine canned crab or tuna with mayo)

2 cups baby spinach (2) with vinaigrette (2)

SUBTOTAL: 8

DINNER

One 8-ounce baked ham steak drizzled with 1 tablespoon sugar-free pancake syrup (1)

½ cup green beans tossed with butter and chopped mint (3)

1 cup mixed greens (1) with vinaigrette (1)

Make a larger portion of ham steak tonight, and you'll have the main ingredient for tomorrow's lunch on hand.

SUBTOTAL: 6

SNACK

½ cup cucumber slices (1) with 1 ounce smoked salmon and 1 tablespoon cream cheese (1)

When purchasing smoked salmon, read the ingredients label carefully.

TOTAL: 20.5 GRAMS

DAY FIVE

BREAKFAST

Atkins® Advantage French Vanilla Ready-to-Drink Shake (2)

2 hard-boiled eggs (1)

SUBTOTAL: 3

SNACK

1 ounce soy nuts (1)

LUNCH

1 cup chicken broth (1)

Open-faced ham sandwich: 1 slice low-carb rye bread (3) with 2 thick slices baked ham and 2 slices American cheese (2), with mayonnaise and mustard

½ cup sliced cucumber (1) served on ½ cup endive (1), with 1 tablespoon vinaigrette

SUBTOTAL: 8

DINNER

2 grilled veal chops seasoned with butter mixed with chopped sage

½ cup sautéed yellow squash (3)

2 cups mixed greens (3), drizzled with vinaigrette (2)

If you prefer, use an equal amount of zucchini in lieu of the yellow squash.

SUBTOTAL: 8

SNACK

1 ounce string cheese (1)

TOTAL: 21 GRAMS

DAY SIX

BREAKFAST

Greek omelet: ½ cup spinach (1), 2 ounces feta cheese (2), and 2 eggs (1)

1 small tomato, sliced (3)

SUBTOTAL: 7

SNACK

Atkins® Advantage Fudge Brownie Bar (2)

LUNCH

1 cup beef broth (1)

8 ounces poached chicken over 2 cups romaine lettuce (2) and ½ cup snow peas (3), drizzled with sesame oil

SUBTOTAL: 6

DINNER

8 ounces panfried halibut

½ cup steamed string beans (3)

1 cup mixed greens (1) with vinaigrette (1)

SUBTOTAL: 5

SNACK

5 black olives (1)

You can have up to 10 olives a day. They're an excellent source of monounsaturated fats during Induction. Also try olive paste to add zip to sandwiches made on low-carb bread.

TOTAL: 21 GRAMS

DAY SEVEN

BREAKFAST

Atkins® Advantage Peanut Butter Granola Bar (3)

1 hard-boiled egg (0.5)

SUBTOTAL: 3.5

SNACK

½ cup sliced cherry tomatoes (2) and 1 ounce mozzarella cheese, sliced (1), drizzled with olive oil

LUNCH

8 ounces cooked shrimp, chopped, mixed with mayonnaise and chopped flat-leaf parsley

2 cups mixed greens (2) with ½ cup sliced bell pepper (3) and vinaigrette (2)

SUBTOTAL: 7

DINNER

8 ounces pork tenderloin seasoned with rosemary, salt, and pepper

1 cup mixed baby greens (1) with ranch dressing (2)

Another name for mixed greens is mesclun, a combination of young small salad greens. Look for prewashed packages in your grocery store.

SUBTOTAL: 3

SNACK

1 cup reduced-carb, whole-milk dairy beverage (3)

TOTAL: 19.5 GRAMS

DAY ONE

BREAKFAST

Atkins® Advantage Morning Peanut Butter Crisp Bar (2)

1 hard-boiled egg (0.5)

SUBTOTAL: 2.5

LUNCH

Veggie pizza: 1 low-carb tortilla (3) topped with ¼ cup tomato sauce (3) and ⅓ cup frozen textured vegetable protein, heated (2); top with 1 ounce mozzarella cheese, shredded (1) and toast

1 cup mixed greens (1) with vinaigrette (1)

Textured vegetable protein, or TVP, is a meatless way to mimic ground beef. You'll find it in the freezer section of most supermarkets, sometimes under the name "burger crumbles."

SUBTOTAL: 11

SNACK

1 ounce almonds (1)

DINNER

Two 4-ounce pork chops, broiled

½ cup kale, sautéed (2)

2 cups mixed greens (2) with ½ cup sliced cucumber (1) and vinaigrette (2)

Chocolate-cheese dessert: Puree 2 ounces ricotta cheese (2) with 1 tablespoon unsweetened cocoa (1) and sucralose, to taste (1)

SUBTOTAL: 11

TOTAL: 25.5 GRAMS

DAY TWO

BREAKFAST

2 poached eggs (1) with 1 small tomato, sliced (3), and 2 tablespoons hollandaise sauce

SUBTOTAL: 4

LUNCH

1 cup chicken broth (1)

Chef salad: 2 slices each thinly sliced ham, turkey, and roast beef, plus 1 hard-boiled egg, chopped (0.5), 1 ounce cheddar cheese, shredded (1), and 1 slice bacon, crumbled, over 3 cups mixed greens (3) with vinaigrette (2)

SUBTOTAL: 7.5

SNACK

½ Hass avocado (2)

DINNER

One 8-ounce grilled salmon fillet

½ cup pea pods (3.5) and ½ cup Chinese cabbage, sautéed and drizzled with sesame oil

2 cups mixed greens (2) with vinaigrette (2)

1 ounce walnuts (1) sprinkled over one 6-ounce cup reduced-carb French vanilla yogurt (2)

SUBTOTAL: 10.5

TOTAL: 23.5 GRAMS

DAY THREE

BREAKFAST
Atkins® Advantage Café Mocha Shake (2)

1 deviled egg (0.5)

SUBTOTAL: 2.5

LUNCH
½ Hass avocado (2) filled with 6 ounces tuna salad (combine canned chunk light tuna with mayonnaise and chopped celery) (1)

2 cups romaine lettuce (2), ½ cup sliced cucumber (1), and ½ cup cherry tomatoes (2) with 2 tablespoons vinaigrette (1)

When selecting avocados, choose the smaller, darker, pebbly textured California Hass variety over the larger shiny and bright green Florida Fuente. The Hass variety is lower in carbs and has a richer flavor.

SUBTOTAL: 9

SNACK
1 slice low-carb multigrain bread (3) with 2 tablespoons soy nut butter (2)

DINNER
8 ounces skirt steak, grilled

1 cup broccoli florets, steamed (2), with 2 ounces cheddar cheese, melted (2)

2 cups mixed greens (2) with Russian dressing (2)

Skirt steak is best known as the choice of beef for fajitas. A long, flat piece of meat, it is also delicious and fast to prepare on the grill. When rolled and braised, it becomes incredibly tender.

SUBTOTAL: 8

TOTAL: 24.5 GRAMS

DAY FOUR

BREAKFAST
Pre-Workout Smoothie (5): Puree in a blender ½ cup unsweetened coconut milk, 3 ounces (⅓ cup) silken tofu, ¼ cup sugar-free vanilla syrup (or more or less to taste), and 1 cup ice cubes.

SUBTOTAL: 5

LUNCH
Open-faced Reuben: 4 ounces corned beef, 2 slices Swiss cheese (2), ¼ cup sauerkraut (1) on 1 slice low-carb rye bread (3)

1 cup butter lettuce (1) with 5 radishes, sliced (0.5), and blue cheese dressing (1)

SUBTOTAL: 8.5

SNACK
2 ounces macadamia nuts (2)

DINNER
8 ounces halibut, topped with ½ cup sautéed scallions (2.5)

2 cups mixed greens (2), ½ cup endive (0.5), and vinaigrette (2)

1 cup sugar-free strawberry gelatin (1) with whipped cream (1)

For flavorful whipped cream without a lot of carbs or sweetener, add a drop or two of your favorite extract to heavy cream before whipping. Almond is particularly nice. A teaspoon of unsweetened cocoa yields a subtly chocolate delight.

SUBTOTAL: 9

TOTAL: 27.5 GRAMS

DAY FIVE

BREAKFAST

Atkins® Advantage Creamy Vanilla Shake (3)

2 hard-boiled eggs (1)

SUBTOTAL: 4

LUNCH

One 8-ounce turkey patty with 1 tablespoon low-carb ketchup (1), ½ dill pickle, sliced (0.5), and ½ small tomato, sliced (1.5)

2 cups mixed greens (2) with 1-ounce goat cheese (1), 5 green olives (1), and vinaigrette (2)

SUBTOTAL: 9

SNACK

1 ounce walnuts (1) and 2 ounces Brie cheese (2)

It's easy to overdo it on portion sizes when it comes to cheese. To avoid taking in too many carbs, remember that 1 ounce is about the size of your thumb or 4 dice.

DINNER

One 8-ounce snapper fillet

8 asparagus spears, steamed with butter (4)

2 cups mixed greens (2), 1 ounce Parmesan cheese, shaved (1), and Caesar dressing (2)

SUBTOTAL: 9

TOTAL: 24 GRAMS

DAY SIX

BREAKFAST

½ cup ricotta cheese (2) mixed with 2 tablespoons flaxseed meal and heated; top with 1 tablespoon natural peanut butter (2)

SUBTOTAL: 4

LUNCH

1 cup chicken broth (1)

Scoop of egg salad (1) made with 1 celery stalk, chopped (1), and mayonnaise over 2 cups mixed greens (2) and 5 black olives, sliced (1)

½ cup chopped cucumber (1) with vinaigrette (1) and chopped dill

1 cup sugar-free lemon gelatin (1) with whipped cream (1)

SUBTOTAL: 10

SNACK

2 celery stalks (2) wrapped with 2 slices proscuitto

Proscuitto is a flavorful ham that has been salt-cured and air-dried. In early phases it is divine around celery or jicama. Wrap a slice around a piece of honeydew melon in later phases.

DINNER

Two 4-ounce lamb chops

½ cup broccoli rabe, steamed (2) and drizzled with olive oil

2 cups mixed greens (2), 1 ounce blue cheese, crumbled (1), and vinaigrette (2)

SUBTOTAL: 7

TOTAL: 23 GRAMS

DAY SEVEN

BREAKFAST
1 slice low-carb rye bread (3) with cream cheese (1) and 2 slices smoked salmon

SUBTOTAL: 4

LUNCH
Roast beef roll-ups: 8 slices roast beef spread with 2 tablespoons jarred no-sugar-added horseradish (2) and rolled up

1 cup mixed greens (1), 1 tablespoon sunflower seeds (1), and vinaigrette (1)

Mascarpone cheese treat: 2 ounces mascarpone (2) mixed with 2 tablespoons whipped cream, sweetened with sucralose to taste (1); garnish with mint sprig

A tablespoon of sunflower seeds packs fiber, protein, and few carbs. Add some to salads, hot dishes, and low-carb baked goods for a bit of crunch and nutrition.

SUBTOTAL: 8

SNACK
½ cup fennel (2) and 1 tablespoon sour cream dip (1)

DINNER
4 ounces cooked low-carb penne (5) with ¼ cup no-sugar-added tomato sauce (3) and two 3-ounce meatballs (made without bread crumbs) and 1 ounce grated Parmesan cheese (1)

1 cup mixed greens (1) with ranch dressing (1)

Low-carb pastas can vary when it comes to grams of carbs. Be sure to choose a brand that totals 5 grams of net carbs or less per serving. Use a measuring cup to serve a proper portion of cooked pasta so you know you're not going overboard.

SUBTOTAL: 11

TOTAL: 26 GRAMS

DAY ONE

BREAKFAST
Atkins® Advantage Morning Cinnamon Bun Bar (2)

2 hard-boiled eggs (1)

SUBTOTAL: 3

LUNCH
One 8-ounce chicken breast, grilled, over 2 cups mixed greens (2), ½ cup sliced cucumber (1), 1 ounce hazelnuts, chopped (1), and vinaigrette (2)

SUBTOTAL: 6

SNACK
½ cup whole-milk cottage cheese (3) with ½ cup raspberries (3)

SUBTOTAL: 6

DINNER
Lobster salad: 8 ounces cold steamed lobster (1) mixed with mayonnaise (1) and served over 2 cups romaine lettuce (2) with ½ cup cherry tomatoes (2) and vinaigrette (2)

½ cup cooked spaghetti squash with butter (4)

Lobster is pricey, so look for specials in your grocery store or fish market and offer your taste buds a treat when it's on sale. But feel free to substitute chopped cooked shrimp or canned crab for the lobster in this salad.

SUBTOTAL: 12

TOTAL: 27 GRAMS

DAY TWO

BREAKFAST
4 pancakes made from soy pancake and waffle mix (3) with ½ cup raspberries (3) and sugar-free pancake syrup

SUBTOTAL: 6

LUNCH
1 cup vegetable broth (1)

Roast beef and blue cheese roll-ups: 4 slices roast beef wrapped around 4 ounces blue cheese, crumbled (4) and 1 cup watercress

One 6-ounce cup reduced-carb French vanilla yogurt (2) with 1 ounce pistachios (1)

SUBTOTAL: 8

SNACK
Atkins® Advantage Strawberry Ready-to-Drink Shake (2)

DINNER
Chicken fajitas: 8 ounces chicken, grilled, ½ cup sliced bell peppers (3), ½ cup onions (5.5), sautéed and served on a low-carb tortilla (3)

2 cups romaine lettuce (2) with ranch dressing (2)

SUBTOTAL: 15.5

TOTAL: 31.5 GRAMS

DAY THREE

BREAKFAST

2 poached eggs (1) with 2 slices Canadian bacon

½ Hass avocado (2)

SUBTOTAL: 3

LUNCH

Monte Cristo sandwich: 2 slices ham, 2 slices Swiss cheese (2), 2 slices turkey breast, and 2 teaspoons mustard on 2 slices low-carb white bread (6), grilled

1 cup mixed greens (1) with vinaigrette (1)

SUBTOTAL: 10

SNACK

1 ounce macadamia nuts (1)

DINNER

Sausage and peppers: 8 ounces Italian sausage, sautéed with ½ cup sliced green bell pepper (3.5) and ½ cup sliced red onion (5.5)

2 cups romaine lettuce (2) with Caesar dressing (2)

½ cup raspberries (3)

SUBTOTAL: 16

TOTAL: 30 GRAMS

DAY FOUR

BREAKFAST
1 soya blueberry muffin (4)

½ cup ricotta cheese (2) with 1 ounce walnuts (1)

SUBTOTAL: 7

LUNCH
Salade Niçoise: 2 cups mixed greens (2) topped with 1 hard-boiled egg (0.5), 6 ounces flaked tuna, 5 black olives (1), ½ cup cold steamed green beans (3), and vinaigrette (2)

Steam some extra green beans today for even easier dinner preparation tomorrow!

SUBTOTAL: 8.5

SNACK
¼ cup blueberries (4) with whipped cream (1)

DINNER
8 ounces pot roast

1 steamed artichoke with aioli (7)

2 cups mixed greens (2) with Russian dressing (2)

SUBTOTAL: 11

TOTAL: 31.5 GRAMS

DAY FIVE

BREAKFAST

¼ cup blueberries (4) with 2 ounces mascarpone cheese (2) and 1 ounce chopped walnuts (1)

1 poached egg (0.5)

SUBTOTAL: 7.5

LUNCH

Meatball sandwich: 2 meatballs (made without bread crumbs) in ¼ cup no-sugar-added tomato sauce (3) on a low-carb roll (5) with 1 ounce Parmesan cheese, grated (1)

2 cups mixed greens (2) with vinaigrette (2)

SUBTOTAL: 13

SNACK

1 stalk celery (1) and 1 ounce mascarpone cheese mixed with chopped anchovies for dipping (1)

For a spicier dip, mix the mascarpone with an equal amount of mustard.

DINNER

8 ounces seared scallops

½ cup yellow squash, sautéed (3)

2 cups arugula (1), ½ cup chopped green beans (3), and Caesar dressing (2)

SUBTOTAL: 9

TOTAL: 31.5 GRAMS

DAY SIX

BREAKFAST

2 eggs scrambled (1) with 2 ounces smoked salmon and ½ cup sautéed scallions (2.5)

1 slice low-carb multigrain toast (3)

SUBTOTAL: 8.5

LUNCH

1 cup vegetable broth (1)

Southwest chicken salad: 8 ounces grilled chicken breast seasoned with cumin and chili powder over 2 cups mixed greens (2), ½ small tomato, chopped (1.5), 1 ounce pepper jack cheese, shredded (1), and ranch dressing (2)

Can't find pepper jack? Combine shredded Monterey Jack cheese and 1 teaspoon chopped jalapeño pepper.

SUBTOTAL: 7.5

SNACK

Atkins® Advantage Peanut Butter Granola Bar (3)

DINNER

One 8-ounce grilled ham steak

½ cup mashed turnips (3)

1 cup cooked collard greens (4)

1 cup mixed greens with vinaigrette (2)

½ cup strawberries, sliced (3), with whipped cream (1)

SUBTOTAL: 13

TOTAL: 32 GRAMS

DAY SEVEN

BREAKFAST

Sausage omelet: 2 eggs (1), 2 links breakfast sausage, chopped (1), and 1 ounce goat cheese (1)

¼ cup blueberries (4)

SUBTOTAL: 7

LUNCH

Shrimp-avocado wrap: 8 ounces grilled shrimp, ½ Hass avocado, chopped (2), and 1 plum tomato, chopped (2), mixed with mayonnaise and wrapped in a low-carb tortilla (3)

2 cups baby greens (2) with 1 cup sliced cucumber (1) and vinaigrette (2)

SUBTOTAL: 12

SNACK

Atkins® Advantage Chocolate Chip Granola Bar (3)

DINNER

8 ounces panfried trout topped with 1 ounce almonds, sliced and toasted (1)

1 cup kale (4), sautéed with 1 clove of garlic (1)

1 cup endive (1) with 1 ounce Brie, sliced (1), and vinaigrette (1)

SUBTOTAL: 9

TOTAL: 31 GRAMS

DAY ONE

BREAKFAST

Atkins® Advantage Morning Oatmeal Raisin Granola Bar (4)

½ cup strawberries (3) with whipped cream (1)

SUBTOTAL: 9

LUNCH

Italian wrap: 2 slices each salami, ham, and provolone (2) with mustard and ½ cup lettuce (0.5), wrapped in a low-carb tortilla (3)

2 cups mixed greens (2), ½ cup fennel, sliced (2), and Italian dressing (2)

SUBTOTAL: 11.5

SNACK

1 ounce almonds (1)

DINNER

Flounder *en papillote:* Place 8 ounces flounder on a sheet of aluminum foil and top with 2 tablespoons low-carb teriyaki sauce (1), ½ cup sliced red bell pepper (3), ½ cup snow peas (3), 1 cup stir-fried bok choy (1), and 1 tablespoon sesame seeds (1); bake at 350°F about 10 minutes

2 cups mixed greens (2), ½ cup bean sprouts (2), and ginger dressing (2)

While the method for preparing the flounder isn't traditional en papillote *(cooking foods inside a wrapping of parchment paper), aluminum foil yields the same result—moist and flaky fish.*

SUBTOTAL: 15

TOTAL: 36.5 GRAMS

DAY TWO

2 poached eggs (1) with 1 cup spinach, sautéed (1), and hollandaise sauce

2 sausage patties (2)

SUBTOTAL: 4

LUNCH

Peanut butter and jelly sandwich: 2 slices low-carb bread (6) with 2 tablespoons natural nut butter (4) and 1 tablespoon fruit only jam (2)

1 cup reduced-carb milk dairy beverage (3)

1 celery stick (1) with ¼ cup whole-milk cottage cheese (1.5)

A traditional PB&J can contain 58 grams of carbs. We shave off 46 grams in this scrumptious version. In later phases, layer on slices of apple for added texture and fiber. Just remember to tack on 9 grams of net carbs per half apple, too.

SUBTOTAL: 17.5

SNACK

½ cup strawberries (3) and 2 tablespoons whipped cream (1)

DINNER

8 ounces Italian sausage, grilled

1 cup broccoli rabe (4), sautéed with 1 clove garlic (1)

3 cups romaine lettuce (3), ½ cup alfalfa sprouts (0.5), and Caesar dressing (2)

SUBTOTAL: 10.5

TOTAL: 32 GRAMS

DAY THREE

BREAKFAST

1 slice high-fiber whole grain bread (7) with cream cheese (1), 2 slices beefsteak tomato (1), 1 slice onion (1), and 1 tablespoon capers (1)

SUBTOTAL: 11

LUNCH

Vegetarian soft tacos: ⅔ cup textured vegetable protein (4) sautéed with ½ cup sliced bell peppers (3) and 2 tablespoons no-sugar-added salsa (2) with sour cream (1)

1 cup mixed greens (1) with ranch dressing (1)

SUBTOTAL: 12

SNACK

½ cup jicama and guacamole: mash ½ ripe Haas avocado (2) with 1 tablespoon of mayonnaise; season with salt and pepper

DINNER

8 ounces pork tenderloin (0)

½ cup mixed mushrooms, sautéed (2)

2 cups romaine lettuce (2) with 1 ounce pine nuts (1), 1 ounce Parmesan cheese, grated (1) and Caesar dressing (2)

1 cup sugar-free lime gelatin (1)

Save the remainder of the pork tenderloin for tomorrow's lunch salad—it's a terrific change from an ordinary grilled chicken salad.

SUBTOTAL: 9

TOTAL: 36.5 GRAMS

DAY FOUR

BREAKFAST

½ cup high-protein, low-carb flake cereal (5) with 1 cup reduced-carb, whole-milk dairy beverage (3) and ½ cup blueberries (4)

Finding a cereal that's acceptable during OWL can be tricky, since whole grains aren't yet permitted. Look for low-carb varieties made from soy with a net carb count of 5 grams or less.

SUBTOTAL: 12

LUNCH

1 cup beef broth (1)

2 cups mixed greens (2) topped with 8 ounces pork tenderloin, sliced, ½ cup fennel, sliced (2), 1 ounce Parmigiano-Reggiano cheese, shaved (1), 1 small tomato, sliced (3), and vinaigrette (2)

SUBTOTAL: 11

SNACK

½ cup ricotta cheese (2) topped with 1 ounce toasted hazelnuts (1)

DINNER

8 ounces baked cod

Cauliflower puree (2) (see recipe with Meal Plan for Day Six, p. 269)

½ cup beet greens, sautéed (4)

3 cups mixed greens (3), 1 ounce blue cheese, crumbled (1), and vinaigrette (2)

SUBTOTAL: 12

TOTAL: 38 GRAMS

DAY FIVE

BREAKFAST

2 scrambled eggs (1) with 2 ounces mozzarella cheese (2)

1 slice low-carb rye toast (3)

SUBTOTAL: 6

LUNCH

Sardine salad: 6 ounces canned sardines mashed with chopped flat-leaf parsley and mayonnaise over 2 cups mixed greens (2), ½ cup sliced red bell pepper (3), ½ cup sliced cucumber (1), and vinaigrette (2)

1 dill pickle (2)

Give sardines a chance. Their fatty flesh and saltiness make them very satisfying. They're also loaded with essential fatty acids.

SUBTOTAL: 10

SNACK

One 6-ounce container low-carb French vanilla yogurt (3)

DINNER

8 ounces roast duck glazed with 1 tablespoon fruit only apricot jam (2)

2 cups mixed greens (2) with 2 ounces blue cheese, crumbled (2), 1 ounce walnuts (1), and lemon vinaigrette dressing (2)

½ cup steamed spaghetti squash with butter (4)

½ cup raspberries (3)

SUBTOTAL: 16

TOTAL: 35 GRAMS

DAY SIX

BREAKFAST

Atkins® Advantage Creamy Vanilla Shake (2)

½ cup strawberries (3) with ½ cup ricotta cheese (2) and 1 ounce sunflower seeds (1)

SUBTOTAL: 8

LUNCH

1 cup chicken broth (1)

Roasted duck wrap: 3 slices roasted duck, 2 ounces Brie cheese (2), wrapped in a low-carb tortilla (3) with mayonnaise and mustard

2 cups mixed greens (2) with ½ cup cherry tomatoes (2), 5 black olives (1), and vinaigrette (1)

Duck for lunch? It's easy when you use leftovers from last night's supper. Add a tablespoon of your favorite fruit only jam for only 2 grams of net carbs.

SUBTOTAL: 12

SNACK

1 tablespoon natural peanut butter (2) and 2 celery sticks (2)

DINNER

Two 4-ounce lamb kebabs

½ cup mashed turnips (2)

2 cups watercress, arugula, and radicchio (2) with 1 small tomato, chopped (3), and blue cheese dressing (1)

½ cup super premium no-sugar-added vanilla ice cream (3)

SUBTOTAL: 11

TOTAL: 35 GRAMS

DAY SEVEN

BREAKFAST

Blueberry smoothie: ¼ cup blueberries (4) pureed with 1 cup reduced-carb whole-milk dairy beverage (3), 2 scoops low-carb vanilla whey protein powder (3), and 4 ice cubes

SUBTOTAL: 10

LUNCH

1 cup beef broth (1)

2 cups mixed greens (2) topped with ⅓ block firm tofu, cubed (2), ½ cup sliced mushrooms (1.5), 1 tablespoon chopped cashews (2.5), and ½ cup chopped broccoli (1), dressed with 2 tablespoons soy sauce and 1 tablespoon sesame oil

Tofu, or soybean curd, comes in several textures, from soft to extra-firm. Firm tofu is best for salads since it can be cubed and tossed. Look for it in the produce section of your supermarket.

SUBTOTAL: 10

SNACK

1 ounce walnuts (1) and 1 ounce Brie cheese (1), melted in microwave about 30 seconds, with 1 celery stalk (1) for dipping

DINNER

Burger taco: 8-ounce turkey patty with 1 tablespoon ketchup (1), 2 ounces cheddar cheese, shredded (2), and 1 cup arugula (0.5) on a low-carb tortilla, folded (3)

½ cup baked spaghetti squash (4)

1 cup mixed greens (1), ½ cup chopped radishes (1), and ranch dressing (1)

SUBTOTAL: 13.5

TOTAL: 36.5 GRAMS

DAY ONE

BREAKFAST
½ cup low-carb high-protein flake cereal (5) and 1 cup reduced-carb, whole-milk dairy beverage (3), topped with 1 tablespoon ground flaxseed

One 4-ounce glass tomato juice (4)

SUBTOTAL: 12

LUNCH
1 cup chicken broth (1)

Bacon, lettuce, and tomato sandwich: 2 slices low-carb multigrain bread, toasted (6), 3 slices bacon, 3 slices tomato (2), and 2 leaves Boston lettuce (0.5) with mayonnaise

½ cup raspberries (3)

When buying berries, shake the container to be sure they're not stuck together, a sign that they have been crushed or are going bad.

SUBTOTAL: 12.5

SNACK
1 deviled egg (0.5)

DINNER
Crab bake: mix 6 ounces crab meat, 2 tablespoons chopped bell pepper (1), and 2 tablespoons mayonnaise, and place in oven-safe dish; sprinkle with ¼ cup low-carb bread crumbs (4) and 1 ounce cheddar cheese, shredded (1); bake at 350° F until warm and cheese is bubbly

2 cups romaine lettuce (2), ½ cup chopped zucchini (1), ½ cup chopped radishes (1), and ranch dressing (2)

8 asparagus spears, steamed (4)

SUBTOTAL: 16

TOTAL: 41 GRAMS

DAY TWO

BREAKFAST

¼ cup cottage cheese (2) with ¼ cup blueberries (4)

1 slice low-carb rye toast (3) with 1 tablespoon natural peanut or other nut butter (2) and 1 tablespoon fruit only apricot jam (2)

Natural nut butters contain no manufactured trans fats (partially hydrogenated oils).

SUBTOTAL: 13

LUNCH

Farm salad: 2 slices roast turkey and 2 slices thick-cut bacon, 2 chopped hard-boiled eggs (1), 6 cherry tomatoes, sliced (4), 1 ounce goat cheese (1), and 3 cups mixed greens (3) with vinaigrette (2)

1 cup broccoli florets (4) with sour cream and herb dip (1)

SUBTOTAL: 16

SNACK

2 asparagus spears (1) wrapped in prosciutto

DINNER

Bean-free beef chili: 6 ounces ground beef seasoned with cumin and chili powder, 2 stalks celery, chopped (2), and ½ cup chopped onion (5.5)

2 cups mixed greens (2) with ranch dressing (2)

SUBTOTAL: 11.5

TOTAL: 41.5 GRAMS

DAY THREE

BREAKFAST

Strawberry smoothie: ½ cup strawberries (3.5) blended with 1 cup reduced-carb, whole-milk dairy beverage (3), 2 scoops low-carb vanilla whey protein powder (3), and 4 ice cubes

SUBTOTAL: 9.5

LUNCH

1 cup vegetable broth (1)

One 6-ounce turkey burger with 2 ounces Swiss cheese (2) on a high-fiber bread roll (5)

1 cup coleslaw: 1 cup green cabbage, shredded (2), with mayonnaise

SUBTOTAL: 10

SNACK

Atkins® Advantage Morning Oatmeal Raisin Granola Bar (5)

DINNER

6 ounces steak, grilled

½ cup red pepper (3.5), sautéed with ½ cup sliced onion (5.5) and ½ cup mushrooms (1.5)

1 cup cauliflower florets (2), steamed and mashed

Caprese salad: 1 small tomato, sliced (3), 2 ounces fresh mozzarella cheese (2), and chopped fresh basil, drizzled with olive oil

There is a reason that tomatoes, basil, and fresh mozzarella are a staple at Italian restaurants. Caprese salad is irresistible and a great low-carb choice when dining out.

SUBTOTAL: 17.5

TOTAL: 42 GRAMS

DAY FOUR

BREAKFAST

One 6-ounce cup reduced-carb French vanilla yogurt (2) with 1 tablespoon ground flaxseed

1 slice high-fiber whole grain bread, toasted (3), with cream cheese (1) and 2 tablespoons fruit only strawberry jam (3)

SUBTOTAL: 9

LUNCH

2-egg omelet (1) with 1 ounce mozzarella cheese (1), 1 cup spinach (1), and ¼ cup scallions (3)

2 cups mixed greens (2), 4 asparagus spears, blanched and sliced (2), and vinaigrette (2)

SUBTOTAL: 12

SNACK

1 cup endive (1) with ¼ cup eggplant appetizer (caponata) (1)

DINNER

Snapper Veracruz: 6 ounces snapper, baked and topped with 2 tablespoons no-added-sugar salsa (2)

1 cup escarole (1), sautéed with 1 clove garlic (1), chopped, in olive oil

2 cups mixed greens (2) and vinaigrette (2)

½ cup low-carb vanilla ice cream (3) with ½ cup raspberries (3)

SUBTOTAL: 14

TOTAL: 37 GRAMS

DAY FIVE

BREAKFAST

2 poached eggs (1) and 2 slices Canadian bacon in a low-carb pita (6)

1 cup tomato juice (8)

SUBTOTAL: 15

LUNCH

1 cup vegetable broth (1)

Chicken salad in a tomato: 6 ounces poached chicken mixed with mayonnaise and 2 stalks celery, chopped (2), served over 1 small tomato, halved (3)

2 cups mixed greens (2) with French dressing (2)

SUBTOTAL: 10

SNACK

1 ounce Brie cheese (1) and 1 ounce almonds (1)

DINNER

6 ounces turkey kielbasa, sautéed with 1 cup green cabbage, shredded (1), and ½ cup sliced onions (5), topped with caraway seeds

½ cup each watercress, spinach, and chopped radishes (1.5), and vinaigrette (2)

¼ cup blueberries (4) with 1 ounce crème fraîche (1)

SUBTOTAL: 14.5

TOTAL: 41.5 GRAMS

DAY SIX

BREAKFAST
4 blueberry-walnut pancakes made from soya flour pancake and waffle mix (3), with ¼ cup blueberries (4) and 2 ounces sugar-free pancake syrup and 1 ounce chopped walnuts (1)

SUBTOTAL: 8

LUNCH
Steak salad: 6 ounces sirloin strips, stir-fried, over 3 cups mixed greens (3) with 2 scallions, chopped (1), 1 small tomato, chopped (3), ½ cup chopped cucumber (1), ¼ red pepper, chopped (1.5), with vinaigrette (2)

SUBTOTAL: 11.5

SNACK
2 tablespoons eggplant appetizer (caponata) (2) and 2 celery sticks (2)

DINNER
Seafood kebabs: 3 ounces shrimp and 3 ounces scallops with 5 cherry tomatoes (3), ½ cup cubed red pepper (3) and ½ onion, cubed (5.5)

1 cup baby greens (1) with vinaigrette (1)

½ cup baked spaghetti squash (4)

SUBTOTAL: 17.5

TOTAL: 40.5 GRAMS

DAY SEVEN

BREAKFAST
Steak and 2 eggs (1)

1 slice low-carb whole grain bread (3), buttered

SUBTOTAL: 4

LUNCH
Large grilled portobello mushroom, sliced (4), with 1 small tomato, sliced (3), 2 ounces mozzarella cheese (2), and 1 tablespoon chopped fresh basil with olive oil and red wine vinegar (1) in a low-carb pita (6)

2 cups arugula and parsley salad (2) with lemon vinaigrette (2)

SUBTOTAL: 20

SNACK
One 6-ounce container reduced-carb French vanilla yogurt (3)

DINNER
6 ounces roasted turkey breast and ½ cup cranberries (4) cooked with ¼ cup water and 1 packet sucralose (1)

½ cup boiled pumpkin (4), mashed with butter and nutmeg

1 cup escarole, sautéed (1)

1 slice sugar-free cheesecake (3)

SUBTOTAL: 13

TOTAL: 40 GRAMS

This week's plans add back legumes such as lentils and chickpeas.

DAY ONE

BREAKFAST

2 scrambled eggs (1), 1 tablespoon chopped flat-leaf parsley, and 2 ounces cheddar cheese, shredded (2)

1 slice low-carb rye toast (3)

SUBTOTAL: 6

LUNCH

1 cup chicken broth (1)

6 ounces chicken strips, grilled, with peanut dipping sauce (mix 2 tablespoons natural peanut butter with 1 tablespoon teriyaki sauce) (5)

3 cups mixed greens (3), ½ small tomato, chopped (1.5), and vinaigrette (2)

1 cup sugar-free raspberry gelatin (1) with whipped cream (1)

SUBTOTAL: 14.5

SNACK

1 ounce macadamia nuts (1) and 1 ounce fontina cheese (1)

DINNER

Crab cakes: Mix 6 ounces crab meat, 2 tablespoons chopped bell pepper (1), ¼ cup low-carb bread crumbs (4), and 2 tablespoons mayonnaise

2 cups Boston lettuce and watercress (2), ½ cup chopped scallions (2.5), ½ cup black beans (13), and vinaigrette (2)

SUBTOTAL: 24.5

TOTAL: 47 GRAMS

DAY TWO

BREAKFAST

½ cup ricotta cheese (4) with 2 tablespoons ground flaxseed, heated

1 slice low-carb rye toast (3)

The ricotta mixed with ground flaxseed has the satisfying consistency of hot cereal.

SUBTOTAL: 7

LUNCH

Chopped salad: 2 slices each thinly sliced ham, turkey, and roast beef, plus 2 hard-boiled eggs, chopped (1), 1 small tomato, chopped (3), and 1 slice crumbled bacon over 3 cups mixed greens, chopped (3), with vinaigrette (2)

SUBTOTAL: 9

SNACK

1 ounce almonds (1)

DINNER

One 6-ounce grilled beef burger

Bean salad: ½ cup chickpeas (17) and ½ cup steamed green beans (3) with ¼ cup chopped red bell pepper (1.5), over 1 cup mixed greens (1) with Italian dressing (2)

¼ cup blueberries (4)

SUBTOTAL: 28.5

TOTAL: 45.5 GRAMS

BREAKFAST

Double berry smoothie: ½ cup raspberries (3) and ¼ cup blueberries (4) blended with 1 cup reduced-carb, milk dairy beverage (3), 2 scoops low-carb whey protein vanilla powder (3), and 4 ice cubes

SUBTOTAL: 13

LUNCH

Asian tuna plate: combine one 6-ounce can light tuna with 2 stalks celery, chopped (2), ½ cup daikon (1), chopped, 1 hard-boiled egg, sliced (0.5), and ½ cup edamame (green soybeans) (6), and mayonnaise, serve over 2 cups mixed greens (2) and ginger dressing (2)

1 slice sugar-free cheesecake (3)

SUBTOTAL: 16.5

SNACK

1 tablespoon macadamia nut butter (1) and 1 celery stalk (1)

DINNER

6 ounces shell steak, grilled

1 steamed artichoke with drawn butter (7)

2 cups romaine lettuce (2), ½ cup sliced cucumber (1), 1 ounce Parmesan cheese, shaved (1), 2 anchovies, chopped, and Caesar dressing (2)

SUBTOTAL: 13

TOTAL: 44.5 GRAMS

DAY FOUR

BREAKFAST

1 slice high-fiber whole grain bread, toasted (5), with cream cheese (1)

1 reduced-carb peach yogurt smoothie (3)

SUBTOTAL: 9

LUNCH

2-egg omelet (1) with 1 ounce mozzarella cheese (1), ½ cup sliced zucchini (1), and ½ cup sliced red bell pepper (3)

2 cups mixed greens (2), ½ cup lima beans (13), with vinaigrette (2)

SUBTOTAL: 23

SNACK

1 ounce pistachios (1)

DINNER

6 ounces pan-seared halibut, seasoned with salt and pepper

½ cup roasted Brussels sprouts (8)

1 cup mixed greens (1) with vinaigrette (1)

½ cup blackberries (5.5)

SUBTOTAL: 15.5

TOTAL: 48.5 GRAMS

DAY FIVE

BREAKFAST
½ cup high-protein flake cereal (5) with 1 cup reduced-carb, milk dairy beverage (3)

¼ cup raspberries (1.5)

SUBTOTAL: 9.5

LUNCH
Low-carb Reuben: 4 ounces corned beef, 2 slices Swiss cheese (2), and ½ cup sauerkraut (2), on 2 slices low-carb rye bread (6), toasted

2 cups leaf lettuce (2) with ½ Hass avocado, chopped (2), and French dressing (2)

SUBTOTAL: 16

SNACK
Sugar-free gelatin with whipped cream (1)

DINNER
6 ounces roasted leg of lamb

1 small tomato, chopped (3), ½ cup eggplant (2), and ¼ cup cannelloni beans (8.5), stewed

2 cups mixed greens (2) with 1 ounce feta cheese, crumbled (1), 5 black olives (1), ½ cup chopped cucumber (1), and vinaigrette (2)

SUBTOTAL: 20.5

TOTAL: 47 GRAMS

DAY SIX

BREAKFAST
2 poached eggs (1) with ½ small tomato (1.5) and 1 slice high-fiber multigrain toast (5)

SUBTOTAL: 7.5

LUNCH
4 slices roast beef and 2 slices Swiss cheese (2) over 2 cups mixed greens (2) and blue cheese dressing (2)

Lentil salad: ½ cup cooked lentils (12), ¼ cup chopped green pepper (1.5), ¼ cup chopped red onion (2.5), and 1 stalk celery (1), chopped, with vinaigrette (2)

SUBTOTAL: 25

SNACK
1 ounce pumpkin seeds (1)

DINNER
Turkey-spinach quesadilla: 6 ounces ground turkey, sautéed with ½ cup chopped bell pepper (3), 2 tablespoons chopped jalapeño, and 1 cup spinach (1), seasoned with chili powder and cumin to taste; serve on low-carb tortilla (3) with 1 ounce Monterey Jack Cheese, melted (1)

1 cup mixed greens (1) with ranch dressing (1)

½ cup steamed yellow squash (3)

1 cup sugar-free lime gelatin (1)

SUBTOTAL: 14

TOTAL: 47.5 GRAMS

BREAKFAST

2 eggs (1) scrambled with ½ cup black beans (13) and 1 ounce cheddar cheese, shredded (1), with 2 tablespoons salsa (2)

2 sausage patties

SUBTOTAL: 17

LUNCH

Salmon salad: 6 ounces canned salmon, mixed with 2 tablespoons mayonnaise, 1 tablespoon each chopped flat-leaf parsley and capers (1), and ½ cup sliced cucumber (1)

2 cups mixed greens (2) with ½ cup bamboo shoots (1), ½ cup pea pods (2), and ranch dressing (2)

SUBTOTAL: 9

SNACK

One 6-ounce container reduced-carb strawberry banana yogurt (3)

DINNER

One 6-ounce pork cutlet with 1 tablespoon fruit only apricot jam (2)

½ cup broccoli rabe (2), sautéed with garlic (1)

½ cup mashed turnip (2)

½ cup blueberries (8) with 1 ounce mascarpone cheese (1)

SUBTOTAL: 16

TOTAL: 45 GRAMS

DAY ONE

BREAKFAST
½ cup tomato juice (4)

2 scrambled eggs (1), ½ cup artichoke hearts (5), and 2 ounces cheddar cheese, shredded (2)

1 slice low-carb rye toast (3)

SUBTOTAL: 15

SNACK
1 ounce walnuts (1)

For a more decadent snack, cream walnuts with blue cheese or cream cheese and stuff into celery sticks or endive "spoons."

LUNCH
Curried chicken salad: 6 ounces poached chicken with ½ Granny Smith apple, chopped (9), 1 stalk celery, chopped (1), and 1 ounce walnuts, chopped (1), seasoned with curry powder to taste.

2 cups mixed greens (2), ¼ cup snap beans (1.5), and vinaigrette (2)

SUBTOTAL: 15.5

DINNER
Seafood and pasta: 6 ounces shrimp, scallops, and white fish over 2 ounces pasta, cooked (5), and ¼ cup tomato sauce (2)

2 cups mixed greens (2), ¼ cup black beans (6.5), and vinaigrette (2)

1 cup sugar-free orange gelatin (1)

SUBTOTAL: 18.5

TOTAL: 50 GRAMS

DAY TWO

BREAKFAST

½ cup cottage cheese (3) with ½ red grapefruit (8)

1 slice low-carb rye toast (3)

SUBTOTAL: 14

LUNCH

Greek fisherman's salad: 6 ounces cod, 5 black olives (1), 2 ounces feta cheese (2) over ½ cup spinach (1) and 2 cups mixed greens (2), with vinaigrette (2)

1 small tomato, chopped (3), and 2 slices onion, chopped (2)

SUBTOTAL: 13

SNACK

1 ounce macadamia nuts (1)

DINNER

6 ounces grilled duck breast

Chickpea salad: ½ cup chickpeas (17) with ¼ cup chopped red bell pepper (1.5), ½ cup chopped broccoli florets (2), and vinaigrette (2)

1 cup mixed greens (1) with vinaigrette (1)

To select the freshest broccoli you can find, avoid bunches with flowering or yellowed bud clusters and dry or woody stems.

SUBTOTAL: 24.5

TOTAL: 52.5 GRAMS

DAY THREE

BREAKFAST

Apricot-raspberry smoothie: 1 fresh apricot, sliced (3), and ½ cup raspberries (3) blended with 1 cup reduced-carb, milk dairy beverage (3), 2 scoops low-carb vanilla whey protein powder mix (3), and 4 ice cubes

SUBTOTAL: 12

LUNCH

½ Hass avocado (2) filled with Asian salmon salad (combine canned salmon with 2 stalks celery, chopped (2), ½ cup chopped radishes (1), ½ cup cooked soybeans (6), and mayonnaise)

2 cups iceberg lettuce (2), 1 ounce cheddar cheese, shredded (1), ½ cup radishes (1), and Italian dressing (2)

½ cup super premium no-sugar-added butter pecan ice cream (3)

SUBTOTAL: 20

SNACK

2 tablespoons hummus (2) with ½ cup jicama (2.5)

DINNER

6 ounce T-bone steak, grilled, and 2 tablespoons steak sauce (1)

½ cup cauliflower (1) mashed with 2 tablespoons tahini (1)

2 cups mesclun (2) with 2 sun-dried tomatoes, chopped (2), 2 ounces pine nuts (2), ½ cup hearts of palm (1), and vinaigrette (2)

The intense flavor of sun-dried tomatoes means that the carbs are also concentrated, so use them sparingly as snacks and in salads or egg dishes.

SUBTOTAL: 12

TOTAL: 48.5 GRAMS

DAY FOUR

BREAKFAST

½ cup high-protein flake cereal (5) and 1 cup reduced-carb, milk dairy beverage (3)

SUBTOTAL: 8

LUNCH

Vegetable and cheese frittata: 2 eggs (1), ½ cup shredded zucchini (1), ½ cup shredded yellow squash (1.5), ½ cup chopped bell pepper (3), ½ small tomato, chopped (1.5), and 2 ounces fontina cheese (2)

2 cups mixed greens (2), ½ fresh orange, sliced (6.5), 1 ounce pecans (1), and vinaigrette (2)

SUBTOTAL: 21.5

SNACK

1 cup broccoli florets (2) with 3 tablespoons sour cream and chopped dill dip (3)

DINNER

8 ounces halibut with 1 ounce chopped hazelnuts (1)

⅔ cup braised leeks (4.5)

2 cups mixed greens (2), ¼ cup lima beans (6.5), and vinaigrette (2)

SUBTOTAL: 16

TOTAL: 48.5 GRAMS

DAY FIVE

BREAKFAST

Atkins® Advantage Strawberry Supreme Shake (2)

1 slice low-carb multigrain toast (3) with 1 tablespoon soy nut butter (1)

SUBTOTAL: 6

LUNCH

1 cup beef broth (1)

Ham and cheese sandwich: 4 ounces baked ham, 2 slices Swiss cheese (2), and mustard on 2 slices low-carb rye bread (6)

2 cups mixed greens (2), 2 celery stalks, chopped (2), ½ cup chopped radishes (1), and blue cheese dressing (2)

SUBTOTAL: 16

SNACK

1 ounce Brie cheese (1)

DINNER

2 lamb chops

Baba ghanoush: ½ cup roasted eggplant (2) mashed with 1 tablespoon tahini (1) and garlic clove (1)

2 cups mixed greens (2), ¼ cup cannellini beans (8.5), 2 ounces feta cheese, crumbled (2), 5 black olives (1), 1 cup chopped cucumber (2), and vinaigrette (1)

½ cup no-sugar-added chocolate ice cream (3), ½ cup raspberries (3)

SUBTOTAL: 26.5

TOTAL: 49.5 GRAMS

DAY SIX

BREAKFAST

Breakfast burrito: 2 scrambled eggs, 2 tablespoons chopped scallion, 1 ounce cheddar cheese, shredded (1), 1 low-carb tortilla (3), and 2 tablespoons salsa

1 medium tomato, grilled (4)

SUBTOTAL: 10.5

LUNCH

One 6-ounce cup low-carb French vanilla yogurt (2) with ½ cup blueberries (8)

Antipasti roll-ups: 2 slices each salami, ham, and Swiss cheese (2), rolled up over 2 cups mixed greens (2), 5 green olives (1), and ½ cup artichoke hearts (5), with Italian dressing (2)

SUBTOTAL: 22

SNACK

1 ounce macadamia nuts, chopped (1), and mixed with 1 ounce mascarpone (1) and 1 cup endive (1)

DINNER

6 ounces spare ribs brushed with 2 tablespoons barbecue sauce (2)

2 cups cooked collard greens (4) and 1 clove garlic (1)

2 cups iceberg lettuce (2), ½ cup sliced cucumber (1), ¼ Hass avocado, diced (1), and blue cheese dressing (2)

SUBTOTAL: 13

TOTAL: 48.5 GRAMS

DAY SEVEN

2 poached eggs (1) with 2 slices smoked salmon and hollandaise sauce

½ cup strawberries (3)

SUBTOTAL: 4

LUNCH

Croque Monsieur: 2 slices French ham and 2 ounces American cheese (2) on 2 slices high-fiber whole grain bread (6), grilled

2 cups mixed greens (2), 1 small tomato, sliced (3), ½ cup bean sprouts (2), and vinaigrette (2)

Get fresh! Pick crisp-looking bean sprouts with buds and store them in a ziplock bag in the fridge for no more than three days.

SUBTOTAL: 17

SNACK

½ plum (4) and 1 ounce cheddar cheese (1)

DINNER

One 6-ounce veal chop with lemon juice, wine, and chopped parsley (2)

Bean salad: ¼ cup black beans (6.5), ¼ cup soybeans (3), and ¼ cup lima beans (6.5) with vinaigrette (2)

1 cup Boston lettuce (1), 2 artichoke hearts, (2) and French dressing (1)

SUBTOTAL: 24

TOTAL: 50 GRAMS

DAY ONE

BREAKFAST
½ cup low-carb flake cereal (3) with 1 fresh peach, sliced (7), and 1 cup reduced-carb, milk dairy beverage (3)

SUBTOTAL: 13

LUNCH
One 6-ounce kielbasa with ½ cup sauerkraut (2) and mustard on a low-carb roll (5)

2 cups mixed greens (2), ½ cup roasted beets (7), and 1 ounce blue cheese, crumbled (1), with vinaigrette (2)

SUBTOTAL: 19

SNACK
½ cup endive (1) with tapenade (1)

Tapenade is a paste made from capers, anchovies, olives, olive oil, and lemon juice. It adds a unique flavor to sandwiches, omelets, and crudités. Look for prepared tapenade in the condiments aisle of your supermarket.

DINNER
Veal parmigiana: 6-ounce veal cutlet with 2 ounces mozzarella, shredded (2), ½ cup tomato sauce (4), and chopped basil, over 2 ounces low-carb penne, cooked (5)

2 cups leaf lettuce (2), ½ cup chopped bell pepper (3), and Italian dressing (2)

1 slice low-carb cheesecake (3)

SUBTOTAL: 21

TOTAL: 55 GRAMS

BREAKFAST

Egg sandwich: 1 sunny-side-up egg (0.5) on 2 slices low-carb rye toast (6) with 1 ounce American cheese (1) and 1 slice pancetta

½ cup cantaloupe cubes (7)

Pancetta is an Italian bacon cured with salt and spices. Chop up a slice and sauté with garlic and olive oil, then add your favorite bitter green for a flavorful low-carb side dish.

SUBTOTAL: 14.5

LUNCH

Sardine salad: 6 ounces sardines over 2 cups arugula (2), 2 tablespoons parsley, 5 kala-mata olives (1), ¼ cup sliced onion (2), ½ cup artichoke hearts (5), 1 small tomato, chopped (3), and vinaigrette (2)

4 asparagus spears, roasted (2)

SUBTOTAL: 17

SNACK

Strawberry milk shake: ½ cup reduced-carb, whole-milk dairy beverage (1.5), ½ cup strawberries (3), and ½ cup no-sugar-added French vanilla ice cream (3)

DINNER

6 ounces pork roast

1 cup steamed green beans (6)

3 cups mixed greens (3), 1 cup shredded red cabbage (2), ½ cup sliced cucumber (1), 1 ounce Gouda cheese (1), 1 ounce walnuts (1), and vinaigrette (2)

SUBTOTAL: 16

TOTAL: 55 GRAMS

DAY THREE

BREAKFAST
Pecan pancakes: 4 pancakes made from soya flour pancake and waffle mix (3), with 2 ounces pecans, chopped (2), and sugar-free syrup

2 slices bacon

½ medium apple, sliced (8.5)

SUBTOTAL: 13.5

LUNCH
6 ounces grilled chicken over 2 cups iceberg lettuce (2), ½ avocado, sliced (2), ½ cup chopped cucumber (1), 1 plum tomato, chopped (2), and 2 ounces feta cheese (2), dressed with 2 tablespoons tahini (2) mixed with 2 tablespoons lemon juice (2)

Enjoy the other half of your avocado as a snack. Simply mash with a fork and add chopped garlic and onions, lime, and salt. Serve with celery sticks, slices of bell pepper, endive "spoons," or toasted low-carb tortillas.

SUBTOTAL: 13

SNACK
2 ounces Brie cheese (2) and 2 celery stalks (2)

DINNER
6 ounces London broil, grilled and topped with ½ cup sautéed shiitake mushrooms (9)

1 cup broccoli florets (2), roasted with 1 clove garlic (1)

2 cups mixed greens (2), ½ cup chopped endive (0.5), 2 stalks celery, chopped (2), 1 ounce walnuts (1), and ranch dressing (2)

One 6-ounce cup reduced-carb blueberry yogurt (3)

Looking for a laid-back lunch? Save the leftover London broil for your midday meal on Day Five.

SUBTOTAL: 22.5

TOTAL: 53 GRAMS

DAY FOUR

BREAKFAST

1 cup tomato juice (8)

Sausage, vegetable, and cheese frittata: 2 eggs (1), ½ cup shredded zucchini (1), ½ cup shredded yellow squash (1.5), ½ cup chopped bell pepper (3), ½ small tomato, chopped (1.5), 2 links breakfast sausage (1), and 2 ounces fontina cheese (2)

Fontina has a mild, nutty flavor and is downright luscious when melted. Add it to your favorite grilled sandwich instead of the usual American.

SUBTOTAL: 19

LUNCH

Grilled-chicken salad sandwich: 6 ounces pregrilled chicken strips mixed with mayonnaise, 2 stalks celery, chopped (2), ¼ cup water chestnuts, chopped (4), and ½ cup leaf lettuce (0.5) on 2 slices high-fiber flax bread (6)

SUBTOTAL: 12.5

SNACK

½ cup jicama (2.5) with 2 tablespoons sour cream and chopped dill dip (2)

DINNER

6 ounces tilapia wrapped in 1 slice prosciutto with chopped sage

1 cup sautéed zucchini (3) with 1 ounce Parmesan cheese, shaved (1)

2 cups mixed greens (2), ¼ cup chickpeas (9), ½ cup cherry tomatoes (2), and vinaigrette (2)

Tilapia is a widely available fine-textured white fish that can be baked, grilled, steamed, or broiled. It is sometimes called St. Peter's fish.

SUBTOTAL: 19

TOTAL: 55 GRAMS

BREAKFAST

2 Belgian waffles made from soya flour pancake and waffle mix (3), with ½ cup straw-berries (3.5) and whipped cream (1)

SUBTOTAL: 7.5

LUNCH

Taco salad: 2 cups mixed greens (2), 2 celery stalks, chopped (2), ½ cup sliced radishes (1), 1 small tomato, chopped (2), 2 ounces cheddar cheese, shredded (2), 6 ounces London broil strips, topped with 2 tablespoons sour cream (4), 2 tablespoons salsa (2), and ½ Hass avocado, chopped (2), in a low-carb tortilla (3) baked over a bowl

Don't forget to use the leftover London broil from dinner two nights ago to whip up this hearty lunch!

SUBTOTAL: 20

SNACK

1 ounce macadamia nuts (1)

DINNER

Crustless ham and leek quiche made with 2 eggs (1), ½ cup leeks (3), 2 slices ham, chopped, ¼ cup heavy cream (2), and 2 ounces Gruyère cheese (2)

2 cups mixed greens (2), ¼ cup cannellini beans (8.5), ½ cup artichoke hearts (5), and French dressing (2)

½ cup low-carb mint chocolate chip ice cream (3)

Smaller is better when it comes to leeks; in this case, a more diminutive vegetable is excep-tionally tender.

SUBTOTAL: 28.5

TOTAL: 57 GRAMS

DAY SIX

BREAKFAST
Beef scramble: 2 scrambled eggs (1), 2 tablespoons chopped scallion (0.5), 1 ounce Monterey Jack, shredded (1), ½ cup pinto beans (12), and 4 ounces ground beef

1 medium tomato, grilled (4)

SUBTOTAL: 18.5

LUNCH
Smoked salmon tea sandwiches: 2 tablespoons cream cheese (2), 4 slices smoked salmon, and ½ cup sliced cucumber (1) on 2 slices low-carb rye bread (6), cut in fours

2 cups mixed greens (2), 1 ounce pine nuts (1), ½ cup raspberries (3), and vinaigrette (2)

SUBTOTAL: 17

SNACK
1 cup sugar-free lime gelatin (1) with whipped cream (1)

DINNER
6 ounces steamed crab, removed from claws, with drawn butter

8 spears asparagus, grilled (4)

1 cup mashed turnips (7)

2 cups iceberg lettuce (2), ¼ cup sliced red onion (2.5), and Caesar dressing (2)

There's nothing simpler than grilled asparagus. Try soaking spears in a marinade of olive oil, lemon juice, and lemon rind, and cook on an indoor or outdoor grill, turning once, until the vegetable looks slightly browned and wilted.

SUBTOTAL: 17.5

TOTAL: 55 GRAMS

DAY SEVEN

BREAKFAST

Morning parfait: ½ cup high-protein flake cereal (3), layered with one 6-ounce container reduced-carb French vanilla yogurt (3) and ½ cup blueberries (8)

SUBTOTAL: 14

LUNCH

½ cup lentil soup (12)

Pastrami on rye: 4 slices pastrami on 2 slices low-carb rye toast (6) with ½ cup sauerkraut (2) and mustard

1 kosher dill pickle (2)

1 cup mixed greens (1), ½ cup chopped cucumber (1), ½ small tomato, chopped (1.5), and Russian dressing (1)

SUBTOTAL: 26.5

SNACK

½ cup ricotta cheese (2), 1 tablespoon ground flaxseed meal, and 1 tablespoon sugar-free pancake syrup

Always select whole-milk ricotta. Not only is it lower in carbs, but it's also far superior in flavor. Because it is also drier, it keeps dishes such as lasagna from getting watery.

DINNER

6 ounces roasted turkey drumsticks

½ cup steamed green beans (3) with 1 ounce almonds, sliced (1)

½ cup cooked pumpkin (5)

1 cup Boston lettuce (1), 2 roasted red peppers (2), and French dressing (1)

SUBTOTAL: 13

TOTAL: 55.5 GRAMS

60-GRAM MEAL PLAN

This week's meal plans introduce higher-glycemic vegetables such as carrots and sweet peas.

DAY ONE

BREAKFAST
2 scrambled eggs (1) with 2 ounces feta cheese (2) and 10 black olives, sliced (2)

2 slices low-carb multigrain toast (6)

1 tangerine (6)

SUBTOTAL: 17

LUNCH
1 cup chicken broth (1)

⅓ block firm tofu, cubed (2), brushed with 2 tablespoons barbecue sauce (2) and then grilled with peanut dipping sauce (mix 2 tablespoons natural peanut butter with 1 table-spoon teriyaki sauce) (5)

3 cups mixed greens (2) with ¼ cup chickpeas (8), ¼ cup sliced red onion (2.5), and vinaigrette (2)

SUBTOTAL: 24.5

SNACK
1 ounce walnuts (1)

DINNER
6 ounces Cornish game hen glazed with fruit only apricot jam (2)

½ cup steamed carrots (6)

½ cup celery root, grated (4), ½ cup jicama, grated (2.5), and ¼ Granny Smith apple, grated (4.5), mixed with 2 tablespoons mayonnaise over 2 cups romaine lettuce (2)

Make an extra game hen to serve for tomorrow's lunch.

SUBTOTAL: 21

TOTAL: 63.5

BREAKFAST

2 slices low-carb rye bread (6) with 1 slice Swiss cheese (2) and 2 strips cooked bacon, toasted

½ red grapefruit (8)

SUBTOTAL: 16

LUNCH

Vegetable broth (1)

½ Cornish game hen with ½ carrot, grated (2.5), 1 small tomato, chopped (3), and ½ cup sliced radishes (1) over 3 cups mixed greens (3)

1 slice no-sugar-added cheesecake (3) topped with ½ cup blueberries (8)

Look for firm bright orange carrots; if the tops are attached, the leaves should be bright green and look fresh, not wilted.

SUBTOTAL: 21.5

SNACK

One 6-ounce cup reduced-carb strawberry banana yogurt (3)

DINNER

One 6-ounce baked grouper with 2 tablespoons teriyaki sauce (1)

½ cup sweet peas (8) with ¼ cup soybeans (3), steamed

3 cups mixed greens (3), 1 ounce shelled pistachios (1),
½ cup rhubarb, lightly poached and then sweetened with sucralose to taste (2),
tossed with vinaigrette (2)

SUBTOTAL: 20

TOTAL: 60.5 GRAMS

DAY THREE

BREAKFAST

Island smoothie: ½ cup chopped mango (12.5) blended with ½ cup reduced-carb, milk dairy beverage (1.5), ½ cup unsweetened coconut milk (4), 2 scoops whey protein powder vanilla shake mix (3), and 4 ice cubes

SUBTOTAL: 21

LUNCH

½ cup lentil soup (12)

½ Hass avocado (2) filled with crunchy egg salad: 2 hard-boiled eggs chopped (1), with 2 stalks celery, chopped (2), ½ cup chopped radishes (1), and mayonnaise

SUBTOTAL: 18

SNACK

2 stalks celery (2) with 2 tablespoons hummus (5)

DINNER

6 sirloin kebabs, marinated in vinaigrette and grilled with ½ onion (5.5), ½ cup cherry tomatoes (2), and 1 cup sliced zucchini (2)

2 cups mixed greens (2) and ½ cup jicama (2.5) with Russian dressing (2)

SUBTOTAL: 16

TOTAL: 62 GRAMS

DAY FOUR

BREAKFAST

1 slice high-fiber flax toast (3)

1 cup unsweetened whole-milk Greek yogurt (8) with 2 tablespoons fruit only strawberry jam (3) and 1 ounce walnuts, chopped (1)

Greek yogurt, which is highly fermented and therefore tart, has the fewest carbs of any regular yogurt. Try it mixed with fruit or sugar-free syrup.

SUBTOTAL: 15

LUNCH

2-egg omelet (1) with 1 ounce mozzarella cheese (1), ¼ cup black beans (7), ½ cup sliced red bell pepper (3), 2 tablespoons chopped parsley, and 1 chipotle en adobo (1)

2 cups mixed greens (2) and ½ cup chopped cucumbers (1) with vinaigrette (2)

½ peach (4)

SUBTOTAL: 22

SNACK

Atkins® Advantage Morning Triple Berry Breakfast Bar (3)

DINNER:

6 ounces haddock, grilled, topped with ½ cup cooked celery root (4), and served with tartar sauce made from ¼ cup mayonnaise and 1 pickle, chopped (2)

3 cups mixed greens (3), 1 ounce walnuts (1), ½ cup cooked beets (7), 1 ounce blue cheese, crumbled (1), and vinaigrette (2)

To tame celery root, trim and discard the hairy bottom end of the root with a sharp, heavy knife and set it flat on your cutting board. Run your knife down the sides of the root to remove the brown skin and expose the creamy white flesh. If you're making thin slices, it's best to halve it first so it's not so unwieldy.

SUBTOTAL: 20

TOTAL: 60 GRAMS

DAY FIVE

BREAKFAST

1 reduced-carb black cherry yogurt smoothie (3)

2 hard-boiled eggs (1)

1 peach, sliced (8)

SUBTOTAL: 12

LUNCH

Sloppy Joe: 2 slices each roast beef, ham, and Swiss cheese (2) and ½ cup coleslaw (7) on 2 slices low-carb rye bread (6)

2 cups romaine lettuce (2) with ½ Hass avocado, chopped (2), ½ cup hearts of palm (2), and French dressing (1)

SUBTOTAL: 22

SNACK

½ cup no-sugar-added chocolate ice cream (3)

DINNER

6 ounces leg of lamb, slow-roasted

½ cup eggplant (2) topped with ¼ cup tomato sauce (2) and 2 ounces mozzarella, shredded (2), baked

2 cups mixed greens (2), ¼ cup cannellini beans (8), 5 black olives (1), and vinaigrette (2)

½ cup raspberries (3)

SUBTOTAL: 22

TOTAL: 59 GRAMS

DAY SIX

BREAKFAST

½ cup ricotta cheese (4) with 2 tablespoons ground flaxseed meal, heated and topped with ¼ cup blueberries (8)

If you have access to a good old-fashioned Italian deli, by all means purchase fresh, home-made ricotta—it's heavenly.

SUBTOTAL: 12

LUNCH

Salmon-avocado salad: Gently toss 6 ounces canned salmon with ½ Hass avocado, chopped (2), 1 cup steamed green beans, sliced (6), with mayonnaise and 2 tablespoons lemon juice (3), and serve over 3 cups mixed greens (3); garnish with ½ cup broccoli sprouts (1)

SUBTOTAL: 15

SNACK

½ cup cantaloupe melon balls (7) with 1 ounce walnuts (1)

DINNER

Turkey-spinach quesadilla: 6 ounces ground turkey sautéed with ½ cup chopped bell pepper (3), ½ cup pinto beans (11), 2 tablespoons chopped jalapeño, and 1 cup spinach (1), seasoned with chili powder and cumin to taste; serve on low-carb tortilla (3) with 1 ounce Monterey Jack, melted (1)

2 cups baby spinach (2), 1 slice bacon, cooked and crumbled, and vinaigrette (2)

SUBTOTAL: 23

TOTAL: 58 GRAMS

DAY SEVEN

BREAKFAST

2 poached eggs (1), 1 ounce American cheese (1), and 2 sausage patties

1 medium tomato, grilled (4)

½ cup raspberries (3)

SUBTOTAL: 9

LUNCH

Thanksgiving sandwich: 4 ounces roasted turkey and cranberry sauce, made with ¼ cup fresh cranberries (2), water, and sucralose to taste (1), on 2 slices low-carb multigrain toast (6)

2 cups mixed greens (2) with ½ cup mushrooms (1), ½ cup pea pods (2), ½ cup red bell pepper (3), and ranch dressing (2)

SUBTOTAL: 19

SNACK

2 endive "spoons" (2) and 2 tablespoons baba ghanoush (see page 317) (5)

DINNER

6-ounce pork cutlet with 2 tablespoons fruit only applesauce (2.5)

½ cup black-eyed peas (12) simmered with 1 slice bacon

2 cups Boston lettuce (2), ½ cup carrots, shredded (6), ½ cup daikon, shredded (1), and vinaigrette (2)

SUBTOTAL: 25.5

TOTAL: 60.5 GRAMS

This week's plans add back whole grains, such as oats, bulgur, corn, and the occasional piece of 100 percent whole grain bread. You can also start using whole milk and whole-milk yogurt.

DAY ONE

BREAKFAST

1 cup cooked oatmeal (21) with 1 tablespoon butter, 1 ounce walnuts, chopped (1), ¼ cup whole milk (3), and cinnamon

SUBTOTAL: 25

LUNCH

1 cup chicken broth (1)

Chicken and bean salad: ½ cup green beans (3), ¼ cup chickpeas (6.5), ¼ cup kidney beans (6), chopped parsley, and vinaigrette (2) over 6 ounces grilled chicken strips and 2 cups mixed greens (2)

SUBTOTAL: 20.5

SNACK

½ cup raspberries (3) with 1 ounce Muenster cheese

DINNER

1 green bell pepper (7) stuffed with 6 ounces ground beef, ¼ cup sliced onion (2.5), and ½ cup cremini mushrooms (4), sautéed together

2 cups romaine lettuce (2), 1 small tomato, chopped (3), and vinaigrette (2)

SUBTOTAL: 20.5

TOTAL: 69 GRAMS

DAY TWO

Fruit salad: ½ kiwi, sliced (4.5), ½ cup strawberries, sliced (3), and ½ red grapefruit, sectioned (9), with ½ cup cottage cheese (4)

1 slice low-carb rye toast (3)

SUBTOTAL: 23.5

LUNCH

Cobb salad: 3 slices each thinly sliced turkey and roast beef, plus 2 chopped hard-boiled eggs (1), 1 ounce blue cheese, crumbled (1), ½ cup corn kernels (13), ½ cup cherry tomatoes (2), ½ cup chopped cucumber (1), and 2 slices cooked bacon, crumbled over 2 cups mixed greens (2), with vinaigrette (2)

SUBTOTAL: 22

SNACK

One 6-ounce cup reduced-carb French vanilla yogurt (2)

DINNER

6-ounce poached salmon fillet topped with ¼ cup pesto sauce (6)

2 cups mixed greens (2), ½ cup steamed soybeans (6), ½ cup artichoke hearts (5), and vinaigrette (2)

1 slice low-carb cheesecake (3)

Although classic pesto calls for basil alone, you can kick things up by adding equal parts parsley and mint.

SUBTOTAL: 24

TOTAL: 71.5 GRAMS

DAY THREE

BREAKFAST

Banana-nut smoothie: ½ small banana (10.5) and 2 tablespoons natural peanut butter (4) blended with 1 cup reduced-carb, milk dairy beverage (3), 2 scoops whey protein vanilla powder (3), and 4 ice cubes

SUBTOTAL: 20.5

LUNCH

1 cup potato leek soup (12)

Tuna salad: 6 ounces light canned tuna combined with mayonnaise in ½ Hass avocado (2)

2 cups romaine lettuce (2), 2 chopped anchovies, and Caesar dressing (2)

A pitted avocado makes the perfect edible "bowl" for a scoop of shrimp, tuna, or chicken salad.

SUBTOTAL: 18

SNACK:

1 ounce walnuts (1)

DINNER

Beef stew: 6 ounces chuck beef, 1 medium carrot, chopped (5), ½ cup chopped onion (5.5), and ¼ cup tomato sauce (4) over ½ cup bulgur (13)

1 cup watercress and arugula (1), with vinaigrette (1)

½ cup no-sugar-added French vanilla ice cream (3)

SUBTOTAL: 32.5

TOTAL: 72 GRAMS

DAY FOUR

BREAKFAST

½ cup Wheatena, cooked (11), with 1 ounce walnuts, chopped (1), ¼ cup whole milk (3), ½ cup raspberries (3), and sugar-free pancake syrup

SUBTOTAL: 18

LUNCH

2-egg omelet (1) with 1 ounce Monterey Jack cheese (1), ½ cup chopped red bell pepper (3), 2 slices ham, chopped, and 2 tablespoons no-added-sugar salsa (2)

1 cup mixed greens (1), ¼ cup black beans (7), ½ Hass avocado (2), and 1 small tomato, chopped (3), with vinaigrette (1)

SUBTOTAL: 21

SNACK

¼ cup ricotta cheese (2) with 1 ounce sunflower seeds (1) and 1 small fresh fig (6)

DINNER

Fish kebabs: 6 ounces swordfish with ½ cup cherry tomatoes (2), ½ cup scallions (2.5), and ½ cup yellow squash (3), marinated in vinaigrette

½ cup baked acorn squash (10)

Goat cheese salad: 2 cups mixed greens (2), 1 ounce goat cheese (1), and vinaigrette (2)

SUBTOTAL: 22.5

TOTAL: 70.5 GRAMS

DAY FIVE

BREAKFAST

2 hard-boiled eggs (1)

1 cup whole-milk plain yogurt (11), topped with ½ cup raspberries (3) and 1 ounce pecans, chopped (1)

SUBTOTAL: 16

LUNCH

Open-faced Reuben: 4 ounces corned beef, 2 slices Swiss cheese (2), ½ cup sauerkraut (2), on 1 slice low-carb rye bread (3), broiled

2 cups mixed greens (2) with ½ cup artichoke hearts (5), 2 tablespoons capers (2), and vinaigrette (2)

SUBTOTAL: 18

SNACK

1 celery stalk (1) with 1 tablespoon soy nut butter (1)

DINNER

One 6-ounce lamb patty served on ¼ cup cannellini beans (8) cooked with 1 small tomato, chopped (3), and ½ cup eggplant, chopped (2)

2 cups iceberg lettuce (1) and Russian dressing (2)

½ cup cooked whole wheat couscous (17)

SUBTOTAL: 33

TOTAL: 69 GRAMS

DAY SIX

BREAKFAST

4 peach pancakes (3) made with soya flour pancake and waffle mix and 1 fresh peach, sliced (7), topped with ¼ cup ricotta cheese (2) and sugar-free pancake syrup

SUBTOTAL: 12

LUNCH

Classic cheeseburger: one 6-ounce beef patty topped with 1 slice American cheese (1) and 1 tablespoon ketchup (1) on a low-carb hamburger roll (5)

1 dill pickle (2)

Coleslaw made with 1 medium carrot, shredded (5), 1 cup green cabbage, shredded (2), and mayonnaise

Half an orange (8.5)

SUBTOTAL: 24.5

SNACK

1½ cups air-popped popcorn (3.5) sprinkled with 1 ounce Romano cheese, grated (1)

DINNER

6 ounces roast duckling with orange glaze made from 2 tablespoons fruit only orange marmalade and ½ teaspoon cinnamon (4)

2 cups watercress (2) with ½ orange, sectioned (8.5), 1 ounce pine nuts (1), and vinaigrette (2)

1 cup kale (4), cooked and mixed with ¼ cup cooked wild rice (8)

Sugar-free lemon gelatin

Don't forget to save the leftover duck for lunch tomorrow!

SUBTOTAL: 29.5

TOTAL: 70.5 GRAMS

DAY SEVEN

BREAKFAST

2 poached eggs (1) on 1 slice whole grain toast (17), 1 ounce American cheese (1)

¼ cup strawberries, sliced (2)

SUBTOTAL: 21

LUNCH

Roast duck wrap: 4 ounces roasted duck, 1 cup leaf lettuce (1), ½ cup sliced red grapes (6.5), and mayonnaise wrapped in a low-carb tortilla (3)

2 cups mixed greens (2), with ½ cup mushrooms (1) and ranch dressing (2)

SUBTOTAL: 15.5

SNACK

1 plum (8) and 1 ounce cheddar cheese (1)

DINNER

6 ounces baked ham with mustard glaze made from 2 tablespoons mustard and 1 table-spoon fruit only apricot jam (2)

½ baked sweet potato (12)

2 cups Boston lettuce (2) and 1 cup radicchio (1), with 2 artichoke hearts (2), ½ cup sliced cucumber (1), and vinaigrette (2)

Chocolate-cheese dessert: Puree 2 ounces ricotta cheese (2) with 1 tablespoon unsweetened cocoa (1) and sucralose (1) to taste

SUBTOTAL: 26

TOTAL: 71.5 GRAMS

DAY ONE

BREAKFAST
½ cup V8 juice (5)

1 cup high-protein flake cereal (6) with 1 cup reduced-carb, milk dairy beverage (3), ½ small papaya, chopped (6), and 1 ounce almonds, sliced (1)

SUBTOTAL: 21

LUNCH
4 ounces grilled beef strips with 1 tablespoon teriyaki sauce (1)

3 cups mixed greens (3) with ½ cup black soybeans (1), ½ small tomato, sliced (3), and ½ cup chopped green pepper (3.5), with vinaigrette (3)

½ cup blackberries (5.5)

SUBTOTAL: 20

SNACK
½ red Delicious apple (9) with 1 ounce cheddar cheese (1)

DINNER
One 1-pound steamed lobster with drawn butter (2)

Coleslaw made with 1 medium carrot, shredded (5), 1 cup green cabbage, shredded (2), and mayonnaise

1 ear steamed corn (17) with butter

1 slice sugar-free cheesecake (3)

Instead of plain butter, work chopped parsley into softened butter and add a little garlic and lemon juice. Roll extra into a log with waxed paper, slice into disks, and freeze.

SUBTOTAL: 29

TOTAL: 80 GRAMS

DAY TWO

BREAKFAST
½ cup cottage cheese (4), 1 ounce almonds, sliced (1), and ½ red grapefruit (8)

2 rye crisp breads (10) with 1 tablespoon fruit only blueberry preserves (2)

Crisp breads vary considerably in carb count. Wasa, Kava, and Ryvita all offer acceptable choices, but check carb counts.

SUBTOTAL: 25

LUNCH
Chef salad: 2 slices each thinly sliced ham, turkey, and roast beef, plus 2 chopped hard-boiled eggs (1), 4 asparagus spears, sliced (2), 1 cup cherry tomatoes (4), and 2 slices cooked bacon crumbled over 3 cups mixed greens (3) and vinaigrette (3)

½ kiwi fruit (4)

SUBTOTAL: 17

SNACK
Hot cocoa: 1 cup reduced-carb milk dairy beverage (3) with 2 tablespoons unsweetened cocoa (2) and 1 packet sucralose (1)

DINNER
Vegetarian stir-fry: Sauté ½ cup tempeh (3.5) with 1 clove garlic (1), 1 teaspoon chopped ginger, ½ cup sliced zucchini (2), 1 cup baby bok choy (0.5), ¼ cup sliced red bell pepper (1.5), and ¼ cup water chestnuts (4) in sesame oil and soy sauce, and top with 1 ounce peanuts, chopped (1)

½ cup cooked brown rice (21)

Tempeh is made of cooked, fermented soybeans and is higher in protein than tofu. It's also more flavorful. With a firm texture, it is well suited to stir-fries.

SUBTOTAL: 34.5

TOTAL: 82.5 GRAMS

DAY THREE

BREAKFAST

Peach-strawberry smoothie: 1 fresh peach, sliced (7), and ½ cup strawberries (3) blended with 1 cup reduced-carb, milk dairy beverage (3), 2 scoops low-carb vanilla whey protein shake mix (3), and 4 ice cubes

SUBTOTAL: 18

LUNCH

Smoked turkey and Brie sandwich: 4 ounces smoked turkey, 2 ounces Brie cheese (2), and ½ Granny Smith apple, sliced (9), with mustard on 2 slices low-carb multigrain bread (6)

2 cups mixed greens (2) with 1 small tomato, chopped (3), ½ cup bean sprouts (2), and French dressing (2)

SUBTOTAL: 26

SNACK

1 ounce walnuts (1)

DINNER

6 ounces lamb chops, grilled

½ cup cooked couscous (17) with 1 ounce almonds, chopped (1), ½ cup chopped red bell pepper (3), and ¼ cup chopped onion (3)

2 cups mixed greens (2) with Russian dressing (2)

½ cup blueberries (8)

SUBTOTAL: 36

TOTAL: 81 GRAMS

DAY FOUR

BREAKFAST
¼ cup hot oat bran cereal (17) with ½ cup pitted cherries (8), 1 ounce almonds, sliced (1), and ½ cup reduced-carb, milk dairy beverage (1.5)

SUBTOTAL: 27.5

LUNCH
2-egg omelet (1) with 1 ounce mozzarella cheese (1), ¼ cup black beans (7), ½ cup chopped red bell pepper (3), and 2 tablespoons salsa (2)

1 slice whole grain bread, toasted (14)

2 cups mixed greens (2) with vinaigrette (2)

SUBTOTAL: 32

SNACK
1 ounce hulled sunflower seeds (1)

DINNER
6 ounces bay scallops sautéed in olive oil with 1 garlic clove (1), ½ cup zucchini (1), ½ cup chopped red pepper (3), and sprinkled with chopped parsley and lemon juice

½ cup pea pods (3.5) and ½ cup carrots (6), steamed

2 cups mixed greens (2), 1 ounce goat cheese (1), and vinaigrette (2)

1 cup no-sugar-added chocolate ice cream (3)

SUBTOTAL: 22.5

TOTAL: 83 GRAMS

DAY FIVE

BREAKFAST

2 ounces mascarpone cheese (2), topped with 1 plum, sliced (8), and 1 ounce almonds (1)

2 hard-boiled eggs (1)

SUBTOTAL: 12

LUNCH

Open-faced roast beef sandwich: 4 ounces roast beef on 1 slice whole rye bread (18), with Russian dressing, ½ small tomato, sliced (1.5), and ½ dill pickle, sliced (1)

1 medium carrot, cut into sticks (5), and 2 celery stalks (2) with 2 tablespoons sour cream and dill dip (2)

SUBTOTAL: 29.5

SNACK

½ cucumber (1.5), hollowed and filled with 2 tablespoons cream cheese (1)

DINNER

One 6-ounce lamb patty

½ cup cooked whole wheat couscous (17) mixed with ½ cup chopped onions (5.5), sautéed, ½ cup cherry tomatoes (2), and ½ cup chopped zucchini (2)

2 cups mixed greens (2) with ½ cup fennel (1.5), 5 black olives (1), and vinaigrette (2)

SUBTOTAL: 33

TOTAL: 77 GRAMS

DAY SIX

BREAKFAST

1 cup oatmeal (21), cooked with 1 ounce walnuts, chopped (1), and ¼ cup whole milk (3)

To add interest to oatmeal, consider adding a teaspoon of vanilla, cinnamon, or nutmeg and a pat of butter.

SUBTOTAL: 25

LUNCH

Antipasti sandwich: 2 slices each salami, ham, provolone (2), 2 roasted red peppers (2), ½ cup artichoke hearts (5), 5 olives, chopped (1), and mustard in a low-carb roll (5)

2 cups romaine lettuce (2), ¼ cup cannellini beans (6.5), 1 small tomato, chopped (3), and Caesar dressing (2)

SUBTOTAL: 28.5

SNACK

1 kiwi (9) with 1 ounce walnuts (1)

DINNER

Turkey–Swiss chard scramble: 6 ounces ground turkey seasoned with chili powder and cumin to taste, sautéed with ½ cup Swiss chard (2) and ½ cup tomato sauce (4)

¼ cup brown rice (10)

1 cup mixed greens (1) with ½ cup hearts of palm (2) and vinaigrette (1)

SUBTOTAL: 20

TOTAL: 83.5 GRAMS

DAY SEVEN

BREAKFAST

2 poached eggs (1), 1 ounce Swiss cheese (1), 1 small tomato (3), and 1 sausage patty on ½ cup cooked kale (2)

½ cup raspberries (3)

1 slice 100 percent whole wheat toast (12)

SUBTOTAL: 22

LUNCH

1 cup beef broth (1) with ½ cup cooked pearl barley (19)

Salmon salad: 6 ounces canned salmon mixed with 2 tablespoons mayonnaise and 1 tablespoon each chopped flat-leaf parsley and capers (1), ½ cup sliced cucumber (1), and 1 cup leaf lettuce (1) in a low-carb pita (6)

SUBTOTAL: 29

SNACK

½ Golden Delicious apple (9) with 1 ounce cheddar cheese (1)

DINNER

One 8-ounce pork cutlet with 1 tablespoon fruit only apricot jam (2)

½ cup baked butternut squash (8)

2 cups mixed greens (2) with ½ cup mushrooms (1), ½ cup pea pods (2), ½ cup baby corn (2), ½ cup chopped red bell pepper (3), and ranch dressing (2)

SUBTOTAL: 22

TOTAL: 83 GRAMS

REFERENCES

The efficacy and safety of Atkins are backed by an ongoing stream of scientific studies, many of which have directly compared Atkins to a low-fat approach. As the findings of these studies reveal, Atkins works as well or better than low-fat approaches. Atkins is the only weight loss approach that has stood up to such intense scrutiny from the medical community. These studies were funded by independent organizations such as the National Institutes of Health, the American Heart Association, and the American Diabetes Association, and the results have been published in such leading journals as the *New England Journal of Medicine* and *Annals of Internal Medicine*. To date there are 46 studies, but more are published regularly. Further studies are available at http://atkins.com/science/researchsupportingatkins.html.

Aude, Y. W., A. S. Agatson, F. Lopez-Jimenez et al., "The National Cholesterol Education Program Diet vs. a Diet Lower in Carbohydrates and Higher in Protein and Monounsaturated Fat," *Archives of Internal Medicine* 164, 2004: 2141–46.

Bailes, J. R., M. T. Strow, J. Werthammer, et al., "Effect of Low-Carbohydrate, Unlimited Calorie Diet on the Treatment of Childhood Obesity: A Prospective Controlled Study," *Metabolic Syndrome and Related Disorders* 1(3), 2003: 221–25.

Boden, G., K. Sargrad, C. Homko, et al., "Effect of a Low-Carbohydrate Diet on Appetite, Blood Glucose Levels, and Insulin Resistance in Obese Patients with Type 2 Diabetes," *Annals of Internal Medicine* 142, 2005: 403–11.

Brehm, B. J., R. J. Seeley, S. R. Daniels, et al., "A Randomized Trial Comparing a Very Low Carbohydrate Diet and a Calorie-Restricted Low Fat Diet on Body Weight and Cardiovascular Risk Factors in Healthy Women," *Journal of Clinical Endocrinology and Metabolism* 88(4), 2003: 1617–23.

Brehm, B. J., S. E. Spang, B. L. Lattin, et al., "The Role of Energy Expenditure in the Differential Weight Loss in Obese Women on Low-Fat and Low-Carbohydrate Diets," *Journal of Clinical Endocrinology and Metabolism* 90(3), 2005: 1475–82.

Dansinger, M. L., J. L. Gleason, J. L. Griffith, et al., "One Year Effectiveness of the Atkins, Ornish, Weight Watchers, and Zone Diets in Decreasing Body Weight and Heart Disease Risk." Presented at the American Heart Association Scientific Sessions, November 12, 2003, in Orlando, Florida.

Dashti, H. M., Y. Y. Bo-Abbas, S. K. Asfar, et al., "Ketogenic Diet Modifies the Risk Factors of Heart Disease in Obese Patients," *Nutrition* 19(10), 2003: 901–02.

Dashti, H. M., C. M. Mathew, T. Hussein, et al., "Long-Term Effects of a Ketogenic Diet in Obese Patients," *Clinical Cardiology* 9(3), 2004: 200–05.

Foster, G. D., H. R. Wyatt, J. O. Hill, et al., "A Randomized Trial of a Low-Carbohydrate Diet for Obesity," *New England Journal of Medicine* 348(21) 2003: 2082–90.

Gann, D., "A Low-Carbohydrate Diet in Overweight Patients Undergoing Stable Statin Therapy Raises High-Density Lipoprotein and Lowers Triglycerides Substantially," *Clinical Cardiology* 27(10), 2004: 563–64.

Gannon, M. C. and F. Q. Nuttall, "Effect of a High-Protein, Low-Carbohydrate Diet on Blood Glucose Control in People with Type 2 Diabetes," *Diabetes* 53(9), 2004: 2375–82.

Goldstein, T., J. D. Kark, E. M. Berry, et al., "Influence of a Modified Atkins Diet on Weight Loss and Glucose Metabolism in Obese Type 2 Diabetic Patients," *Israel Medical Association Journal* 6, 2004: 314.

Greene, P. J., J. Devecis, and W. C. Willett, "Effects of Low-Fat Vs Ultra-Low-Carbohydrate Weight-Loss Diets: A 12-Week Pilot Feeding Study." Abstract presented at Nutrition Week 2004, February 9–12, 2004, in Las Vegas, Nevada.

Gutierrez, M., M. Akhavan, L. Jovanovic, et al., "Utility of a Short-Term 25% Carbohydrate Diet on Improving Glycemic Control in Type 2 Diabetes Mellitus," *Journal of the American College of Nutrition* 17(6), 1998: 595–600.

Hays, J. H., A. DiSabatino, R. T. Gorman, et al., "Effect of a High Saturated Fat and No-Starch Diet on Serum Lipid Subfractions in Patients with Documented Atherosclerotic Cardiovascular Disease," *Mayo Clinic Proceedings* 78(11), 2003: 1331–36.

Hays, J. H., R. T. Gorman, and K. M. Shakir, "Results of Use of Metformin and Replacement of Starch With Saturated Fat in Diets of Patients With Type 2 Diabetes," *Endocrinology Practice* 8(3), 2002: 177–83.

Hickey, J. T., L. Hickey, W. S. Yancy, et al., "Clinical Use of a Carbohydrate-Restricted Diet to Treat the Dyslipidemia of the Metabolic Syndrome," *Metabolic Syndrome and Related Disorders* 1(3), 2003: 227–32.

Husain, A. M., W. S. Yancy, Jr., S. T. Carwile, et al., "Diet Therapy for Narcolepsy," *Neurology* 62(12), 2004: 2300–02.

Kossoff, E. H., G. L. Krauss, J. R. McGrogan, et al., "Efficacy of the Atkins Diet as Therapy for Intractable Epilepsy," *Neurology* 61(12), 2003: 1789–91.

McAuley, K. A., C. M. Hopkins, K. J. Smith, et al., "Comparison of High-Fat and High-Protein Diets with a High-Carbohydrate Diet in Insulin-Resistant Obese Women," *Diabetologia* 48(1), 2005: 8–16.

Meckling, K. A., C. O'Sullivan, and D. Saari, "Comparison of a Low-Fat Diet to a Low-Carbohydrate Diet on Weight Loss, Body Composition, and Risk Factors for Diabetes and Cardiovascular Disease in Free-Living, Overweight Men and Women," *Journal of Clinical Endocrinology and Metabolism* 89(6), 2004: 2717–23.

Nickols-Richardson, S. M., J. J., Volpe, and M. D. Coleman, "Premenopausal Women Following a Low-Carbohydrate/High-Protein Diet Experience Greater Weight Loss and Less Hunger Compared to a High-Carbohydrate/Low-Fat Diet." Abstract presented at FASEB Meeting on Experimental Biology: Translating the Genome, April 17–21, 2004, in Washington, D.C.

O'Brien, K. D., B. J. Brehm, and R. J. Seeley, "Greater Reduction in Inflammatory Markers with a Low Carbohydrate Diet than with a Calorically Matched Low-Fat Diet." Presented at American Heart Association's Scientific Sessions 2002 on Tuesday, November 19, 2002. Abstract ID: 117597.

Samaha, F. F., N. Iqbal, P. Seshadri, et al., "A Low-Carbohydrate as Compared with a Low-Fat Diet in Severe Obesity," *New England Journal of Medicine* 348(21), 2003: 2074–81.

Segal-Isaacson, C. J., M. Ginsberg, et. al., "One-Year Data from A Prospective Cohort of Low-Carbohydrate Dieters," 2004 North American Society for the Study of Obesity Conference, Las Vegas, Nevada.

Seshadri, P., N. Iqbal, L. Stern, et al., "A Randomized Study Comparing the Effects of a Low-Carbohydrate Diet and a Conventional Diet on Lipoprotein Subfractions and C-Reactive Protein Levels in Patients with Severe Obesity," *American Journal of Medicine* 117(5), 2004: 398–405.

Sharman, M. J., A. L. Gomez, W. J. Kraemer, et al., "Very Low-Carbohydrate and Low-Fat Diets Affect Fasting Lipids and Postprandial Lipemia Differently in Overweight Men," *Journal of Nutrition* 134(4), 2004: 880–85.

Sharman, M. J. and J. S. Volek, "Weight Loss Leads to Reductions in Inflammatory Biomarkers After a Very Low-Carbohydrate and Low-Fat Diet in Overweight Men," *Clinical Science (London)*, 2004.

Sharman, M. J., W. J. Kraemer, D. M. Love, et al., "A Ketogenic Diet Favorably Affects Serum Biomarkers for Cardiovascular Disease in Normal-Weight Men," *Journal of Nutrition* 132(7), 2002: 1879–85.

Sondike, S. B., N. Copperman, and M. S. Jacobson, "Effects of a Low-Carbohydrate Diet on Weight Loss and Cardiovascular Risk Factor in Overweight Adolescents," *Journal of Pediatrics* 142(3), 2003: 253–58.

Stadler, D. D., V. Burden, W. Connor, et al., "Impact of 42-Day Atkins Diet and Energy-Matched Low-Fat Diet on Weight and Anthropometric Indices," *FASEB Journal* 17(4–5). Abstract of the 12th Annual FASEB Meeting on Experimental Biology: Translating the Genome; Abstract #453.3, San Diego, CA, April 11–15, 2003.

Stern, L., N. Iqbal, P. Seshadri, et al., "The Effects of Low-Carbohydrate Versus Conventional Weight Loss Diets in Severely Obese Adults: One-Year Follow-up of a Randomized Trial," *Annals of Internal Medicine* 140(10), 2004: 778–85.

Vernon, M. C., J. Mavropoulos, M. Transue, et al., "Clinical Experience of a Carbohydrate-Restricted Diet: Effect on Diabetes Mellitus," *Metabolic Syndrome and Related Disorders* 1(3), 2003: 233–37.

Volek, J. S., A. L. Gómez, and W. J. Kraemer, "Fasting Lipoprotein and Postprandial Triacylglycerol Responses to a Low-Carbohydrate Diet Supplemented with N-3 Fatty Acids," *Journal of the American College of Nutrition* 19(3), 2000: 383–91.

Volek, J. S., M. J. Sharman, A. L. Gomez et al., "An Isoenergetic Very Low-Carbohydrate Diet Improves Serum HDL Cholesterol and Triacylglycerol Concentrations, the Total Cholesterol to HDL Cholesterol Ratio and Postprandial Lipemic Responses Compared with a Low-Fat Diet in Normal Weight, Normolipidemic Women," *Journal of Nutrition* 133(9), 2003: 2756–61.

Volek, J. S., M. J. Sharman, and A. L. Gomez, "Comparison of a Very Low-Carbohydrate and Low-Fat Diet on Fasting Lipids, LDL Subclasses, Insulin Resistance, and Postprandial Lipemic Responses in Overweight Women," *Journal of the American College of Nutrition* 23(2), 2004: 177–84.

Volek, J. S., M. J. Sharman, A. L. Gomez, et. al., "Comparison of Energy-Restricted Very Low-Carbohydrate and Low-Fat Diets on Weight Loss and Body Composition in Overweight Men and Women," *Nutrition and Metabolism (London)* 1(1), 2004: 13.

Volek, J. S., M. J. Sharman, D. M. Love, et al., "Body Composition and Hormonal Responses to a Carbohydrate Restricted Diet," *Metabolism* 51(7), 2002: 864–70.

Volek, J. S. and E. C. Westman, "Very-Low-Carbohydrate Weight-Loss Diets Revisited," *Cleveland Clinic Journal of Medicine* 69(11), 2002: 849–62.

Westman, E. C., J. Mavropoulos, W. S. Yancy, et al., "A Review of Low-Carbohydrate Ketogenic Diets," *Current Atherosclerosis Reports* 5(6), 2003: 476–83.

Westman, E. C., W. S. Yancy, J. S. Edman, et al., "Effect of 6-Month Adherence to a Very Low Carbohydrate Diet Program," *American Journal of Medicine* 113(1), 2002: 30–36.

Westman, E. C., W. S. Yancy, J. Hepburn, et al., "A Pilot Study of a Low-Carbohydrate, Ketogenic Diet for Obesity-Related Polycystic Ovary Syndrome," *Journal of General Internal Medicine* 19(1S), 2004: 111.

Yancy, W. S., Jr., M. E. Foy, E. C. Westman, "A Low-Carbohydrate, Ketogenic Diet for Type 2 Diabetes Mellitus," *Journal of General Internal Medicine* 19(1S), 2004: 110.

Yancy, W. S., Jr., M. K. Olsen, J. R. Guyton, et al., "A Low-Carbohydrate, Ketogenic Diet Versus a Low-Fat Diet to Treat Obesity and Hyperlipidemia," *Annals of Internal Medicine* 140(10), 2004: 769–77.

Yancy, W. S., Jr., D. Provenzale, E. C. Westman, "Improvement of Gastroesophageal Reflux Disease After Initiation of a Low-Carbohydrate Diet: Five Brief Case Reports," *Alternative Therapies in Health and Medicine* 7(6):120, 2001: 116–19.

Yancy, W. S., Jr., M. C. Vernon, E. C. Westman, "A Pilot Trial of a Low-Carbohydrate, Ketogenic Diet in Patients with Type 2 Diabetes," *Metabolic Syndrome and Related Disorders* 1(3), 2003: 239–43.

SOURCES

Many publications have been used for reference in this work. The following have been especially useful.

1: WHAT YOU CAN ACHIEVE

Allison, D. B. and F. X. Pi-Sunyer (eds.), "Obesity Treatment: Establishing Goals, Improving Outcomes and Reviewing the Research Agenda," *NATO ASI Series A: Life Sciences*, 1995, vol. 278.

American College of Sports Medicine, *ACSM's Guidelines for Exercise Testing and Prescription*, 2000, B. Franklin (ed.), Lippincott, Williams & Wilkins, pages 5, 6, 138, 237–39.

Bassey, E. J., and S. J. Ramsdale, "Increase in Femoral Bone Density in Young Women Following High-Impact Exercise," *Osteoporosis International* 4(2), 1994: 72–75.

Beitz, R., and M. Doren, "Physical Activity and Postmenopausal Health," *Journal of the British Menopause Society* 10(2), 2004: 70–74.

Campbell, W. W., M. C. Crim, "Increased Protein Requirements in the Elderly: New Data and Retrospective Reassessments," *American Journal of Clinical Nutrition* 60(1), 1994: 160–75.

Campbell, W. W., W. Evans. "Protein Requirements of Elderly People," *European Journal of Clinical Nutrition* 50(1), 1996: S180–S185.

Chernoff, R., "Protein and Older Adults," *Journal of the American College of Nutrition* 23(6), 2004: 627S–630S.

Clarkson, T. B., R. Anthony, "Phytoestrogens and Coronary Heart Disease," *Baillieres Clinical Endocrinol Metabolism* 12(4), 1998: 589–604.

Donnelly, J. E., B. Smith, D. J. Jacobsen, et al., "The Role of Exercise for Weight Loss and Maintenance," *Best Practice and Research: Clinical Gastroenterology* 18(6), 2004: 1009–29.

Hakim, A. A., H. Petrovitch, C. M. Burchfiel, et al., "Effects of Walking on Mortality Among Nonsmoking Retired Men," *New England Journal of Medicine* 338(2), 1998: 94–99.

Hassmen, P., N. Koivula, and A. Uutela, "Physical Exercise and Psychological Well-Being: A Population Study in Finland," *Preventive Medicine* 30(1), 2000: 17–25.

Hill, J. O. and H. Wyatt, "Outpatient Management of Obesity: A Primary Care Perspective," *Obesity Research* 10(2S), 2002: 124S–130S.

Hu, F. B., M. J. Stampfer, C. Solomon, et al., "Physical Activity and Risk for Cardiovascular Events in Diabetic Women," *Annals of Internal Medicine* 134(2), 2001: 96–105.

Hunter, G. R., J. P. McCarthy, and M. M. Bamman, "Effects of Resistance Training on Older Adults," *Sports Medicine* 34(5), 2004: 329–48.

Johnson, C. S. "Postprandial Thermogenesis Is Increased 100% on a High-Protein Low-Fat Diet vs. a High-Carbohydrate, Low-Fat Diet in Healthy, Young Women," *Journal of the American College of Nutrition* 21 (1), 2002: 55–61.

Lane, A. M., and D. J. Lovejoy, "The Effects of Exercise on Mood Changes: The Moderating Effect of Depressed Mood," *Journal of Sports Medicine and Physical Fitness*, 41(4), 2001: 539–45.

Layman, D. K., "Increased Dietary Protein Modifies Glucose and Insulin Homeostasis in Adult Women During Weight Loss," *Journal of Nutrition* 133 (2), 2003: 405–10.

Layman, D. K., "Protein Quantity and Quality at Levels above the RDA Improves Adult Weight Loss," *Journal of the American College of Nutrition* 23: 6, 2004: 631S–636S.

Layman, D. K., "A Reduced Ration of Dietary Carbohydrate to Protein Improves Body Composition and Blood Lipid Profiles During Weight Loss in Adult Women," *Journal of Nutrition* 133 (2), 2003: 411–17.

Leon, A. S., J. Connett, D. R. Jacobs, Jr., et al., "Leisure-Time Physical Activity Levels and Risk of Coronary Heart Disease and Death: The Multiple Risk Factor Intervention Trial," *Journal of the American Medical Association* 258(17), 1987: 2388–95.

Manson, J. E., P. Greenland, A. Z. LaCroix, et al., "Walking Compared with Vigorous Exercise for the Prevention of Cardiovascular Events in Women," *New England Journal of Medicine* 347(10), 2002: 716–25.

McCarthy, J. P., J. C. Agre, B. K. Graf, et al., "Compatibility of Adaptive Responses with Combining Strength and Endurance Training," *Medicine and Science in Sports and Exercise* 27(3), 1995: 429–36.

Myers, J., M. Prakash, V. Froelicher, et al., "Exercise Capacity and Mortality Among Men Referred for Exercise Testing," *New England Journal of Medicine* 346(11), 2002: 793–801.

Nieman, D. C., "Current Perspective on Exercise Immunology," *Current Sports Medicine Reports* 2(5), 2003: 239–42.

NIH Technology Assessment Conference Panel, "Methods for Voluntary Weight Loss and Control," *Annals of Internal Medicine* 119(7 Pt 2), 1993: 764–70.

Noakes, M., F. Paul, and K. J. Keogh, "High Protein Snack Bars Can Reduce Food Intake and Improve Glucose and Insulin Metabolism in Overweight Women," *Obesity Research* 12(S), 2004: A55.

Pratley, R., B. Nicklas, M. Rubin, et al., "Strength Training Increases Resting Metabolic Rate and Norepinephrine Levels in Healthy 50- to 65-Year-Old Men," *Journal of Applied Physiology* 76(1), 1994: 133–37.

Press, V., I. Freestone, and C. F. George, "Physical Activity: The Evidence of Benefit in the Prevention of Coronary Heart Disease," *QIM* 96(4), 2003: 245–51.

Ross, R., D. Dagnone, P. J. Jones, et al., "Reduction in Obesity and Related Comorbid Conditions After Diet-Induced Weight Loss or Exercise-Induced Weight Loss in Men: A Randomized, Controlled Trial," *Annals of Internal Medicine* 133(2), 2000: 92–103.

Shephard, R. J., S. Rhind, and P. N. Shek, "The Impact of Exercise on the Immune System: NK Cells, Interleukins 1 and 2, and Related Responses," *Exercise and Sport Sciences Reviews* 23, 1995: 215–41.

Stefanick, M. L., S. Mackey, M. Sheehan, et al., "Effects of Diet and Exercise in Men and Postmenopausal Women with Low Levels of HDL Cholesterol and High Levels of LDL Cholesterol," *New England Journal of Medicine* 339(1), 1998: 12–20.

Stern, L., N. Iqbal, P. Seshadri, et al., "The Effects of Low-Carbohydrate Versus Conventional Weight Loss Diets in Severely Obese Adults: One-Year Follow-up of a Randomized Trial," *Annals of Internal Medicine* 140(10), 2004: 778–85.

Stuifbergen, A. K., H. Becker, G. M. Timmerman et al., "The Use of Individualized Goal Setting to Facilitate Behavior Change in Women with Multiple Sclerosis," *Journal of Neuroscience Nursing* 35(2), 2003: 94–106.

Weinberg, R. S., and D. Gould, *Foundations of Sport and Exercise Psychology*, 3rd ed. Human Kinetics, 2003, p. 251.

Wessel, T. R., C. B. Arant, M. B. Olson, et al., "Relationship of Physical Fitness vs. Body Mass Index with Coronary Artery Disease and Cardiovascular Events in Women," *Journal of the American Medical Association* 292(10), 2004: 1179–87.

Westman, E. C., W. S. Yancy, J. S. Edman, et al., "Effect of 6-Month Adherence to a Very Low Carbohydrate Diet Program," *American Journal of Medicine* 113(1), 2002: 30–36.

Yamazaki, S., S. Ichimura, J. Iwamoto, et al., "Effect of Walking Exercise on Bone Metabolism in Postmenopausal Women with Osteopenia/Osteoporosis," *Journal of Bone and Mineral Metabolism* 22(5), 2004: 500–08.

2: WHY ATKINS WORKS

American Heart Association Meeting report on Dietary Fatty Acids and Cardiovascular Health, 2000.

Bjorntorp, P., "Do Stress Reactions Cause Abdominal Obesity and Comorbidities?" *Obesity Review* 2(2), 2001: 73–86.

Fife, B., "Saturated Fat May Save Your Life," *HealthWise*, 1999: 207.

German, J. B., and C. J. Dillard, "Saturated Fats: What Dietary Intake?" *American Journal of Clinical Nutrition* 80(3), 2004: 550–59.

Kris-Etherton, P. M., W. S. Harris, L. J. Appel, "Fish Consumption, Fish Oil, Omega-3 Fatty Acids, and Cardiovascular Disease," *Arteriosclerosis, Thrombosis, and Vascular Biology* 23(2), 2003: e20–30.

Kris-Etherton, P. M., T. A. Pearson, Y. Wan, et al., "High-Monounsaturated Fatty Acid Diets Lower Both Plasma Cholesterol and Triacylglycerol Concentrations," *American Journal of Clinical Nutrition* 70(6), 1999: 1009–15.

Lichtenstein, A. H., "Dietary Trans Fatty Acid," *Journal of Cardiopulmonary Rehabilitation* 20(3), 2000: 143–46.

Liu, S., W. C. Willett, M. J. Stampfer, et al., "A Prospective Study of Dietary Glycemic Load, Carbohydrate Intake, and Risk of Coronary Heart Disease in U.S. Women," *American Journal of Clinical Nutrition* 71(6), 2000: 1455–61.

Matthiessen, J., S. Fagt, A. Biltoft-Jensen, et al., "Size Makes a Difference," *Public Health Nutrition* 6(1), 2003: 65–72.

Natow, A., and J. Heslin, "The Cholesterol Counter," 1998, Pocket Books, 5th ed., p. 633.

Ovalle, F., and R. Azziz, "Insulin Resistance, Polycystic Ovary Syndrome, and Type 2 Diabetes Mellitus," *Fertility and Sterility* 77(6), 2002: 1095–105.

Putnam, J. J., and J. E. Allshouse, "Food Consumption, Prices, and Expenditures, 1970–1997," Economic Research Service, USDA, Statistical Bulletin no. 965, 1999: 196.

Ravnskov, U., "The Questionable Role of Saturated and Polyunsaturated Fatty Acids in Cardiovascular Disease," *Journal of Clinical Epidemiology* 51(6), 1998: 443–60.

Sacks, F. M., and M. Katan, "Randomized Clinical Trials on the Effects of Dietary Fat and Carbohydrate on Plasma Lipoproteins and Cardiovascular Disease," *American Journal of Medicine* 113 S(9B), 2002: 13S–24S.

Taubes, G., "Nutrition. The Soft Science of Dietary Fat," *Science* 291(5513), 2001: 2536–45.

Taubes, G., "What if It's All Been a Big Fat Lie?" *New York Times Magazine*, 2002, p. 22.

Willett, W. C., M. J. Stampfer, J. E. Manson, et al., "Intake of Trans Fatty Acids and Risk of Coronary Heart Disease Among Women," *Lancet* 341(8845), 1993: 581–85.

3: ATKINS 101

Westman, E. C., W. S. Yancy, J. S. Edman, et al., "Effect of 6-Month Adherence to a Very Low Carbohydrate Diet Program," *American Journal of Medicine* 113(1), 2002: 30–36.

4: GET READY, GET SET

Bailostosky, K., et al. "Dietary Intake of Macronutrients, Micronutrients, and Other Constituents: United States, 1988–94," *Vital Health Statistics* 11 (245), 2002.

Barringer, T. A., J. K. Kirk, A. C. Santaniello, et al., "Effect of a Multivitamin and Mineral Supplement on Infection and Quality of Life: A Randomized, Double-Blind, Placebo-Controlled Trial," *Annals of Internal Medicine* 138(5), 2003: 365–71.

Fletcher, R. H., K. M. Fairfield, "Vitamins for Chronic Disease Prevention in Adults: Clinical Applications," *Journal of the American Medical Association* 287(23), 2002: 3127–29.

Institute of Medicine of the National Academies, "Dietary Reference Intakes for Energy, Carbohydrates, Fiber, Fat, Fatty Acids, Cholesterol, Protein, and Amino Acids." Available at: http://books.nap.edu/books/0309085373/html/index.html; accessed on December 13, 2004.

Lupton, J. R. and N. D. Turner, "Dietary Fiber and Coronary Disease: Does the Evidence Support an Association?" *Current Atherosclerosis Reports* 5(6), 2003: 500–05.

Marlett, J. A., M. I. McBurney, and J. L. Slavin, "Position of the American Dietetic Association: Health Implications of Dietary Fiber," *Journal of the American Dietetics Association* 102(7), 2002: 993–1000.

Trepel, F., "Dietary Fibre: More Than a Matter of Dietetics. II. Preventative and Therapeutic Uses," *Wiener Klinische Wochenschrift* 116(15–16), 2004: 511–22.

5: WEEK ONE: INDUCTION

Anderson, B. and J., *Stretching*, 1981, Shelter Publication, pp. 10–11.

Bixler, B., and R. L. Jones, "High-School Football Injuries: Effects of a Post-Halftime Warm-up and Stretching Routine," *Family Practice Research Journal* 12(2), 1992: 131–39.

Fredette, D., "Exercise Recommendation for Flexibility and Range of Motion," *ACSM's Resource Manual for Guidelines for Exercise Testing and Prescription*, Lippincott, Williams & Wilkins, 1998, pp. 456–65.

Gimeno, E., M. Fito, R. M. Lamuela-Raventos, et al., "Effect of Ingestion of Virgin Olive Oil on Human Low-Density Lipoprotein Composition," *European Journal of Clinical Nutrition* 56(2), 2002: 114–20.

Keys, A., A. Menotti, M. J. Karvonen, et al., "The Diet and 15-Year Death Rate in the Seven Countries Study," *American Journal of Epidemiology* 124(6), 1986: 903–15.

Tzonou, A., A. Kalandidi, A. Trichopoulou, et al., "Diet and Coronary Heart Disease: A Case-Control Study in Athens, Greece," *Epidemiology* 4(6), 1993: 511–16.

Willett, W. C., "Diet and Coronary Heart Disease," *Monographs in Epidemiology and Biostatistics* 15, 1990: 341–79.

Witvrouw, E., N. Mahieu, L. Danneels, et al., "Stretching and Injury Prevention: An Obscure Relationship," *Sports Medicine* 34(7), 2004: 443–49.

Yeung, E. W. and S. S. Yeung, "A Systematic Review of Interventions to Prevent Lower Limb Soft Tissue Running Injuries," *British Journal of Sports Medicine* 35(6), 2001: 383–89.

6: WEEK TWO: ANYTHING IS POSSIBLE

Westman, E. C., W. S. Yancy, J. S. Edman, et al., "Effect of 6-Month Adherence to a Very Low Carbohydrate Diet Program," *American Journal of Medicine* 113(1), 2002: 30–36.

Witvrouw, E., N. Mahieu, L. Danneels, et al., "Stretching and Injury Prevention: An Obscure Relationship," *Sports Medicine*, 34(7), 2004: 443–49.

7: WEEK THREE: INTRODUCING ONGOING WEIGHT LOSS

ACSM FITNESS BOOK, 3rd ed., American College of Sports Medicine, Human Kinetics, 2003, pp. 4–5.

Bassey, E. J., and S. J. Ramsdale, "Increase in Femoral Bone Density in Young Women Following High-Impact Exercise," *Osteoporosis International* 4(2), 1994: 72–75.

Campbell, W. W., M. C. Crim, V. R. Young, et al., "Increased Energy Requirements and Changes in Body Composition with Resistance Training in Older Adults," *American Journal of Clinical Nutrition* 60(2), 1994: 167–75.

Evans, W. and I. Rosenberg, *Biomakers*, Simon & Schuster, 1992.

Fraser, G. E., "Nut Consumption, Lipids, and Risk of a Coronary Event," *Clinical Cardiology* 22(7S), 1999: 11–15.

Hunter, G. R., J. P. McCarthy, and M. M. Bamman, "Effects of Resistance Training on Older Adults," *Sports Medicine* 34(5), 2004: 329–48.

Keyes, A, H. L. Taylor, and F. Grande, "Basal Metabolism and Age of Adult Man," *Metabolism* 22, 1973: 579–87.

Koffler, K. H., A. Menkes, and R. A. Redmond, et al., "Strength Training Accelerates Gastrointestinal Transit in Middle-Aged and Older Men," *Medicine and Science in Sports and Exercise* 24(4), 1992: 415–19.

Menkes, A., S. Mazel, and R. A. Redmond, et al., "Strength Training Increases Regional Bone Mineral Density and Bone Remodeling in Middle-Aged and Older Men," *Journal of Applied Physiology* 74(5), 1993: 2478–84.

Morgan, W. P., "Affective Beneficence of Vigorous Physical Activity," *Medicine and Science in Sports and Exercise* 17(1), 1985: 94–100.

Singh, R. B., G. Dubnov, M. A. Niaz, et al., "Effect of an Indo-Mediterranean Diet on Progression of Coronary Artery Disease in High-Risk Patients (Indo-Mediterranean Diet Heart Study): A Randomized Single-Blind Trial," *Lancet* 360(9344), 2002: 1455–61.

Stewart, K. J., "Weight Training in Coronary Artery Disease and Hypertension," *Progress in Cardiovascular Diseases* 35(2), 1992: 159–68.

Stewart, K. J., "Role of Exercise Training on Cardiovascular Disease in Persons Who Have Type 2 Diabetes and Hypertension," *Cardiology Clinics* 22(4), 2004: 569–86.

Taylor, C. B., J. F. Sallis, and R. Needle, "The Relation of Physical Activity and Exercise to Mental Health," *Public Health Reports* 100(2), 1985: 195–202.

Yamazaki, S., S. Ichimura, J. Iwamoto, et al., "Effect of Walking Exercise on Bone Metabolism in Postmenopausal Women with Osteopenia/Osteoporosis," *Journal of Bone and Mineral Metabolism* 22(5), 2004: 500–08.

8: WEEK FOUR: FREE SPEED

Anderson, R. A., "Chromium, Glucose Intolerance and Diabetes," *Journal of the American College of Nutrition* 17(6), 1998: 548–55.

Anderson, R. A., "Chromium in the Prevention and Control of Diabetes," *Diabetes and Metabolism*, 26(1), 2000: 22–27.

Anderson, R. A., N. Cheng, N. A. Bryden, et al., "Elevated Intakes of Supplemental Chromium Improve Glucose and Insulin Variables in Individuals with Type 2 Diabetes," *Diabetes* 46(11), 1997: 1786–91.

Cao, G., E. Sofic, and R. L. Prior, "Antioxidant Capacity of Tea and Common Vegetables," *Journal of Agriculture and Food Chemistry* 44, 1996: 3426–31.

Ducros, V., "Chromium Metabolism: A Literature Review," *Biological Trace Element Research* 32, 1992: 65–77.

Greenwald, P., "Clinical Trials in Cancer Prevention: Current Results and Perspectives for the Future," *Journal of Nutrition* 134(12), 2004: 3507S-3512S.

Raphael, T. J., and G. Kuttan, "Immunomodulatory Activity of Naturally Occurring Monoterperies Carvone, Limonene, and Perillic Acid," *Immunopharmacology and Immunotoxicology* 25(2), 2003: 285–94.

Seddon, J. M., U. A. Ajani, R. D. Sperduto, et al., "Dietary Carotenoids, Vitamins A, C, and E, and Advanced Age–Related Macular Degeneration: Eye Disease Case-Control Study Group," *Journal of the American Medical Association*, 272(18), 1994: 1413–20.

Yang, Y. M., C. C. Conaway, J. W. Chiao, et al., "Inhibition of Benzo(a)Pyrene-Induced Lung Tumorigenesis in a/J Mice by Dietary N-Acetylcysteine Conjugates of Benzyl and Phenethyl Isothiocyanates During the Postinitiation Phase Is Associated with Activation of Mitogen-Activated Protein Kinases and P53 Activity and Induction of Apoptosis," *Cancer Research* 62(1), 2002: 2–7.

9: WEEK FIVE: GET MOVING!

ACSM FITNESS BOOK, 3rd ed., American College of Sports Medicine, Human Kinetics, 2003, p. 5.

Greene, P. J., J. Devecis, and W. C. Willett, "Effects of Low-Fat vs. Ultra-Low-Carbohydrate Weight-Loss Diets: A 12-Week Pilot Feeding Study." Abstract presented at Nutrition Week 2004, February 9–12, 2004, in Las Vegas, Nevada.

Sellappan, S., C. C. Akoh, and G. Krewer, "Phenolic Compounds and Antioxidant Capacity of Georgia-Grown Blueberries and Blackberries," *Journal of Agricultural and Food Chemistry* 50(8), 2002: 2432–38.

Sondike, S. B., N. Copperman, and M.S. Jacobson, "Effects of a Low-Carbohydrate Diet on Weight Loss and Cardiovascular Risk Factor in Overweight Adolescents," *Journal of Pediatrics* 142(3), 2003: 253–58.

10: WEEK SIX: LOOK AT YOU!

Erhardt, J. G., C. Meisner, J. C. Bode, et al., "Lycopene, Beta-Carotene, and Colorectal Adenomas," *American Journal of Clinical Nutrition* 78(6), 2003: 1219–24.

Fairfield, K. M., and R. H. Fletcher, "Vitamins for Chronic Disease Prevention in Adults: Scientific Review," *Journal of the American Medical Association* 287(23), 2002: 3116–26.

Kelly, D., and P. E. Wischmeyer, "Role of L-Glutamine in Critical Illness: New Insights," *Current Opinion in Clinical Nutrition and Metabolic Care* 6(2), 2003: 217–22.

11: WEEK SEVEN: SUCCESS—NO MATTER WHAT

Weinberg, R. S., and D. Gould, *Foundations of Sport and Exercise Psychology*, 3rd ed., Human Kinetics, 2003, p. 365.

12: WEEK EIGHT: CHALLENGE YOURSELF!

Gregg, E. W., J. A. Cauley, K. Stone, et al., "Relationship of Changes in Physical Activity and Mortality Among Older Women," *Journal of the American Medical Association* 289(18), 2003: 2379–86.

Hercberg, S., P. Galan, P. Preziosi, et al., "The Su. Vi.Max Study: A Randomized, Placebo-Controlled Trial of the Health Effects of Antioxidant Vitamins and Minerals," *Archives of Internal Medicine* 164(21), 2004: 2335–42.

Lee, I. M., "No Pain, No Gain? Thoughts on the Caerphilly Study," *British Journal of Sports Medicine* 38(1), 2004: 4–5.

Myers, J., M. Prakash, V. Froelicher, et al., "Exercise Capacity and Mortality Among Men Referred for Exercise Testing," *New England Journal of Medicine* 346(11), 2002: 793–801.

Paffenbarger, R. S., Jr., R. T. Hyde, A. L. Wing, et al., "Physical Activity, All-Cause Mortality, and Longevity of College Alumni," *New England Journal of Medicine* 314(10), 1986: 605–13.

United States Department of Health and Human Services, *Physical Activity and Health: A Report of the Surgeon General*, Atlanta, Georgia, U.S. Department of Health and Human Services, Centers for Disease Control and Prevention, National Center for Chronic Disease Prevention and Health Promotion, 1996.

13: WEEK NINE: THE PRE-MAINTENANCE PHASE

Baquet, G., E. van Praagh, and S. Berthoin, "Endurance Training and Aerobic Fitness in Young People," *Sports Medicine* 33(15), 2003: 1127–43.

Ciccolo, J. T., E. M. Jowers, J. B. Bartholomew, "The Benefits of Exercise Training for Quality of Life in HIV/AIDS in the Post-Haart Era," *Sports Medicine* 34(8), 2004: 487–99.

Duthie, G. G., "Parsley, Polyphenols and Nutritional Antioxidants," *British Journal of Nutrition* 81(6), 1999: 425–26.

Rennie, K. L., N. McCarthy, S. Yazdgerdi, et al., "Association of the Metabolic Syndrome with Both Vigorous and Moderate Physical Activity," *International Journal of Epidemiology* 32(4), 2003: 600–06.

Thomas, N. E., J. S. Baker, and B. Davies, "Established and Recently Identified Coronary Heart Disease Risk Factors in Young People: The Influence of Physical Activity and Physical Fitness," *Sports Medicine* 33(9), 2003: 633–50.

Torti, D. C., and G. O. Matheson, "Exercise and Prostate Cancer," *Sports Medicine* 34(6), 2004: 363–69.

14: WEEK TEN: SPICE IT UP

Cao, G., E. Sofic, and R. L. Prior, "Antioxidant Capacity of Tea and Common Vegetables," *Journal of Agriculture and Food Chemistry* 44, 1996: 3426–31.

O'Hara, M., D. Kiefer, K. Farrell, et al., "A Review of 12 Commonly Used Medicinal Herbs," *Archives of Family Medicine* 7(6), 1998: 523–36.

Olson, M. B., S. F. Kelsey, V. Bittner, et al., "Weight Cycling and High-Density Lipoprotein Cholesterol in Women: Evidence of an Adverse Effect: A Report from the NHLBI-Sponsored Wise Study. Women's Ischemia Syndrome Evaluation Study Group," *Journal of the American College of Cardiology* 36(5), 2000: 1565–71.

Shade, E. D., C. M. Ulrich, M. H. Wener, et al. "Frequent Intentional Weight Loss Is Associated with Lower Natural Killer Cytocity in Postmenopausal Women: Possible Long-Term Immune Effects." *Journal of the American Dietetic Association* 104(6), 2004: 903–12.

15: WEEK ELEVEN: ATKINS YOUR WAY

Lambert, E. V., D. P. Speechly, S. C. Dennis, et al., "Enhanced Endurance in Trained Cyclists During Moderate Intensity Exercise Following 2 Weeks' Adaptation to a High-Fat Diet," *European Journal of Applied Physiology and Occupational Physiology* 69(4), 1994: 287–93.

INDEX

berries, 104, 127

beverages, in Induction phase, 30–31

Biceps Curl, 97, 201

binges

    recognizing when you're on the brink of one, 190, 193

    resisting urge for one more, before starting Atkins, 42

    on trigger foods, 105

blood chemistry

    establishing baseline of, 39–40

    rechecking, 153–54

blood cholesterol, 153–54

blood sugar, carbohydrates' effect on, 11–15

blueberries, 127, 261

body, paying attention to warning signs from, 244

Body Mass Index (BMI), 42, 138

boot camp programs, 214

boredom, 204

    in exercising, 213–15

    in food, cure for, 208–10

breakfast, protein in, 176

breathing, 76

broccoli, 113, 261

Broom Builder, 238

buddy support in doing Atkins, 71–72

"But" Busters, writing them down, 56–58

"But Now" busters, writing them down, 140–43

Butterfly, 65

caffeine, 30 *note*, 49–50

calcium, 53

Calf Lift, 119

Calf Stretch, 151

calorie-controlled diets, failure of, 19

calories

    counting not necessary when following the meal plans, 51, 260

    daily minimum and maximum requirements for losing weight, 126

carb creep, 158

Carbohydrate Ladder (ACL), 14–15, 158, 188

carbohydrates, 10–15

    added allowance of, as reward for exercise, 202

    addiction to, 50–51

    and blood sugar, 11–15

    control of amount eaten, 6

    favorites in the Atkins Nutritional Approach, 261

    "good" and "bad," 10, 188

    limiting and then reintroducing, in the four phases of Atkins Nutritional Approach, 23–25

    in proportion to other nutrients in a meal, 139–40

    quality of, in terms of fiber and nutrients, 189, 223, 225

    reintroducing, in Ongoing Weight Loss phase, 106, 138–40, 160

    reintroducing, in Pre-Maintenance phase, 189, 222–23

carbs. *See* hidden carbs; net carbs

cardiovascular exercise, 131–33

    avoiding boredom by taking up new activities, 213–15

    building endurance, 152

    gym equipment for, 248

    sports as part of, 230–31

cardiovascular fitness, 130–31

    levels of, 131

carrots, 174, 261

Cat and Dog, 64

Chair Ab Lift, 183

challenging yourself, 171–86

cheating

    not letting it become a habit, 191

    "smart" way of, 191–93, 226

checkpoints

    for Induction phase, 66–67, 82–84

    for Lifetime Maintenance phase, 255

    for Ongoing Weight Loss phase, 101–2, 123–24, 136, 153–54, 170, 186

    for Pre-Maintenance phase, 203, 221, 239

    for Week One, 66–67

    for Week Two, 82–84

    for Week Three, 101–2

    for Week Four, 123–24

    for Week Five, 136

    for Week Six, 153–54

    for Week Seven, 170

    for Week Eight, 186

    for Week Nine, 203

    for Week Ten, 221

    for Week Eleven, 239

    for Week Twelve, 255

cheese

    in Induction phase, 27

    types to avoid, 27 *note*

chewing, 126

child care, obtaining, to make time for Atkins, 57

children, should not follow Atkins Advantage Program without medical supervision, 33

cholesterol

    blood, 18, 153–54

    dietary, 18

chromium, 107

clothing, exercise, 81, 230
Combined Biceps Curl/Overhead Press, 201
constipation, 76
contracting with yourself, 43–44, 144
convenience foods, 31
cookbooks, Atkins, 128
cooking meals
  adding variety to, 127–28, 208–10
  Atkins style, 263
  challenging yourself with new recipes, 172–73
  tips for efficiency in, 109–10
core (body), strength training of, 182–85
cortisol, 12
counting your blessings, 143
cravings, 11, 50–51, 133
  conquering, 50–51, 141
Critical Carbohydrate Level for Losing (CCLL), 24, 138–39
cycling off and on Atkins (don't do it), 69

dance classes, 214
date, making one with yourself, to accomplish a task, 177
dedicating your practice to someone or something else, 165
diabetes, 12, 36
dieting, yo-yo, 206
"diet" products, 19
diets, calorie-controlled, failure of, 19
dining out, strategies for avoiding forbidden foods when, 112–14
disease, due to overeating, 10
doctors, enlisting their help when doing Atkins, 39, 153–54, 157
"draping the elephant," 164
dressings for salads, 259–60
drinking alcohol, 87
drinking water, 30, 70
dumbbells, 94–95

eating
  pleasure of, 18–19
  slowly, 126
  till full, but not stuffed, 49, 70, 127, 139
  unconscious, don't do it, 126
eggs, in Induction phase, 27
empowerment, 3, 68, 240
endurance, building, with exercise, 152
essential fatty acids (EFAs), 36–37
Essential Strengtheners, 96–100, 118–22
excuses, not accepting from yourself, 228
exercise

benefits of, 5–7, 201–2
challenging yourself in, 179–81, 186, 213–15
clothing for, 81, 230
cutting back on, in Induction phase, 50
fitting it into your life, 59
at the gym, 195
increasing it, when experiencing setbacks, 156, 159, 165
individualized in Atkins Advantage Program, 6
while traveling, 135
and weight loss, 201–2
exercise (term used in strength training), 96
exercise equipment
  gym, 249–54
  home, 214–15
exertion
  levels of, 116
  maximizing but not overdoing, 115–16

family
  cooking for, but eating lower-carb food beforehand, 57
  support or resistance from, to Atkins Advantage Program, 33
farmers' markets, 208
fat (body), burning of, 24
fat (dietary), 18–21
  appropriate amount at meals, 70–71
  balance of, in diet, 20
  demonization of, and obesity epidemic, 18
  eating sufficient, 49, 226
  helping digestion of vegetables, 260
  in Induction phase, 29
  need for, in diet, 18, 50
  in proportion to other nutrients in a meal, 139–40
  types of, "good" and "bad," 19–21
Feel the Burn, 180–81
fiber
  benefits of, 37–38
  grams of, and computation of net carbs, 15
  recommended amount, 37
  supplement forms of, 38
fish, in Induction phase, 27
fitness
  as basic to Atkins Advantage Program, 5–7, 226
  full spectrum plan of, 6–7
  in Induction phase, 59–65, 75–81
  in Lifetime Maintenance phase, 247–55
  in Ongoing Weight Loss phase, 91–100, 115–22, 130–35, 144–52, 164–69, 179–86
  in Pre-Maintenance phase, 195–202, 213–20, 230–38

Fitness Rewards, 201–2
flexibility, levels of, 60–61
focused, staying, 163
focus string, 41, 246
Follow Your Hand, 80
food(s)
    acceptable, 26–31, 262–63
    keeping pantry and refrigerator stocked with, 107–9
    making a list of your ten favorite, 43
    preparing ahead of time, 109–10
    seasonal and local, 208
    shopping for, 35, 107–9, 208
    staples to have on hand, 108–9
    tempting, saying no to, 114, 173–74
    that you should never eat, 192, 243
    trigger, 72, 104–5, 114, 192, 226
    typical portion sizes, 261
    whole foods better than "low-carb" products, 25
    See also eating; meals
food journal, 105, 158, 160, 190
Ford, Henry, on obstacles, 155
Forward Lunge, 149
fowl, in Induction phase, 27
free speed, 103
freezing food, 109
fruits
    Atkins Glycemic Ranking (AGR) chart of, 224
    glycemic impact of, 14

garlic, 209, 261
garnishes, 29
glycemic impact, 12–14
    glycemic index (GI) to measure, 13–14
    glycemic load (GL) to measure, 13–14
goals, personal
    getting started by writing them down, 74–75
    taking steps to accomplish them, 88–90
    thinking big, 210–11
goal weight
    being realistic, 211
    establishing, before starting Atkins, 42
group exercise classes, 214
gyms and health clubs, 247–54
    tips for choosing, 247–48

habits, replacing old with new, in twelve-week program, 7–8
Half Squats, 219
Hamstring Curls equipment, 253
Head Up, Chest Out, 63

heart disease, exercise to diminish risk of, 6
heart rate, target, 145–47
heart rate monitor, 147
"heart" that wins games, 125
Heel Walking, 120
herbs, 29, 208–9
hidden carbs, 49, 158
humans, natural diet and weight control of, 9
hunger
    decreasing it with hot tea or broth, 110, 189
    forestalling with a protein breakfast, 176
hydrogenated and partially hydrogenated fats (trans fats), 20–21

"I don't want to" excuse, 228
Induction phase of Atkins Nutritional Approach, 23, 47–84, 85, 123
    acceptable foods in, 26–31, 262
    checkpoints for, 66–67, 82–84
    determining when to leave and move on, 82–84
    meal plans for, 260–61
    no cheating during, 191
    nutrition rules of, 48–49
    returning to, in case of weight gain, 242
    staying in or returning to, 206–7
insulin, and blood sugar level, 11–12
interval training, 131–33

job hunting (as example of a goal), 88–89
jogging, 132–33, 231
journal, Atkins, 34, 244
journaling exercises, 56–58, 72–75, 88–91, 105, 140–44, 175–77, 210
junk food, discarding from kitchen, 32–34

ketoacidosis, 24
ketosis, 24

labels, reading them for forbidden ingredients, 189, 243–44
Lat Pull Down equipment, 250
leftovers, 110
    saving, rather than cleaning the plate of, 127
Leg Press equipment, 251
lentils, 226, 261
L-glutamine, 141
life
    empowerment for, with Atkins, 240, 255–56
    quality of, 3
    stop procrastinating with, 193–95

nutrition rules (*continued*)
    of Lifetime Maintenance phase, 241–44
    of Ongoing Weight Loss phase, 86
    of Pre-Maintenance phase, 188–90, 224–26
nuts, 85–86

oats, 244, 261
obesity, 10
    epidemic of, 18
object of desire, choosing a, 75
Oblique Ab Lift, 184
obstacles, 155–64
    getting past, 155–62
    what Henry Ford said about, 155
oils
    helping digestion of vegetables, 260
    in Induction phase, 29
"old you," discarding items connected with, 34
olives, 54, 261
omega-3 fatty acids, 19, 36–37
omega-6 fatty acids, 19, 37
omega-9 fatty acids, 19
One-Legged Stand, 236–37
Ongoing Weight Loss (OWL) phase of Atkins Nutritional
    Approach, 23–24, 48, 69, 82, 84, 85–186, 188, 222, 255
    acceptable foods in, 262
    adding net carbs in, 106–7, 138–39
    checkpoints for, 101–2, 123–24, 136, 153–54, 170, 186
    customizing it, 106–7
    moving on to, 84, 126
    nutrition rules of, 86
overeating
    breaking the habit of, 126–27
    in modern diet, 9–10
    obesity and disease due to, 10
Overhead Press, 98, 201

parsley, 192
parties, eating at, 113, 225
pasta, 227
Pectoral Fly equipment, 252
Personal Goals List, 74–75, 90
personal trainers, 249
Phelps, Michael, 128
Pilates, 214
plate, adjusting ratio of foods on your, 139–40, 158–59, 226
plateau (in weight loss program), 159, 161–62
play, as part of a fitness program, 91–92

polyunsaturated fats, 19
portion control, 126–27
portions, size of, for typical foods, 261
potassium, 53–54
Pre-Maintenance phase of Atkins Nutritional Approach,
    24–25, 48, 67, 69, 84, 85, 86, 101, 104, 123, 156,
    187–239, 241, 255
    acceptable foods in, 263
    adding net carbs in, 188–90
    checkpoint for, 203, 221, 239
    customizing it, 205–7
    moving on to, 188
    nutrition rules of, 188–90, 224–26
Press Up, 78
problem solving, examples of, 57–58, 141–43
processed meat, 27
procrastination
    about life, 193–95
    overcoming, 175–77
protein, 15–17
    in breakfast, 176
    complete, from animal sources, 16
    daily requirement, 17, 139, 226
    need for, in diet, 16–17
    in proportion to other nutrients in a meal, 139–40, 261
    sources of, 16
protein bars and shakes, 17
pulse, taking your, 146

Quad Stretch, 77

recipes, Atkins, 113, 128, 262–63
Reclining Ankle-to-Knee Stretch, 150
relationships, family and friends, that may interfere with
    sticking with Atkins, 142
relaxation techniques, 54–56, 245–47
repetition (rep) (term in strength training), 96
restaurants, dining at, 113
ricotta cheese, 161
running
    a mile, how fast can you do it? 186
    proper form in, 133

salads, garnishes for, 29
salad vegetables, 28
satiety (feeling of satisfaction), 18–19
saturated fats, 19–20
sauces, 209–10